MEDICAL
BREAKTHROUGHS
2001

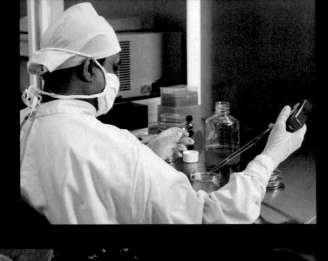
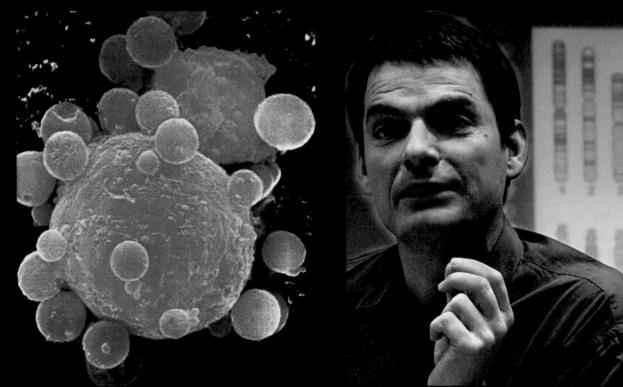

MEDICAL
BREAKTHROUGHS
2001

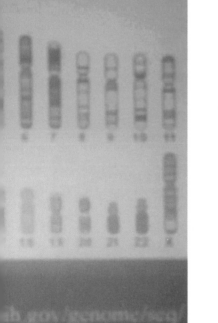

The latest advances in preventing, treating, and curing nearly 100 common diseases

The Reader's Digest Association, Inc.
Pleasantville, New York • Montreal

MEDICAL BREAKTHROUGHS PROJECT STAFF

Senior Editor
Marianne Wait

Senior Designer
Susan Welt

Contributing Editors
John Poppy
Annie Stine

Production Technology Manager
Douglas A. Croll

READER'S DIGEST HEALTH PUBLISHING

Editorial Director
Christopher Cavanaugh

Art Director
Joan Mazzeo

Marketing Director
James H. Malloy

Vice President and General Manager
Shirrel Rhoades

THE READER'S DIGEST ASSOCIATION, INC.

Editor-in-Chief
Eric W. Schrier

*President,
North American Books
and Home Entertainment*
Thomas D. Gardner

ISBN 0-7621-0305-1
ISSN 1537-0674

Address any comments about
Medical Breakthroughs 2001 to:
    Reader's Digest
    Editorial Director, Reader's Digest Health Publishing
    Reader's Digest Road
    Pleasantville, NY 10570-7000

To order additional copies of *Medical Breakthroughs 2001*, call 1-800-846-2100.

Visit us on our website at: rd.com.

Printed in the United States of America

1 3 5 7 9 10 8 6 4 2

NOTE TO OUR READERS
The information in this book should not be substituted for, or used to alter, medical therapy without your doctor's advice. For a specific health problem, consult your physician for guidance.

Any references in this book to any products or services do not constitute or imply an endorsement or recommendation.

IE 0088A/IC-US

PRODUCED BY CMD PUBLISHING

President
Dan Salomone

Executive Vice President
Steve Abramson

Vice President
Sarah Butterworth

Managing Editor
Donna Balopole

Editor
Anita Vanca

Editorial Assistant and Picture Research
Stacey Sharaby

Art Department
Rob Crow, Christine Dawydiak, Jim Kieffer, Patrick Walsh

CONTRIBUTORS

Design
Mindy Lang
Wendy Talvé Reingold

Writers and Editors
Andrea Balinson, David Biello, Debra Fulghum Bruce, Constance Buchanan, Susan Carleton, Lisa Davis, Karen de Seve, Brooke Dramer, Scott Gottlieb, Laird Harrison, Larry Katzenstein, Aileen Love, John McCormick, Robert Somerville, Annie Stuart, Rebecca Taylor, Kirk Walsh, Lyn Yonack

Picture Research
Jean Marie Wasilik
Sarah Wilson

Copy Editor
Deslie Lawrence

Indexers
Ann Cassar
Deborah E. Patton

Contents

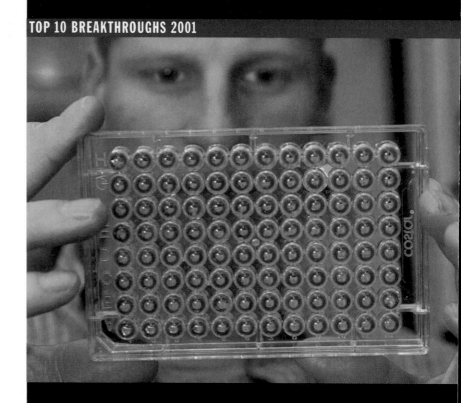

TOP 10 BREAKTHROUGHS 2001

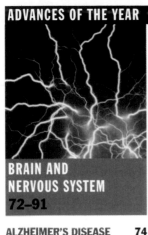

BRAIN AND NERVOUS SYSTEM
72–91

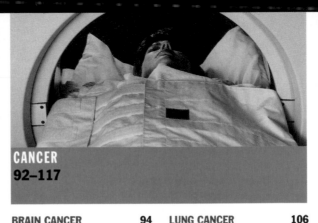

CANCER
92–117

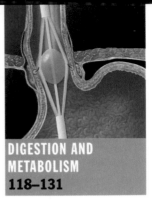

DIGESTION AND METABOLISM
118–131

ADVANCES OF THE YEAR

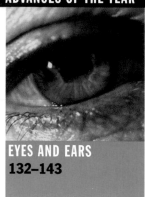

EYES AND EARS
132–143

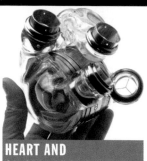

HEART AND CIRCULATORY SYSTEM
144–167

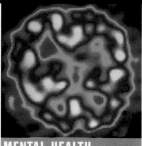

MENTAL HEALTH
168–181

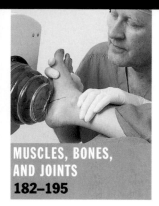

MUSCLES, BONES, AND JOINTS
182–195

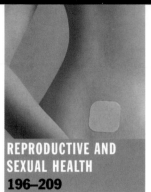
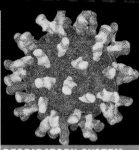
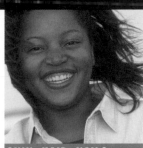
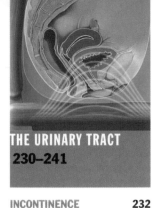

REPRODUCTIVE AND SEXUAL HEALTH
196–209

RESPIRATORY SYSTEM
210–217

SKIN, HAIR, NAILS, AND TEETH
218–229

THE URINARY TRACT
230–241

About This Book

How many times have you caught fragments of a news clip about an exciting new treatment for ——— that will cut ——— weeks off the recovery time, or a brand-new surgery to correct ——— with fewer side effects? Perhaps you wanted to write the information down but couldn't find a pen or a scrap of paper in time. Maybe you heard months ago about an experimental new Alzheimer's drug or a new way to lower high blood pressure and now you want to tell a friend about it but can't remember the details.

In the new millennium, medicine is changing at warp speed. Yesterday's tests, treatments, and cures are being replaced by faster and more effective ones every day. While some of the tried-and-true protocols are still the best option, there are better ways to diagnose or treat many conditions or avoid them in the first place. Now you can find this information all in one place—and all in plain English.

Medical Breakthroughs 2001 brings you the most important advances in health care. Our writers and editors consulted with leading physicians and researchers in every field. We sifted through medical journals, news articles, and technical briefings—every bit of health information we could find—and identified the most exciting developments. Doctors then read every word of each article to ensure accuracy.

All of the articles are conveniently arranged by body system (for example, Heart and Circulatory) and within each system, by ailment (such as Coronary Artery Disease), so you can easily find information that may help you or a loved one make a health-related decision or cope with a chronic health problem.

In the first section, Top Ten Breakthroughs, you'll find the ten biggest health stories of the year, from the first reading of the human genetic code to the advent of inhaled insulin to the dawn of new vaccines that may one day treat or prevent diabetes, and even certain cancers. Even if your health is perfectly fine, you'll be amazed by the medical marvels scientists have engineered, like artificial retinas that may help the blind to see and the tiny video camera that you swallow to help your doctor diagnose problems in your intestinal tract.

This book is not intended as a general medical reference; it's possible that for your condition there are older treatments that may work just as well as, or even better than, some you'll find here. But many of the advances you'll read about, including those still in the development or testing stage (see the chart at right to understand the different stages of testing a drug goes through), may one day become the accepted practice. Gleevec, the headline-grabbing leukemia drug, was studied for more than a decade before it was approved by the U.S. Food and Drug Administration in 2001. Some of the drugs in *Medical Breakthroughs 2001* may very well be the next Gleevec but may not be available for several years to come; others may never get approved.

You might not want to wait for a drug or procedure to be approved. Depending on your health and your medical condition, you may be able to join a clinical trial that is testing a new way to treat

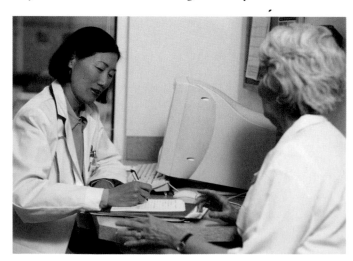

your disease. To learn about clinical trials in the United States, log on to the clinical trials page on the National Institutes of Health (NIH) website at www.clinicaltrials.gov. If you do not have Internet access at home, try your public library; many allow you to search the Internet for free.

Use *Medical Breakthroughs 2001* as a tool to ensure you get the best possible treatment for your condition. Talk to your doctor about whether a device, drug, diagnostic test, or surgery mentioned here might benefit you. If you'd like to share the cutting-edge medical information in this book with a friend or loved one, order an extra copy by calling 1-800-846-2100. Turn to the resource directory on page 242 for a list of organizations you can contact for more information on a variety of topics. And don't miss next year's edition of *Medical Breakthroughs*, where you'll find updates on many of the articles in this edition—plus brand-new discoveries that are just around the corner.

Drug Development and Approval Process

An experimental drug's journey from lab to medicine chest takes 12 years on average. Of every 5,000 compounds that enter pre-clinical testing, only 5 make it to human testing. Of these 5, one is approved by the FDA. Clinical trials—that is, testing on people—advance through three phases, with an additional phase of testing on animals beforehand and one phase of testing after the drug is marketed.

	PRECLINICAL TESTING		PHASE I	PHASE II	PHASE III		FDA APPROVAL	PHASE IV
YEARS	3.5		1	2	3		2.5	
TEST POPULATION	Laboratory and animal studies		20 to 80 healthy volunteers or patients	100 to 300 patient volunteers	1,000 to 3,000 patient volunteers			
PURPOSE	Assess safety and biological activity	File IND at FDA	Determine safety and dosage and identify side effects	Evaluate effectiveness and further evaluate safety	Verify effectiveness, monitor adverse reactions from long-term use, and compare drug with commonly used treatments	File NDA at FDA	Review process culminating in approval	Additional post-marketing testing required by FDA
SUCCESS RATE	5,000 compounds evaluated		5 enter trials				1 approved	

SOURCES Pharmaceutical Research and Manufacturers Association and National Institutes of Health
ABBREVIATIONS FDA: U.S. Food and Drug Administration; IND: Investigational New Drug Application; NDA: New Drug Application

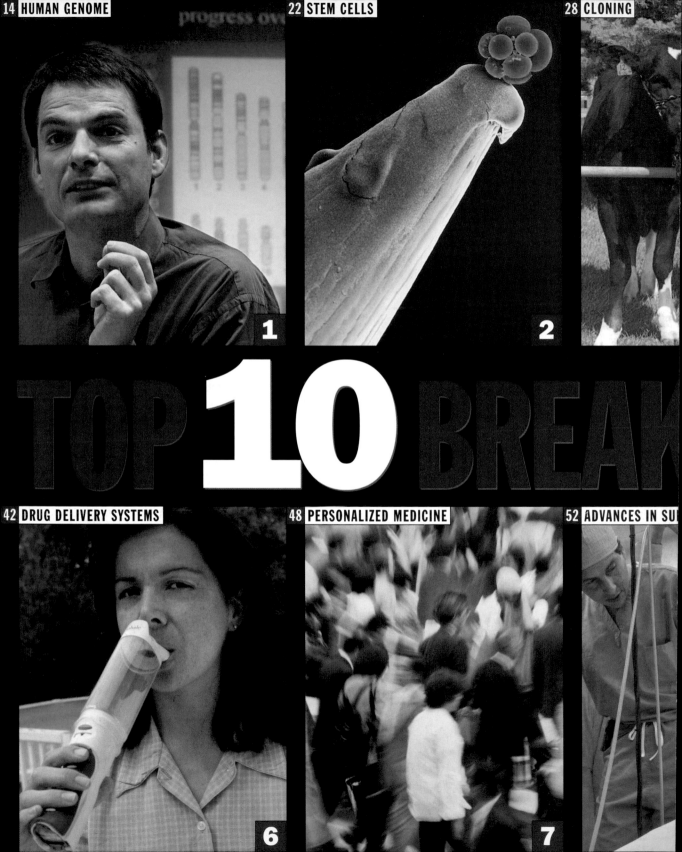

TOP 10 BREAK

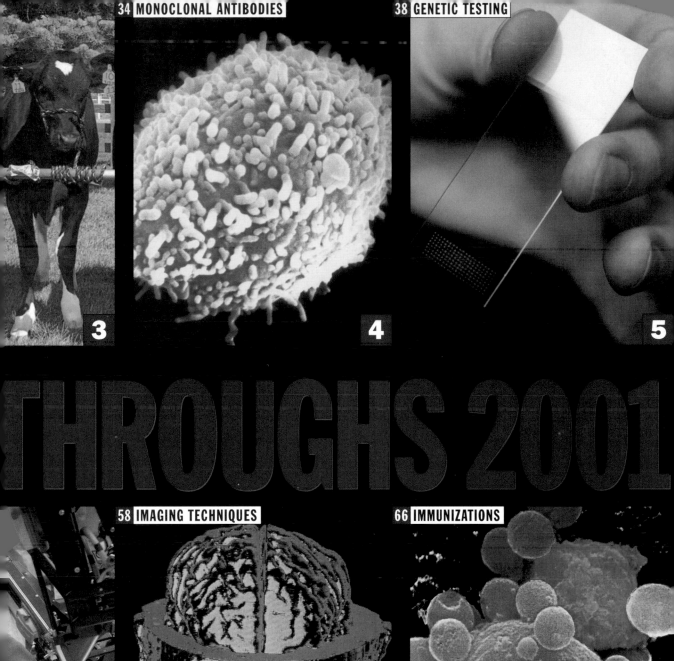

THROUGHS 2001

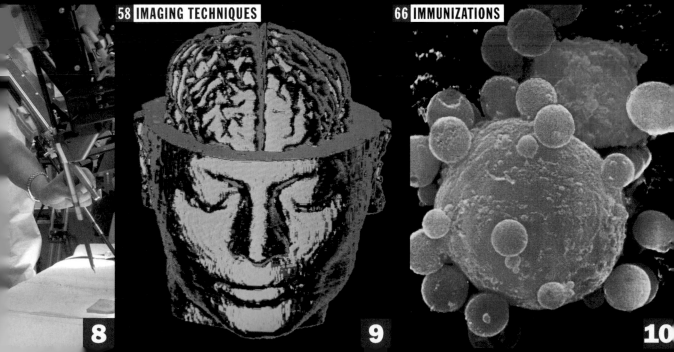

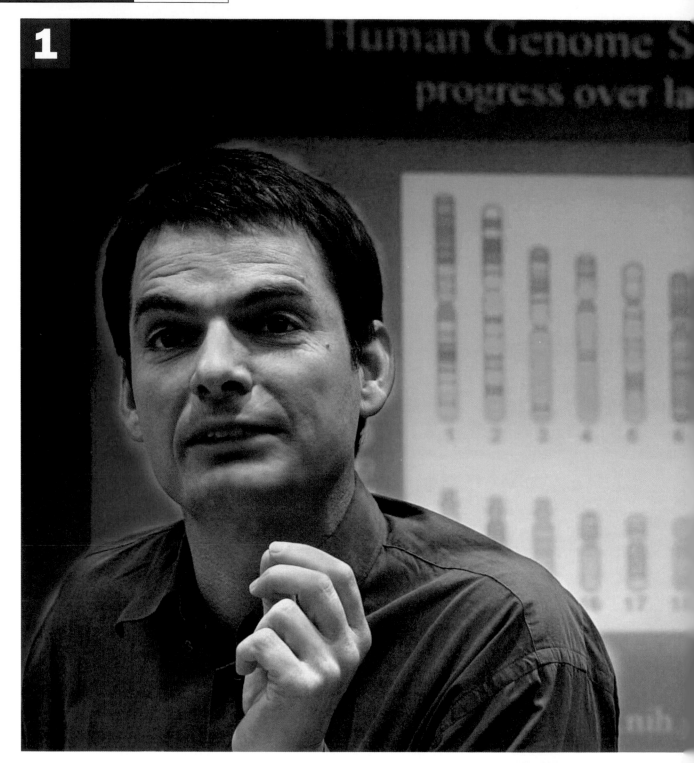

Scientists Read

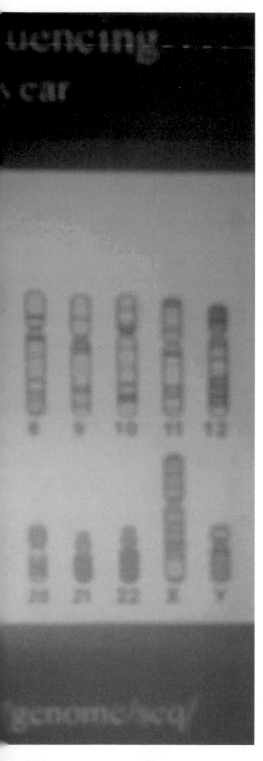

Early in 2001, scientists published the instruction manual that comes with every one of us. This was not merely the biggest medical breakthrough of the year; the sequencing and analysis of the human genome—the full package of genetic instructions for a human being—is one of the greatest advances of the past millennium, indeed of all history.

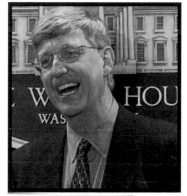

Dr. Francis Collins

"We've read the letters of our own instruction book," Collins says.
"It's something that we human beings will do only once in the entire course of history."

◀ Andre Rosenthal of the public German Human Genome Project explains the genome sequencing in front of a slide projection during a news conference in Berlin on June 26, 2000.

The genome is a shop manual that carries the blueprint for each cell in our bodies, said Francis Collins, director of the National Human Genome Research Institute, at the ceremony on February 12 marking a major milestone in a 15-year effort—and it is more than that. It's a history book that tells the story of our species' journey from slimy primordial soup to skyscraper and spaceship. And it is the most detailed medical text ever written. Most likely, the sequencing of the genome will affect our notion of what it means to be human. Certainly, the project will change nearly everything about the way we treat and even prevent disease.

"We've read the letters of our own instruction book," stated Collins. "It's something that we human beings will do only once in the entire course of history."

These are lofty statements about what looks to be a pretty modest list of parts. How many mind-boggling stories, how much crucial instruction, what life-changing discoveries can a book contain when it's written with just four letters—A, T, G, and C—in endless, and endlessly monotonous, variation? Plenty, in fact, because those letters stand for the four chemical building blocks of life, the so-called nucleotide bases: adenine, thymine, guanine, and cytosine. A, T, G, and C are the crucial ingredients of deoxyribonucleic acid (DNA), the molecule in every living cell of the body that carries your genetic

the Letters of Life

code. That code is simply the pattern of those As, Ts, Gs, and Cs—the way they line up—and it conveys all the biochemical information needed to build and maintain a person's body.

Segments of DNA called genes regulate the function of your cells, controlling the way they build the proteins that make up skin, bone, blood, and the rest of you. And not just your structural components: Genes directed the manufacture of the proteins that are sending neurochemical messages from your eyeballs to your brain right now so you can read these words, for example, and others that may be rousing immune cells to attack a cold virus in your nose. Your DNA does all this while working at 5 percent capacity: 95 percent of it, the so-called "junk DNA," apparently doesn't code for much of anything, though it may turn out to perform other important tasks.

The information encoded in DNA does more than keep a living body going, of course. It also allows one body to make another. James D. Watson and Francis H. C. Crick discovered in 1953 that each base always pairs up with the same partner—A with T and G with C—to form the steps of a spiral staircase, the famous double helix structure of DNA. Their realization that the helix could "unzip," with each side a template for the formation of a new helix, solved the puzzle of how DNA could transmit genetic instructions from one cell to the next cell it forms, and from parent to child.

Some Surprises Emerge

In an engineering feat akin to fitting an elephant into a thimble, just about every cell in the human body contains roughly six feet of DNA, spiraled and accordioned onto 23 pairs of chromosomes—structures in the nucleus of each cell that contain the

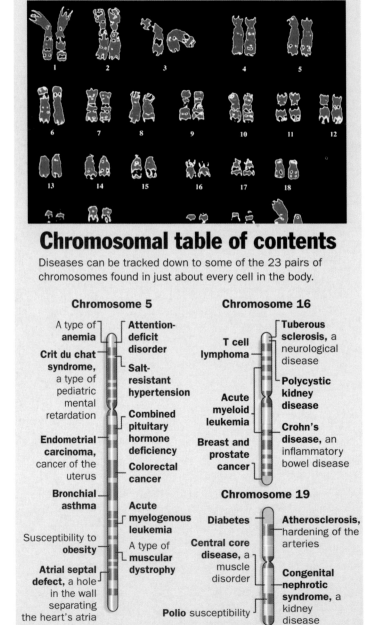

Chromosomal table of contents

Diseases can be tracked down to some of the 23 pairs of chromosomes found in just about every cell in the body.

Chromosome 5

- A type of anemia
- Crit du chat syndrome, a type of pediatric mental retardation
- Endometrial carcinoma, cancer of the uterus
- Bronchial asthma
- Susceptibility to obesity
- Atrial septal defect, a hole in the wall separating the heart's atria
- Attention-deficit disorder
- Salt-resistant hypertension
- Combined pituitary hormone deficiency
- Colorectal cancer
- Acute myelogenous leukemia
- A type of muscular dystrophy

Chromosome 16

- T cell lymphoma
- Acute myeloid leukemia
- Breast and prostate cancer
- Tuberous sclerosis, a neurological disease
- Polycystic kidney disease
- Crohn's disease, an inflammatory bowel disease

Chromosome 19

- Diabetes
- Central core disease, a muscle disorder
- Polio susceptibility
- Atherosclerosis, hardening of the arteries
- Congenital nephrotic syndrome, a kidney disease

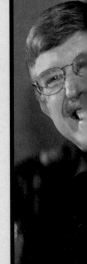

genes. It was in October 1990 that an international, publicly funded consortium of researchers set out to unpack the cell and give its DNA a good read. Another group of researchers formed a private U.S. company called Celera Genomics in May 1998 to start an independent attempt, and they later joined the public group as competitive allies. The scientists chopped DNA into small pieces, then determined the sequence of bases on each piece and fitted the pieces back together.

From the moment the first snippets of DNA were sequenced and the results posted on the Internet, scientists in labs around the world have been working to glean information from the patterns.

The public researchers set themselves a goal of completing a rough draft of the entire genome by 2005 and will probably end up beating their own deadline by 2003. By June 2000, they and Celera had sequenced better than 90 percent of the genome, and in February 2001, the two groups together released their analysis. The work is by no means over. If you think of the genome as a house, the researchers have finished the frame; it is infinitely better than living out in the open, but there's lots of stucco work, sanding, and cleaning still to be done. But all along, from the moment the first snippets of DNA were sequenced and double-checked and the results posted on the Internet—the public consortium published their data as they got it, within 24 hours—scientists in labs around the world have been working to glean information from the patterns. So just what do we know, now that we know how the As and Ts and Gs and Cs line up?

We know, for one thing, that it takes remarkably few genes to make a human—an estimated 30,000 to 60,000, far fewer than the 80,000 to 120,000 that some researchers had anticipated at the start. In fact, humans seem to have only about twice as many genes as the fly or the worm.

On the other hand, it's clear that our genes are extremely hardworking. Although scientists used to assume that each gene makes a single protein, genome analysis reveals that each produces three proteins, on average, by rearranging the parts of the protein during assembly, like so many Lego blocks. The process is called alternative splicing.

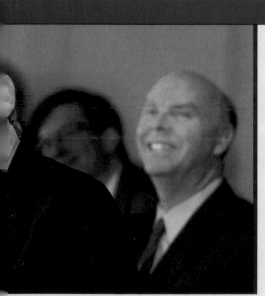

Francis Collins, M.D., (left) and Craig Venter, Ph.D., at the February 12, 2001, news conference.

into larger maps. The project was on schedule to meet its deadline of 2005.

Meanwhile, molecular biologist Craig Venter rounded up funding, facilities, and brainpower to start a private sequencing project. He and his wife, Claire Fraser, founded The Institute for Genomic Research in 1991, using sophisticated technology that read the individual A, T, G, C components of the genetic code. Venter put pressure on the HGP in 1995 when his team published the genome of the bacterium *Haemophilus influenzae,* consisting of nearly 2 million DNA base pairs. Turning up the heat in 1998, he announced that his new company, Celera Genomics, would use a "whole genome shotgun" method—cutting the human genome into several hundred thousand fragments, sequencing the fragments, then reassembling them on the basis of overlaps—to finish the job by 2001.

The race was on. The HGP stepped up its pace, still piecing the genome together one chromosome at a time. Celera kept using its shortcut, firing big chunks through sequencing machines all at once. By June 2000, both groups had a working draft of the human genome. In February 2001, they published their results on the same day in competing scientific journals, *Science* and *Nature.*

Some six months later, both Celera and the HGP began the next phase in their study of the genetic code: sequencing the individual genomes of several people. This moves us a step closer to developing truly personalized medical diagnoses based on scans of a person's genomic profile, perhaps in digital form on a convenient card.

Dr. Collins said in his 2001 publication announcement, "We are profoundly humbled by the privilege of turning the pages that describe the miracle of human life, written in the mysterious language of all the ages, the language of God."

Dr. Venter, speaking to television interviewer Charlie Rose, said, "This has to be the most exciting phase in the history of human endeavor, in the history of science. The next 10 years are going to be extraordinary."

We've also learned that men are driving the evolution of the species, though you might say they're doing it with their eyes closed. One of the genome's surprising revelations is that a sperm cell is more than twice as likely as a woman's egg to contain the genetic mistakes called mutations. People have tended to presume that eggs are the weak sisters because a woman's full complement of eggs has already been assembled and stored away for later use by the time she is born. Given their age, the theory has been, no wonder the occasional egg goes bad; sperm, on the other hand, is continually made fresh.

Now, it's true that an older woman is more likely than a younger one to harbor eggs with genetic defects; nothing in the genome analysis undermines the logic of a woman over 35 getting amniocente-

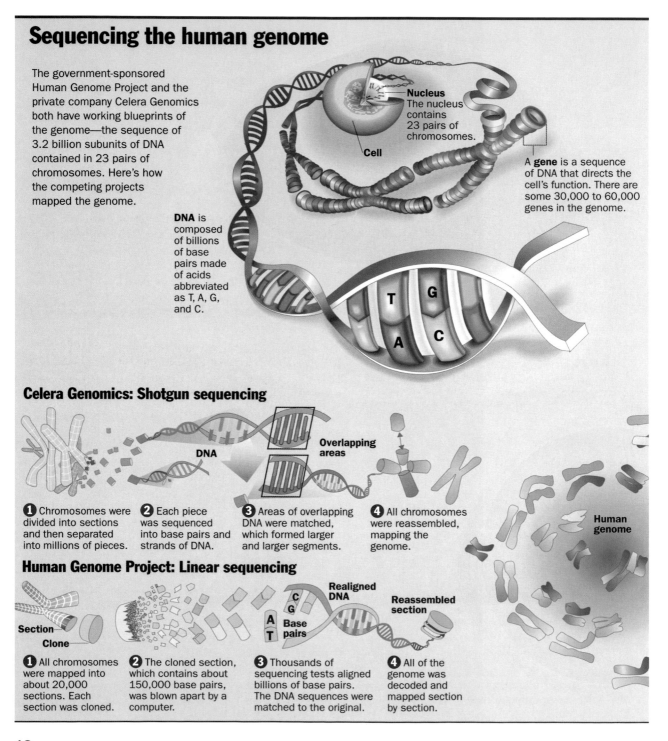

Sequencing the human genome

The government-sponsored Human Genome Project and the private company Celera Genomics both have working blueprints of the genome—the sequence of 3.2 billion subunits of DNA contained in 23 pairs of chromosomes. Here's how the competing projects mapped the genome.

Nucleus
The nucleus contains 23 pairs of chromosomes.

Cell

A **gene** is a sequence of DNA that directs the cell's function. There are some 30,000 to 60,000 genes in the genome.

DNA is composed of billions of base pairs made of acids abbreviated as T, A, G, and C.

Celera Genomics: Shotgun sequencing

DNA

Overlapping areas

Human genome

❶ Chromosomes were divided into sections and then separated into millions of pieces.

❷ Each piece was sequenced into base pairs and strands of DNA.

❸ Areas of overlapping DNA were matched, which formed larger and larger segments.

❹ All chromosomes were reassembled, mapping the genome.

Human Genome Project: Linear sequencing

Realigned DNA

Reassembled section

Section

Clone

Base pairs

❶ All chromosomes were mapped into about 20,000 sections. Each section was cloned.

❷ The cloned section, which contains about 150,000 base pairs, was blown apart by a computer.

❸ Thousands of sequencing tests aligned billions of base pairs. The DNA sequences were matched to the original.

❹ All of the genome was decoded and mapped section by section.

Within the decade, Collins estimates, physicians will be able to test for genes involved in up to a dozen common diseases, just as they currently can check for the mutated BRCA genes that raise the risk of breast cancer.

sis or another test to check the chromosomal normality of her fetus. But the genome data show that the frantic cell divisions that produce 300 million sperm per day frequently go awry. The mutations that a sperm may carry are most likely to prove lethal to any embryo it fathers, but occasionally the embryo grows into a flourishing human with a kink in its DNA. Over vast periods of time, those mutations can start to pile up. Add some random environmental "pressure" in the form of an Ice Age, say, and these events may actually give the DNA an advantage. Voilà: That's the way a species can take a step down the evolutionary path.

All of this is strange and interesting—fun trivia to take to a cocktail party. But what in the genome analysis can you take to the doctor's office? For starters, how about your genetic profile?

A Guide to Strengths—and Weak Spots

The sequencing of the genome is already making it much easier for researchers to uncover genes that raise the risk of illness. Before sequencing began, it took nine years of painstaking labor to identify the gene for cystic fibrosis. In 1997, it took just nine days to identify a gene for Parkinson's disease, and an additional mere nine months to fully analyze the gene, base by base.

Finding the genetic roots of other illnesses will generally prove more challenging, since most are likely to result from the combined small effects of many damaged genes, not to mention the environmental hazards that work on those weak points. Still, scientists believe that fairly soon they will identify the genes that increase a person's vulnerability to diabetes, heart disease, Alzheimer's, asthma—virtually every medical problem besides accidents and trauma that sends people to the doctor. Indeed, within the decade, Collins

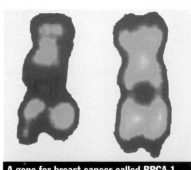

A gene for breast cancer called BRCA-1 has been found on chromosome 17.

estimates, physicians will be able to test for genes involved in up to a dozen common diseases, just as they currently can check for the mutated BRCA genes that raise the risk of breast cancer, or for the genetic mutation that makes Huntington's disease a grim near-certainty.

What this means is that at some point in the not-too-distant future, you'll be able to go to your doctor for a baseline genome scan that will highlight any significant glitches in your DNA. And that means preventive medicine is likely to get much more individualized and much more effective. It will go beyond the earnest speech—"Don't smoke, get some exercise, and quit eating so many fatty foods"—and get personal. Your genetic profile may show that you're at relatively low risk for Alzheimer's disease, say, but particularly vulnerable to lung cancer or heart disease. That doesn't mean those diseases are hardwired into your genes, but it does suggest that there are some bad habits you really can't afford. It may also alert you to the need to start getting screened for cancer at a younger age than is normally recommended, or get you thinking about starting preventive treatment for your heart, such as taking cholesterol-lowering drugs.

These kinds of advances are all but guaranteed to alter medical care in diverse ways that will affect society deeply. Not all of the changes, however, are guaranteed to be for the better.

Who's Watching over Your Shoulder?

Even before February 2001, we got a peek at the way lengths of DNA could be used to tie up a sense of ethics and hide it in a closet.

A railroad worker named Gary Avary, who handles track maintenance for Burlington Northern Santa Fe Railroad, had developed a bad case of carpal tunnel syndrome after 27 years on the job. His bosses agreed to pay for wrist surgery but after the procedure, they asked him to see the company doctor to help determine if the workplace was responsible for his injury. Another worker who had been through the drill told Avary to expect to give up seven vials of blood for various lab tests. "That just made no sense to me," said Janice Avary, Gary's wife, a registered nurse by profession. "Three vials is normal. And what could an exam after treatment tell you? Nothing added up."

As it turned out, the company wanted Avary's blood for a genetic

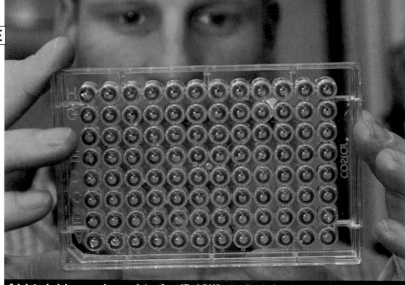

A lab technician examines a plate of purified DNA samples to be sequenced.

CRACKING THE CODE OF LIFE

Gregor Mendel, the grandfather of genetics, studied color traits of pea plants to reveal how characteristics are passed from parents to offspring.

Swiss chemist Johan Miescher identified the genetic material found in the nucleus of each cell as "nuclein." At first, Miescher did not know exactly how this substance worked, but he could see that it was important in passing along traits from one generation to the next.

A research team led by the scientist Oswald Avery described the chemical deoxyribonucleic acid (DNA), which carries genetic information.

James Watson and Francis Crick unveiled the chemical structure of DNA: a double helix of nucleotide bases that scientists abbreviate as A, T, G, and C. Watson and Crick reported modestly, "This structure has novel features which are of considerable biological interest." Rosalind Franklin's X-ray photographs of DNA led Watson and Crick to their discovery, for which they received the Nobel Prize in 1962, four years after Franklin's death.

The Human Genome Project (HGP), an international consortium of research institutes, began to sequence the genetic code. Its deadline was 2005.

Celera Genomics, a private company, announced it had the technology to sequence the human genome by 2001.

The HGP and Celera together announced that each had a "working draft" of the human genome: the sequence of the 3.2 billion A, T, G, C units that make up the DNA needed to create and maintain a human being.

The HGP and Celera each published the results of the first draft of their genome sequencing. They also reported that humans have about 30,000 genes, far fewer than expected.

test. They planned to test for a syndrome known as hereditary neuropathy with liability to pressure palsies (HNPP), which can cause a variety of problems, including a kind of carpal tunnel disorder. People who have HNPP generally develop symptoms in their teens; it's extremely unlikely that carpal tunnel syndrome caused by HNPP would make its first appearance decades into the career of a railroad worker. More to the point, testing a patient without his consent is unethical, and when an employer is doing it to see whether a currently healthy worker might have a predisposition to any type of problem, it's flat out illegal, as the Equal Employment Opportunity Commission informed the railroad in an injunction given just a few days before the genome researchers released their analysis.

"The science was wrong, the approach by the company of testing employees without their knowledge was profoundly wrong, the motivation, which presumably was to try to avoid paying compensation, or worse yet to fire the people who were at risk, was profoundly unjust," Collins says. "Everything about this makes your hair stand on end. And yet it happened."

A number of states have already outlawed the use of genetic information to hire or fire or to deny health coverage. But state-by-state protection is spotty and not always effective. Congress is considering federal legislation now. Meanwhile, nervousness on the part of the public is slowing the pace of scientific discovery. About a third of the people who consider getting a genetic test as part of studies funded by the National Institutes of Health decide to opt out because they're not sure about who will be allowed to peruse their personal operating code.

A More Perfect Prescription

That's a pity, because genetic profiling offers more than risk analysis. Whether you're considering preventive drugs like a cholesterol-lowering statin or medicine to treat an established illness, from foot fungus to cancer, having your genetic profile in hand may well increase the prescription's safety and effectiveness.

The genome project has given rise to a field called pharmacogenomics, which is where genes and drugs intersect to produce the most personalized approach possible to medicine (see Drugs Get Personal, page 48, and Better Ways to Take Your Medicine, page 42). Mutated genes are behind many of the hundreds of thousands of bad drug reactions that occur each year because genes determine how fast or slowly you metabolize a drug, among other things. If you metabolize it very slowly, a dose that is safe for most people may be dangerous for you. If you're a fast metabolizer the standard dose may be ineffective. Pharmacogenomics can make it possible to customize your prescriptions to fit your genes.

One drug highlights a different way the genome project is paying off. The leukemia drug Gleevec was approved by the U.S. Food and Drug Administration in 2001 amid great fanfare, with headlines heralding a new era in cancer treatment. For once, it seems the celebration was warranted. Most cancer drugs—in fact, most drugs, period—are found pretty much through luck and nearly blind grunt-work, with heaps upon heaps of compounds being screened in hopes of finding one that works. It's the opposite of what's known as rational drug design, but there hasn't been much alternative, simply because scientists haven't known enough about their target diseases. (We know that in diabetes there's something wrong with the way

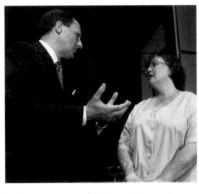

▲ The president of Novartis AG speaks with a Gleevec trial patient on the day Gleevec's approval by the FDA was announced.

the body handles insulin and glucose, for instance, but we don't have a clue as to why.)

But with Gleevec, some crucial discoveries helped researchers aim their efforts. They knew that in chronic myelogenous leukemia, a gene makes a deformed version of a certain protein that then signals white blood cells to divide wildly. Cancer specialist Brian Druker at Oregon Health and Science University devised Gleevec to fit into the business end of the deformed molecule and block it. Simple, and effective. Once Druker determined the right dose, every patient in the early tests got better.

More than 100 designer drugs now in the pipeline have been sculpted to fix the genetic flaw behind a given cancer. "If even a few of those drugs turn out to be as successful as Gleevec, it's going to change the way cancer is treated," said Francis Collins. "Not 30 years from now, but much sooner." The American Medical Association, after studying this issue, has concluded that the sequencing and analysis of the human genome is going to bring about the largest paradigm shift of all time in medicine. It has already become the core of biomedical research. Collins says, "The momentum is unstoppable. By 2025 we won't recognize medicine."

The genome project has been compared to the space effort in terms of sheer ambition and importance. The attempt to know ourselves has been costly, and like the space initiative it has required a certain hubris to imagine that humans could accomplish so much. The analogy raises a thrilling question. It took just 66 years for humans to travel from Kitty Hawk to the moon. In 2067, propelled by the knowledge of the genome, in what strange and wonderful terrain will we find ourselves?

GENOMIC GLOSSARY

Chromosome A tightly wound bundle of DNA, wrapped up in protective proteins, that forms when cells divide.

Deoxyribonucleic acid (DNA) A twisting chain of molecules in the form of a double helix that contains an organism's genetic information.

Gene Parts of the human genome that oversee body growth, maintenance, and function.

Gene therapy Correcting a mistake in the genetic code by inserting new genetic material.

Genetic mutation A mistake in the A, T, G, C sequence along the DNA.

Genome All the genetic information needed to create, run, and maintain an organism. Humans have two copies of every chromosome, for a total of 46, in the nucleus of nearly every cell.

Nucleotide bases The chemical components that pair up to create the structural "rungs" of the DNA double helix. Adenine (A) pairs with thymine (T) and guanine (G) pairs with cytosine (C).

Protein Fundamental components of all living cells. Major types of proteins include enzymes, which boost the rate of chemical reactions; antibodies, which fight viruses and bacteria; hemoglobin, which carries oxygen through the blood; and the various hormones.

Single nucleotide polymorphism (SNP) A single letter variation along the genetic code, such as an A in the place of a G.

Trait The physical manifestation of a gene, as interpreted by the body and influenced by the environment.

2

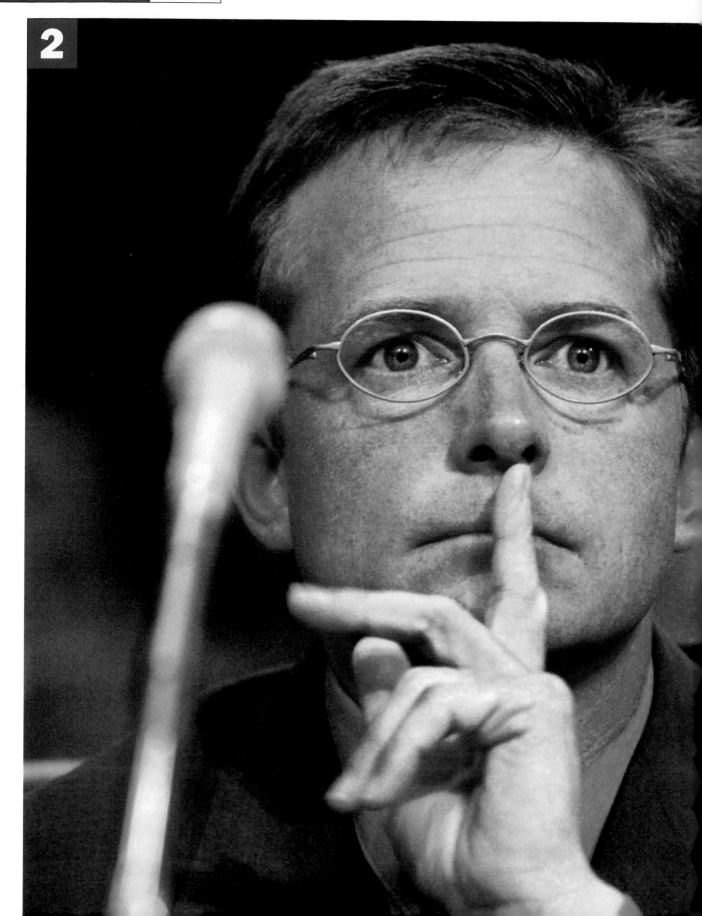

Stem Cells Raise Hopes and Fears

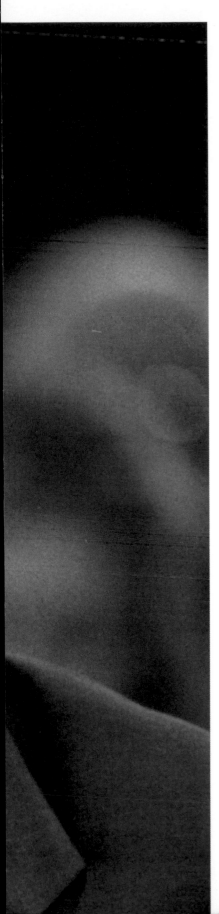

◀ Actor Michael J. Fox, who has Parkinson's disease, has testified before the U.S. Senate in support of stem cell research.

Actor Michael J. Fox took on a new role a couple of years ago. Every six months or so Fox appears as a witness in hearings before the U.S. Senate, pressing Congress to fund research on embryonic stem cells. These amazingly versatile cells, Fox testified, could be the keys to a cure for his Parkinson's disease.

And that's not all. Researchers believe stem cells can help cure an array of other ailments, including ALS (amyotrophic lateral sclerosis, or Lou Gehrig's disease), Alzheimer's disease, arthritis, cancer, diabetes, and heart disease. Furthermore, they may help heal damage from burns, spinal cord injury, and stroke. "This research," according to a report from the U.S. National Institutes of Health (NIH), "has the potential to revolutionize the practice of medicine and improve the quality and length of life."

What is it about stem cells that raises such hopes? Just this: At their earliest stage, in an embryo, they are master cells, able to produce almost every other type of cell in the body. In science-speak they are "pluripotent." And they're something else. In a laboratory, cultures of these cells are immortal; a colony can produce generation after generation of identical stem cells poised to specialize as new skin, brain, nerve, blood, or whatever cells are needed.

Revolutionary Medicine: Embryonic Stem Cells

Just three years ago, two researchers shocked the scientific world with announcements that they had isolated human pluripotent stem cells and had started growing them in laboratory dishes. James Thomson, V.M.D., Ph.D., of the University of Wisconsin-Madison, got his cells from embryos donated by couples at an in vitro fertilization (IVF) clinic. John D. Gearhart, Ph.D., of Johns Hopkins University, used cells from fetuses donated by women who had undergone abortions.

Medical hopes—and political passions—rose to new heights in 2001 as one scientist after another reported fresh uses for stem cells, and as private biotechnology companies announced plans to create human embryos for the sole purpose of harvesting stem cells.

Most of the action swirls around stem cells from embryos, for several reasons. Certain types of cells from a fetus—which an embryo becomes after developing for eight weeks in a uterus—also posses therapeutic potential, but they can't escape the context of abortion. Embryonic stem cells show up about four days after an egg is fertilized, and they

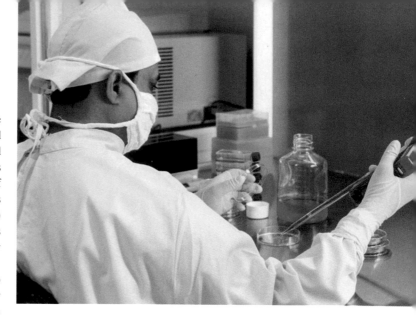

▲ **The NIH has identified 10 labs around the world that have developed 64 embryonic stem cell colonies, or "lines."**

keep their master-cell status for a few weeks at most. Then they become "adult" stem cells committed to a particular function—forming blood cells, say, or brain cells. Adult stem cells are called multipotent. They can continue to divide without producing tumors, each time making a new specialized cell and a new adult stem cell ready to repeat the process. However, no adult stem cell has yet proven to be as versatile as its younger self.

Harvesting cellular building blocks

Stem cells, taken from human embryos, can potentially be used to produce any type of cell in the body, such as a nerve cell, red blood cell, or liver cell.

Removing stem cells

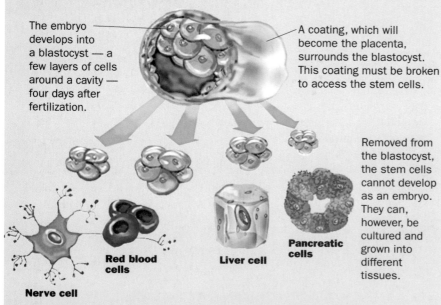

The embryo develops into a blastocyst — a few layers of cells around a cavity — four days after fertilization.

A coating, which will become the placenta, surrounds the blastocyst. This coating must be broken to access the stem cells.

Removed from the blastocyst, the stem cells cannot develop as an embryo. They can, however, be cultured and grown into different tissues.

Nerve cell

Red blood cells

Liver cell

Pancreatic cells

Miracles in Animals

So far, all of the excitement springs from visions of what might be. You can't go to a hospital yet for treatment based on embryonic stem cells. (You can find a small handful of therapies based on adult stem cells. For instance, transplanting bone marrow, which contains blood stem cells, is a common way to generate healthy blood cells in people with some forms of cancer.) Even the first clinical trials of embryonic cells in humans are probably at least three years or more in the future. The clearest results so far have shown up in research on lab animals. Gearhart reported in July 2001 that after transplants of human stem cells, rats with spinal cord injuries could move their legs and partially stand.

The work of other researchers enabled rats that had strokes in motor regions of the brain to move again. In both cases, stem cells took

Medical hopes—and political passions—rose to new heights in 2001 as one scientist after another reported fresh uses for stem cells.

cues from their new surroundings and transformed themselves into nerve cells (neurons). Mice with heart disease have improved after transplants of healthy cells into their failing heart muscle. And scientists have used chemicals to coax embryonic cells from mice into becoming pancreatic islet cells—the cells a mouse (or a person) needs to produce insulin. "It's a startling finding," says Ronald McKay, Ph.D., of NIH, who led the mouse-pancreas research. "When we put glucose on these cells, they release insulin. That's astonishing. It reflects the 'self-assembly' of living systems. They know what to do."

By the same token, Fox and researchers pursuing a cure for Parkinson's disease hope that stem cells can revive the brain's ability to produce dopamine, a chemical that helps coordinate movement. Parkinson's destroys dopamine-releasing cells. Doctors want to see if embryonic stem cells can replace them.

Scientists came a long way in 2001 in their ability to isolate and experiment with stem cells. Three major paths are now open for stem cell research:

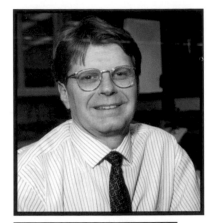

John D. Gearhart, Ph.D

"We still have a lot to learn about how stem cells work, but given time, stem cell research could lead to the development of cell-based therapies for many devastating diseases and injuries, such as Parkinson's disease, Lou Gehrig's disease, and spinal cord injury."

■ **Transplants and cell therapies.** Stem cells prompted to develop into specialized cells could be a renewable source of spare parts, compensating for the fact that there are far too few donated organs and tissues available for transplants. And cells damaged or destroyed by disease could be replaced by healthy ones derived from stem cells.

■ **Basic cell behavior.** Studying stem cells may help researchers understand the complex series of events that occur during normal human development—including the specialization of cells—and what happens when these events take a wrong turn, resulting in birth defects and cancer. By scrutinizing the genes that turn on and off during specialization, they could potentially learn to control and treat these diseases.

■ **Drug testing.** New medications could be tested on an endless supply of living, normal human cells developed from stem cells before the drugs are given to animals and people. Benefits would include lower costs, greater accuracy, and testing in a broader variety of cell types.

Science Meets Politics

There's a catch to all this: getting the stem cells from the embryos. Fertility centers join eggs and sperm in petri dishes, producing more embryos than would-be mothers can use and routinely discarding the extra ones unless a researcher takes them. Whether discarded or used for research, the embryos die, and for many people that is unacceptable. Pope John Paul II, in a July 2001 meeting with U. S. President George W. Bush, denounced "practices that devalue and violate human life at any stage from conception until natural death."

The pace of research in the United States was slowed—at least temporarily—by President Bush's decision in August 2001 to restrict federal funding to work done with cells that had already been taken

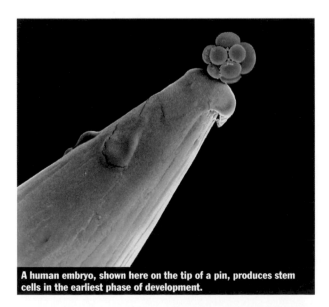

A human embryo, shown here on the tip of a pin, produces stem cells in the earliest phase of development.

before his decision. In his opinion, in this case "the life-and-death decision has already been made."

Objections to embryonic stem cell research echo the objections to abortion. But, say defenders of the research, abortion is not the issue here. They point out that a four- or five-day-old embryo in a lab is not a fetus, and instead of being discarded its cells should be used to help people. Be that as it may, government policy prevents the NIH, the main source of funding for biomedical research in the United States, from supporting any work on fresh

supplies of stem cells taken from human embryos. At least one scientist, Roger Pederson, a top researcher at the University of California, San Francisco, announced in 2001 that he would move to England to continue his work. Hundreds of others, including 80 Nobel Prize winners, have petitioned the U.S. federal government to fund embryonic stem cell research.

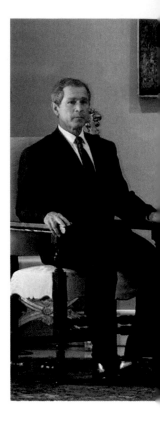

Polls show that Americans support stem cell research by a two-to-one margin and say it should have federal funding; that margin holds up even among Roman Catholics. And some conservative politicians who strongly oppose abortion, including U.S. Human Services Secretary Tommy Thompson and Senators Trent Lott, Strom Thurmond, and Orrin Hatch, regard embryonic stem cell research as an important way to save lives. Hatch has said that "a frozen embryo stored in a refrigerator in a clinic" is nothing like "a fetus developing in a mother's womb."

Another Candidate: Adult Stem Cells

As an alternative to cells from embryos, some scientists look to their offspring, the more specialized stem cells that are committed to forming particular cell types. These adult cells exist in grownups (and, despite the name, in children), so they don't raise the religious and political questions that surround embryonic cells.

In theory, adult stem cells should be able to repair damaged parts that their family built in the first place. But can these cells go beyond producing more of their own kind? Are they flexible enough to change course and make other types of tissue?

Scientists thought not—until experiments with animals produced a surprise: At least some adult stem cells can be retrained. Bone marrow cells implanted in the hearts of mice that had suffered heart attacks became cardiac tissue. And researchers at Stanford University reported in December 2000 that bone marrow stem cells from rats could become nerve cells.

The NIH, however, cautions that adult stem cells may have "limited potential." In humans, no adult

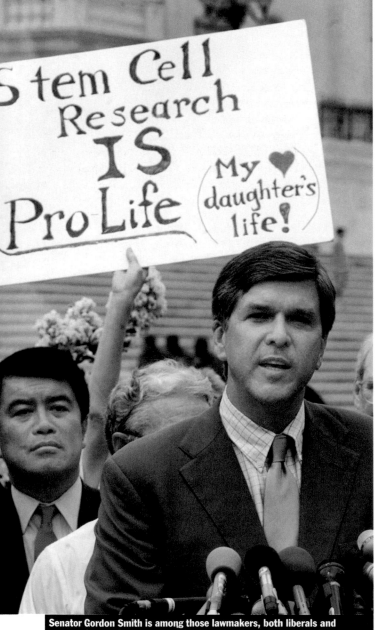

Senator Gordon Smith is among those lawmakers, both liberals and conservatives, who have urged President Bush to allow stem cell research to continue at the National Institutes of Health.

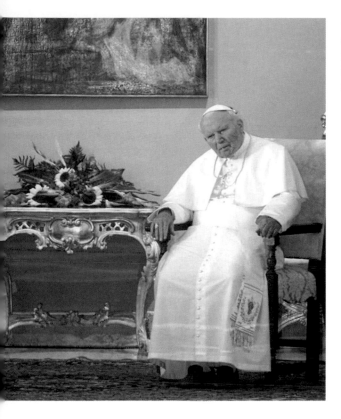

◄ George Bush discussed stem cell research with Pope John Paul II in July 2001 before reaching a decision on funding.

Still, any adult stem cells that can be harnessed should be a safe bet for organ repairs and other cell therapies. If doctors could take stem cells from you, coax them to produce the type of cell you need, then transplant them back, your immune system—already familiar with the stem cells—should not reject the new cells. Because of this added safety, the use of adult stem cells is being explored for children with problems such as osteogenesis imperfecta, a rare disease in which bones become brittle and break easily.

Whatever the source of these magnificently helpful cells, one thing is certain: All the revelations of the past year are just a hint of the developments to come. Cutting-edge researchers, political and religious leaders, investors, and ordinary people all over the world, both healthy and ill, are fascinated by the potential of stem cells.

There's no way of knowing whether the promise the cells hold will become reality and whether the cures that emerge will last for months, years, or lifetimes. But for Michael J. Fox and millions of other people who see help within reach, sometimes for the first time in their lives, there is everything to gain and no time to waste.

stem cells have yet been found for certain crucial types of tissue—heart muscle, for example, and insulin-producing islets in the pancreas. Except for blood stem cells, most of the adult cells that have been found are very scarce, become even scarcer as we age, and are difficult to isolate and purify. So far, nobody has shown that they can develop into more than a few different cell and tissue types. And the adult stem cells seem to have a life span that is much shorter than that of pluripotent cells.

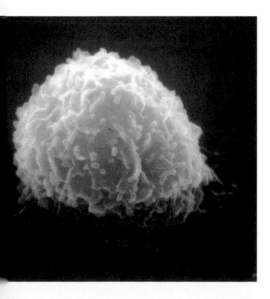

◄ Adult stem cells like this one skirt the ethical issues—but how useful are they to medicine? Only time will tell.

WHAT DOES IT MEAN TO YOU?

Stem cells can grow into healthy tissue that could one day restore any part of the body that has been damaged by accident, age, or disease. They could be used to reverse:

■ **Brain and nervous system damage.** Cells destroyed by Alzheimer's, Parkinson's, strokes, or spinal cord injuries could be replaced with healthy nerve cells produced by stem cells.

■ **Burns.** New skin grown from stem cells could put an end to skin grafts.

■ **Cancer.** Infusions of stem cells could repair tissue damaged by the disease and by toxic treatments.

■ **Diabetes.** New insulin-producing islet cells in the pancreas, grown from embryonic stem cells, could reduce or eliminate insulin injections for people with type 1 diabetes.

■ **Heart disease.** Stem cells programmed to become heart muscle cells could replace heart muscle killed in a heart attack. Other stem cells could repair damaged arteries.

■ **Kidney and liver disease.** Infusions of healthy kidney or liver cells grown from a patient's own stem cells could make organ transplants unnecessary.

■ **Vision problems.** Aging cells in the retina of the eye could be restored.

Cloning Promises Cures and Conflict

"**I**t's totally unacceptable, irresponsible and reckless, and these people need to be stopped," says Rudolf Jaenisch, M.D., professor of biology at the Massachusetts Institute of Technology. The target of his condemnation? An international group of fertility experts who announced in January 2001 that they intended to clone a human being.

The expressed purpose of the attempt—to help men who have no sperm be able to father children—did nothing to quench the flames of controversy surrounding the issue of human cloning. To critics such as Jaenisch, a scientist who has made important contributions to cloning technology, these experiments cross the line between responsible science and dangerous tinkering with human life.

Just where does the line lie? That was the question behind the new wave of controversy in 2001. Since the arrival in 1997 of Dolly the sheep, the first cloned mammal, scientists have successfully cloned mice, goats, cows, and pigs while critics and supporters— politicians,

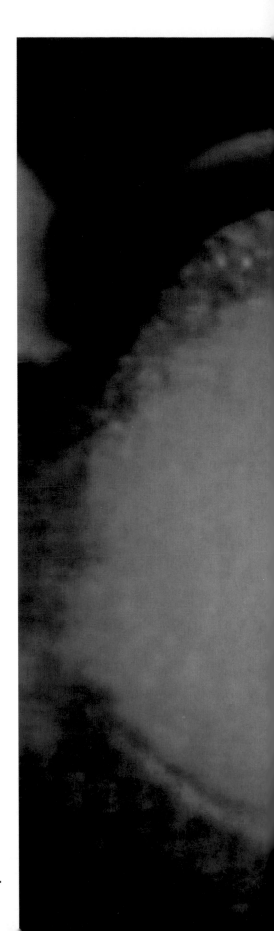

▶ **To make a clone, an egg's nucleus — including its DNA — must first be removed.**

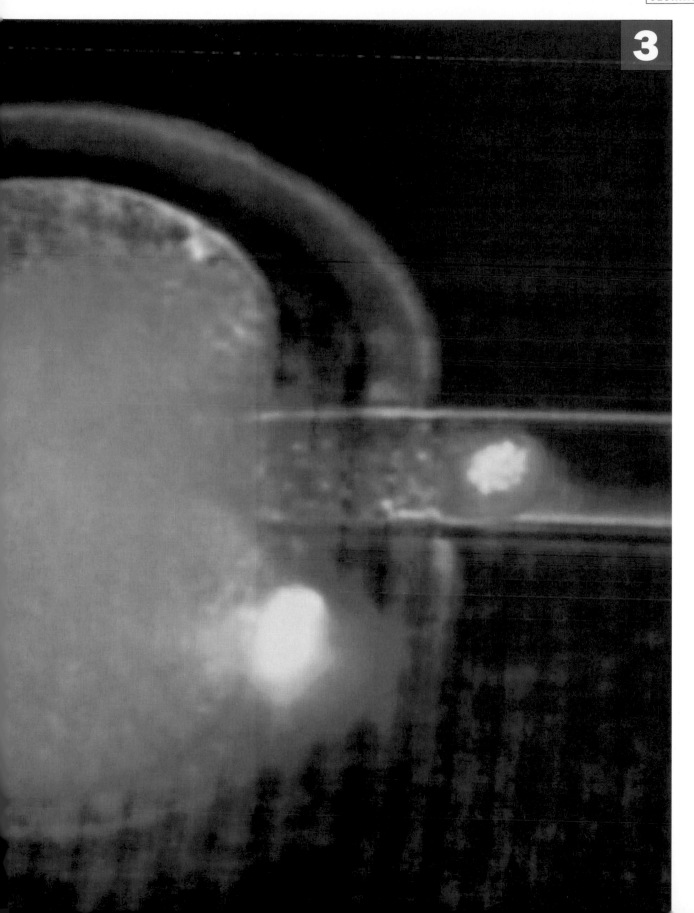

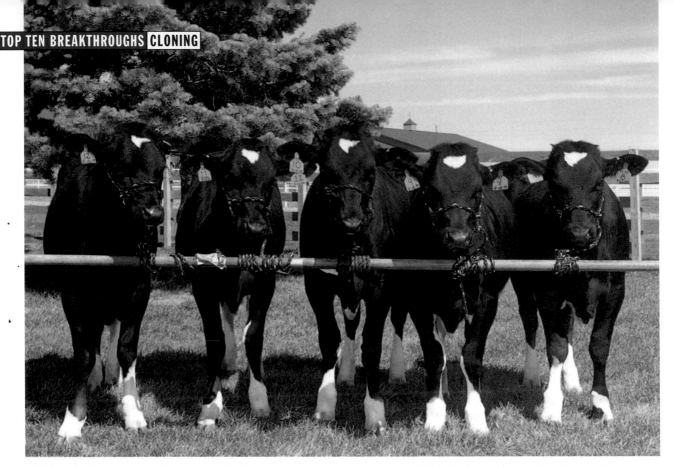

religious leaders, experts in medical ethics, and other scientists—have wrestled with the ultimate implications of letting this genie out of the bottle.

▲ These cows were cloned succesfully in 2000, but many more efforts to clone a complete animal fail.

Many countries have passed laws against human cloning. In July 2001, the U.S. House of Representatives voted to ban the cloning of human embryos for any purpose, whether to make babies or to use cells from the embryos to pursue cures for disease. Political and scientific debate rages even as researchers continue to explore new ways in which cloning—not necessarily of complete bodies but of human components, for example, entire organs such as the liver or kidney or certain types of cells such as stem cells—could prove beneficial. It seems that as the science behind cloning improves, the ethical problems become more complex.

Sex 101

Cloning alters one fundamentally important step in the normal reproductive process. Understanding precisely what that alteration is and the different ways cloning might be applied can clarify what the controversy is all about.

Your own personal genetic code—the DNA containing the genetic instructions that define you—resides in the nucleus of each one of your cells. It was created when a sperm cell from your father and an egg cell from your mother united and their genetic material combined. The resulting embryo thus contained a mixture of DNA from both of your parents.

As that embryo divided again and again to create the new cells that would make up your whole body, your basic instructions—packaged in 46 chromosomes, 23 from each parent—were passed along to every new cell, eventually coming into play to produce your own set of biological characteristics. You may have your father's chin and your mother's eyes, but in your entirety, you are a genetically distinct individual because your particular combination of genetic material is unique.

You end up with a mixture of traits because each sperm cell and each egg cell, unlike other cells in the body, contains just 23 chromosomes, or one half of the genetic code. Only when the egg and the sperm join together do they form an embryo that contains a whole set of genes.

This is where cloning differs from ordinary conception: Instead of combining the DNA from two individuals, cloning uses the DNA from only one individual. The resulting offspring is, genetically speaking, an exact copy of the single individual from which the DNA came.

To Make a Clone

The process is far simpler to describe than it has been to accomplish. To create a clone of, say, a sheep, scientists first remove the nucleus from an unfertilized egg cell. Then they take the nucleus from one of the sheep's adult cells (or they use a whole cell) and place it next to the egg cell. Finally they fuse the two cells with the help of an electric current and transfer the resulting embryo to a surrogate mother's uterus. There it grows to term, developing into a genetic duplicate of the original sheep.

In Dolly's case, the cloning team took the nucleus from an udder cell in a six-year-old ewe, but researchers have also transferred nuclei from skin and other adult cells.

The process of removing an egg cell's nucleus and inserting new material is laborious and often has to be repeated hundreds of times before it's successful. Even then, more than 95 percent of the attempts to clone animals have ended in failure. The genes are all there but some of them don't work right, and consequently many animal clones abort spontaneously. So far, nobody knows why these errors occur. Of those fetuses that make it to term, many come out deformed or monstrously big. Others die soon from problems with the immune system, heart, blood vessels, lungs, or other organs.

But let's say the process could be perfected someday. What would be the point of making a clone? If you could somehow set aside ethical and religious considerations for a moment, you might see a number of possibilities. Farmers, for example, could benefit economically from creating whole herds of genetically identical animals: Find the perfect cow with just the right combination of qualities, and make thousands of identical copies. Although genetically identical mice have been created by breeding methods, scientists would love the chance to study a new treatment using other identical groups of mammals; with a cloned control group literally identical in every way, the results in the test group could be produced only by the treatment being studied. Environmentalists might relish the ability to create clones of a species whose numbers are dwindling or even to bring back those species recently extinct.

As for human cloning, you can forget about the science-fiction scenario of madmen creating armies of perfect replicas. Even if the technology were good enough (it certainly is not,

Debate rages even as researchers continue to explore new ways in which cloning—not necessarily of complete bodies but of human components, for example, entire organs or certain types of cells such as stem cells—could prove beneficial.

experienced cloners point out, and it won't be for a long time, if ever), its proponents envision more benign uses. The main possibility they have outlined so far is enabling infertile couples or those in which one partner has a genetic defect to have children genetically identical to the healthy parent instead of using sperm or eggs donated by a stranger. Proponents stress that such procedures could be restricted to couples who can't conceive healthy offspring naturally. But opponents see a slippery

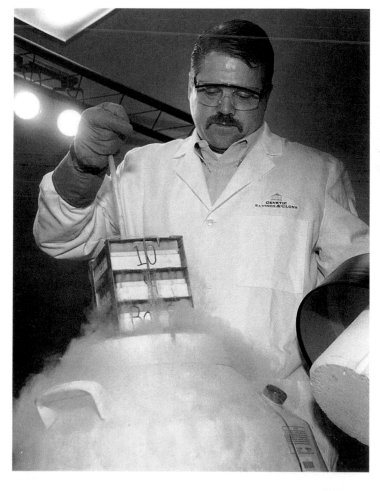

▶ Animal cells being saved for future cloning must be stored in liquid nitrogen, which keeps them at a temperature of −320°F (−196°C).

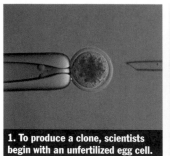

1. To produce a clone, scientists begin with an unfertilized egg cell.

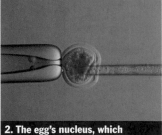

2. The egg's nucleus, which contains its DNA, is removed.

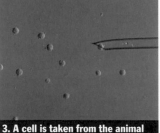

3. A cell is taken from the animal being cloned.

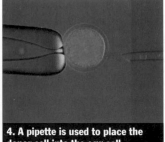

4. A pipette is used to place the donor cell into the egg cell.

slope. As evidence, they point to a private company's announcement in the fall of 2000 that an unidentified American couple was investing $1 million in an attempt to clone a child using cells from their 10-month-old daughter, who died in an accident.

Growing Only So Far

There is, however, another aspect of cloning that brings the controversy closer to home: the fact that the goal of most cloning work now under way is *not* to copy a whole person. Instead, serious researchers are concentrating on growing cloned embryos only to a certain point and then harvesting early cell forms, called stem cells, that show considerable promise in treating various illnesses. This approach is known as therapeutic cloning, and it may offer the best hope for millions of people who suffer from diseases such as Alzheimer's, cancer, cystic fibrosis, diabetes, heart failure, and Parkinson's, among others. (See Stem Cells Raise Hopes and Fears, page 22.)

In two separate studies published in the journal *Science* in the spring of 2001, researchers describe how they cloned cells from mice to make embryos that they could use to create cells of certain specialized types. The first experiment produced nerve cells; the second produced cells that secrete insulin. The hope is that when these cells are implanted back into the mice they came from, they will replace cells damaged by injury or disease. The great advantage of their being clones is that they won't be rejected as for-

To its strongest defenders, therapeutic cloning seems little different from banking your own blood, and it stirs few pangs of conscience.

eign bodies by the animals' immune systems.

In theory, the same process should work with human cells. Researchers even envision the possibility of growing entire replacement organs (such as hearts and livers) from cloned cells, making it possible for transplant patients to receive healthy copies of organs that are in every respect their own.

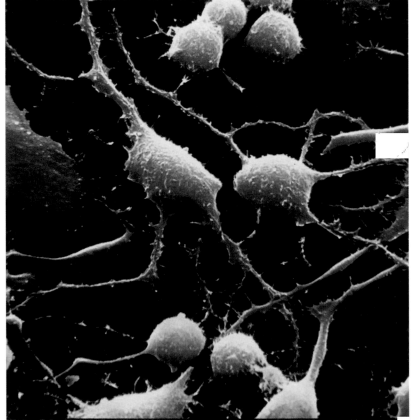

In the future, stem cells from cloned embryos may be used to grow new nerve cells (above) offering a possible cure for neurological diseases such as Parkinson's disease.

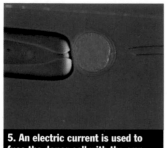

5. An electric current is used to fuse the donor cell with the egg.

In early July 2001, researchers at the Jones Institute for Reproductive Medicine, a private laboratory in Virginia, announced that they had begun to clone human embryos as sources of stem cells. The following day a company in Massachusetts called Advanced Cell Technology reported that it hoped to do so soon. The announcements sparked a new firestorm of debate fed by hope and fear about therapeutic cloning.

The Great Debate

To its strongest defenders, therapeutic cloning seems little different from banking your own blood, and it stirs few pangs of conscience. But some people who are fiercely opposed see any kind of experiment with—let alone harvesting of—human embryos as a totally unacceptable creation and destruction of life. "Human embryo farms" would be a "ghoulish industry," said Douglas Johnson, legislative director of the National Right to Life Committee, in applauding the House of Representatives vote to ban all cloning of embryos. The dispute—over points of science, ethics, religion, and practicality—is unlikely to simmer down soon.

On August 7, 2001, a spirited debate on the subject of cloning took place at a daylong conference held at the U.S. National Academy of Sciences (NAS), in Washington, D.C. The NAS, charged with the task of advising the U.S. government on what direction to take with human cloning experiments, convened the Panel on Scientific and Medical Aspects of Human Cloning to foster discussion and gather information. Among those speaking were three who reiterated their previously announced plans to clone a human being. Severino Antinori, M.D., from Rome, Italy—the controversial fertility doctor who gained fame in 1994 for helping a 62-year-old woman have a child—was one of them.

Antinori defended his plans to use cloning to allow infertile couples to have children, noting that there were hundreds of couples ready to volunteer for the experiments he and his co-panelist Panayiotis Zavos, M.D., an infertility expert from Lexington, Kentucky, plan to perform. Opponents,

including Dr. Jaenisch and Ian Wilmut, Ph.D., the creator of Dolly, stressed the inherent dangers in the technique, including the possibility of genetic abnormalities, miscarriage, and stillbirth.

Ethical aspects of cloning and the use of therapeutic cloning were also among the hot topics discussed by the international group of experts. The recommendations of the NAS will help to shape cloning policy in the United States, and perhaps elsewhere in the world. And as lawmakers try to determine ethical and legal boundaries for society as a whole, researchers continue to make the task more complicated—some by pushing for experiments that approach the realm of fantasy, others by working more modestly to expand the possibilities for breakthroughs in everyday medicine.

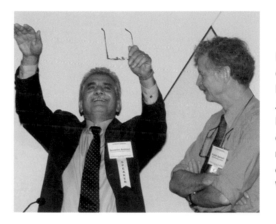

◀ Severino Antinori, M.D. (left), a proponent of human cloning from Rome, Italy, and Rudolf Jaenisch, M.D., from Massachusetts, a human cloning opponent, met at an August 2001 conference in Washington, D.C.

WHAT DOES IT MEAN TO YOU?

Some forms of cloning—such as the creation of monoclonal antibodies (see Smart Drugs Zero In on Cancer, page 34)—are already widely accepted and being put to use. Other cloning techniques that may be possible in the future include:

■ Growing genetically matched tissues for skin grafts and complete organs, such as hearts and livers, for transplants.
■ Cloning colonies of human stem cells capable of turning into insulin-producing pancreatic cells to cure diabetes, dopamine-producing brain cells to cure Parkinson's disease, heart cells to reverse heart disease and heal tissue damaged by heart attacks, and other cells for a variety of other therapies. (See Stem Cells Raise Hopes and Fears, page 22.)
■ Creating cloned human embryos to enable infertile couples or those with genetic defects to have healthy children.

Smart Drugs Zero

4

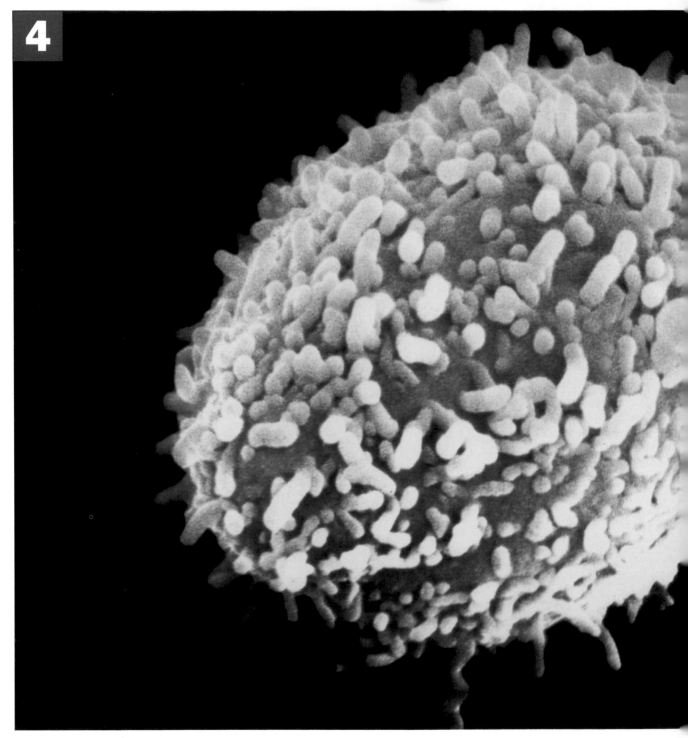

in on Cancer

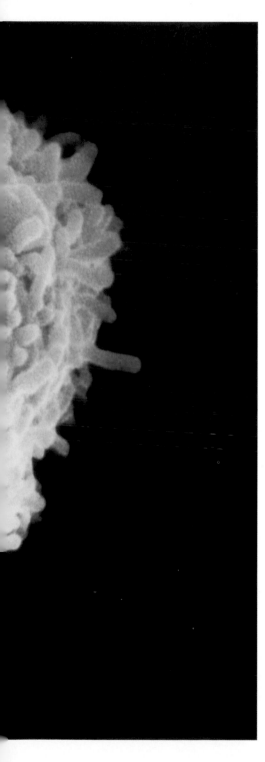

Most of the time, the immune system does a terrific job of fighting disease. Among the key troops in the body's defending army are tiny Y-shaped molecules called antibodies, whose role is to identify invaders—such as viruses or bacteria—and neutralize them. Some antibodies bind to the invaders, marking them for destruction by other immune system forces; others do the job themselves. And once the antibodies have done their work, it's only a matter of time until the foe is conquered.

Researchers are using genetically engineered antibodies to target tumors with razor-sharp precision.

But when they come up against an enemy such as cancer, the body's defenders face a bigger challenge. Because cancer cells are normal cells that have gone awry, they carry markers on their surface that identify them as "self." Antibodies don't see them as a threat, therefore, and they leave them alone. Cancer-fighting drugs typically have the same problem distinguishing friend from foe; as a result, they kill indiscriminately. That's what makes chemotherapy so miserable and potentially harmful: The assault against cancer cells damages healthy cells, too.

A New Breed of Antibodies

◀ **Monoclonal antibodies (left) are made-to-order weapons against cancer and other diseases.**

Now, medicine has a remarkable new trick up its sleeve: precision laboratory-engineered forms of that front-line defender, the antibody. These new weapons, called monoclonal antibodies, can target cancer cells for attack, allowing the immune system to recognize them as the enemy. And by putting a finger on the bad guys, they can help chemotherapy drugs zero in on just the cancer cells, leaving healthy cells alone.

Herceptin and breast cancer cells

Cell division in the breast cancer cell below could be stopped by the monoclonal antibody Herceptin. It works by attaching itself to extra HER2 receptors that cause the abnormally rapid growth of cancerous cells.

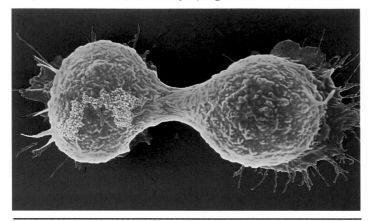

What are monoclonal antibodies? In simple terms, they're perfect copies, or clones, of antibodies that have been genetically engineered to bind to, and thus mark for identification, any kind of cell one desires to find.

That means monoclonals—unlike the ordinary antibodies our body produces—can be custom designed to recognize specific diseases, including cancer and other conditions that involve malfunctions of the body's own cells or systems. Instead of just distinguishing between what's "self" and what's not, they set their sights on very specific targets, enabling the immune system to attack what it would otherwise ignore and helping drugs to do only good, and no harm.

Most drugs affect a variety of different functions in the body—just look at the list of side effects on your next prescription. You may know of a child with leukemia who is shorter than her classmates and perhaps you thought that her cancer had somehow affected her growth. But did you know that the reason for this was not the cancer itself but the very treatment that has given her the possibility of an enjoyable, normal life? Cancer drugs that stop cancer cells from growing also stop healthy cells from growing, and the result can be that a child's overall growth slows down considerably.

The great news about monoclonal antibodies is that someday they'll be able to make good drugs better—by keeping them tightly focused on the problem at hand. The possibilities are exciting, and they grow more so almost every day.

In the fall of 2000, researchers announced successful clinical trials of a monoclonal-based drug for non-Hodgkin's lymphoma, a cancer of the lymphatic system, which may join a similar type of drug, rituximab, as a treatment option. A few months later, in May of 2001, researchers revealed at the American Cancer Society's Science Writers Seminar that they had developed a monoclonal antibody capable of recognizing metastatic prostate cancer cells—ones that have already spread beyond the prostate and in the past have been nearly impossible to treat. The good news promises to keep on coming.

A Trojan Horse for Toxic Payloads

The customized nature of monoclonal antibodies means they may eventually be used to treat an enormous range of diseases, from arthritis to heart disease. Many would argue that monoclonals offer the greatest promise against cancer, especially if they can be turned into delivery trucks for toxic payloads such as radiation-laden molecules or anti-cancer drugs. This approach offers the great appeal of delivering fatal packages right to the cancer cells' door while leaving healthy cells alone.

OF MICE AND MONOCLONALS

In 1975, Georges Köhler, Ph.D., and César Milstein, Ph.D., created the first genetically engineered antibodies and, along with Niels Jerne, M.D., won a Nobel Prize in 1984 for their efforts. They created specific immune reactions in mice, developed a technique for cloning the antibody-containing immune cells from the mice, and then harvested those antibodies to create therapeutic drugs for human use.

Although it was comparatively easy to do this in mice, there turned out to be one big problem: The resulting drugs were rejected by human patients' immune systems, which identified the drugs as foreign bodies. Patients who received these medications on a trial basis often suffered life-threatening reactions.

Researchers then began to "humanize" the antibodies by replacing at least half of the mouse DNA in the antibodies with DNA from humans. The most successful effort to date has been Genentech's trastuzamab (brand name Herceptin), approved in 1999 for the treatment of breast cancer; it's 5 percent mouse and 95 percent human.

Scientists Niels Jerne (left) and Georges Köhler. Jerne's work on the immune system led to the development of the first monoclonal antibodies by Köhler and Milstein.

The customized nature of monoclonal antibodies means they may eventually be used to treat an enormous range of diseases, from arthritis to heart disease.

Monoclonal antibodies have the potential not only to destroy cancerous and other diseased cells but also to control virtually any system in which cells send signals to one another using proteins as messengers. When this communication breaks down, or the proteins send the wrong signals, the result can be inflammatory diseases such as rheumatoid arthritis and Crohn's disease (an inflammatory bowel disease). If monoclonals could identify and then block errant messages, they could become a highly effective treatment for these problems and others.

Monoclonals continue to unite the latest medical advances with the best of the body's own medicine. As the focus of the Human Genome Project moves to identifying which proteins are created by each of the 30,000-plus human genes—and, more important, what these proteins do—researchers anticipate finding a burgeoning host of new targets for the little Y-shaped wonders.

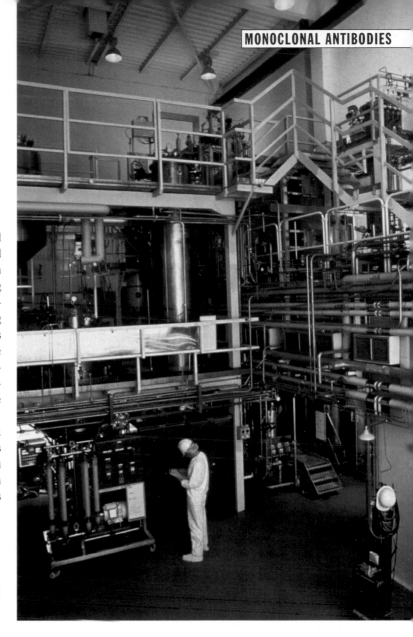

▶ Monoclonal antibodies are multiplied in a fermenter to produce large quantities of genetically identical copies.

WHAT DOES IT MEAN TO YOU?

In the not-too-distant future, monoclonal antibodies will be helping people overcome a wide variety of health problems. These new medicines may bring the added benefit of fewer side effects than the drugs patients are currently taking. Monoclonal-based medications currently on the market or undergoing major clinical trials offer the promise of breakthroughs in treatment for diseases including:

■ Rheumatoid arthritis. D2E7, a drug that is undergoing advanced-phase trials now, could treat rheumatoid arthritis by blocking an inflammatory response that leads to joint destruction.

■ Breast cancer. Trastuzamab (Herceptin), approved in 1999, inhibits the growth of breast cancer cells.

■ Non-Hodgkin's lymphoma (NHL). Rituximab (brand name Rituxan), approved in 1997 for the treatment of NHL, attacks potentially cancerous cells directly. Rituximab also acts as a delivery truck for anticancer drugs.

■ Clot-related heart problems. Abciximab (brand name ReoPro), approved for pharmaceutical use in 1995, attacks blood clots by targeting platelets; it has reduced the risk of death during angioplasty (a procedure used to open blocked coronary arteries) by 57 percent.

■ Acute myeloid leukemia. Mylotarg, approved in May 2000, uses a monoclonal antibody (anti-CD33) to deliver a potent anticancer antibiotic (calicheamicin) directly to the white blood cells affected by the cancer while sparing healthy white blood cells. Mylotarg can be prescribed in patients over the age of 60 who are not candidates for other forms of chemotherapy.

Biochips Tell Your Genetic Fortune

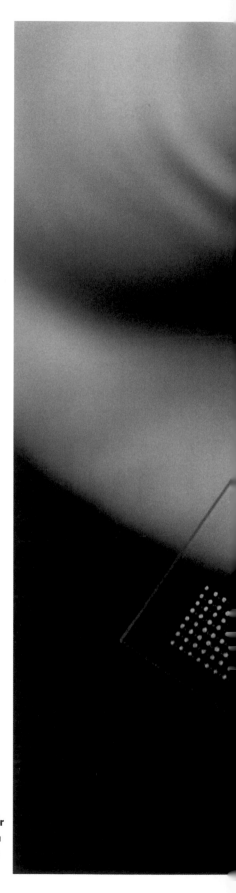

A new family of microchips made news in 2001 because they are no ordinary computer chips. Instead of crunching 0s and 1s, they read the molecular letters of life—the As, Ts, Gs, and Cs of our DNA. These new chips, called biochips, have a mission unlike any ever before: to scan a person's genes, looking for DNA sequences that warn of tendencies to develop such diseases as breast cancer, Alzheimer's, and Parkinson's.

Biochips resemble computer chips in one respect: They are small and flat. But instead of carrying tiny transistors on their surface, these thin wafers of glass or plastic are peppered with spots of DNA, called probes, that serve as samples against which your own DNA can be tested for mutations that increase your risk of disease.

In the spring of 2001, researchers announced the development of a particularly powerful biochip. Capable of analyzing up to 10,000 genes at one time, it offers the potential to distinguish or diagnose many different disorders in short order. Although not yet available commercially, this biochip and others promise to accelerate what is

▶ **These glass wafers, with their dots of DNA, can read the secrets of your genes.**

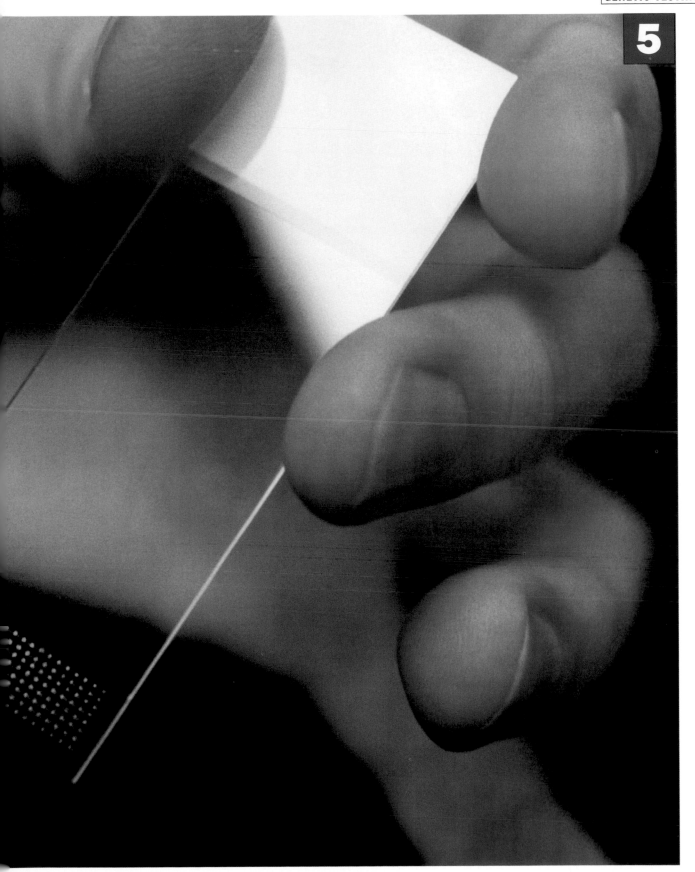

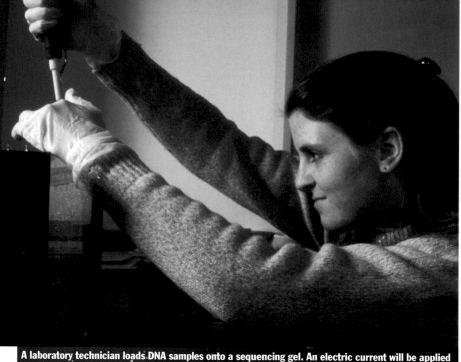

5

A laboratory technician loads DNA samples onto a sequencing gel. An electric current will be applied to the gel to separate the fragments of DNA so the gene sequence can be read.

Birds of a feather flock together

When the solution of the DNA being tested is washed over the biochip, only those strands that share the genetic profile of the disease being tested for will bind to the probes. The probes for DNA's four molecular building blocks (T, A, C, and G) are shown on the left. The DNA being tested is shown on the right.

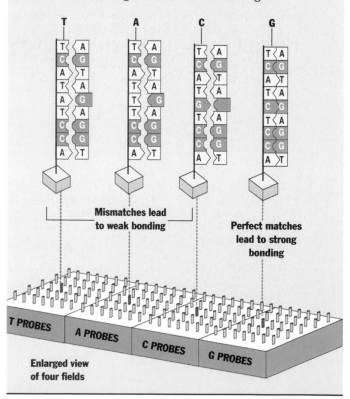

Mismatches lead to weak bonding

Perfect matches lead to strong bonding

T PROBES
A PROBES
C PROBES
G PROBES

Enlarged view of four fields

already an astounding revolution in the diagnosis, treatment, and prevention of disease.

Getting the Jump on Disease

The best treatment for almost every progressive disease—hereditary or not, depends on early detection. The sooner a cancer can be identified, for example, the better the chances of survival. Screening tests of all kinds are designed for just this purpose: to find evidence of a disease before it has progressed far enough to make symptoms appear.

Some tests, like the tuberculin skin test for tuberculosis or the HIV blood test for AIDS, look for precursor factors that might eventually cause a specific disease—a bacteria for tuberculosis, a virus for AIDS. Other tests, including many for various cancers, can detect only the presence of the disease itself. The PSA (prostate-specific antigen) test for prostate cancer is a case in point; it identifies a protein produced by prostate cells that have already started to grow out of control.

Genetic testing goes one giant step further. It tracks a disease down to its genetic source, potentially long before it begins to cause trouble. Doctors and patients couldn't ask for a better head start.

Reading "Mistakes" in the Code

We've known for years that certain hereditary diseases can be traced to abnormalities in our genes. Until recently, though, for most diseases, doctors could do little better than guess, based on family history, whether someone was genetically predisposed to a given illness. All that has changed with the sequencing of the human genome, an astonishing feat just completed in 2001. (See Scientists Read the Letters of Life, page 14.) Scientists now have access to the entire 3.2-billion-letter arrangement of DNA's four building-block molecules: adenine (A), thymine (T), guanine (G), and cytosine (C).

By examining DNA sequences carefully—in some cases comparing the DNA of healthy individuals with the DNA of people in whom a genetic illness has shown up—researchers have begun to link specific arrangements of As, Ts, Gs, and Cs with specific diseases. What they've started to find, in other words, are differences in the coding that tells the body how to function properly. Some of these differences (called variants) are associated with an increased risk of disease. Researchers are now developing a battery of screening tests for these variants that will one day take the guesswork out of predicting some people's risk of disease. Whereas in the past such genetic tests might have been prohibitively expensive and time-consuming—with some tests taking months and even years to show results—biochips will make them infinitely more practical for routine clinical use.

The verdict is in as soon as the chip is analyzed: If the probe has made any matches, the patient has a seven-fold risk of developing Alzheimer's.

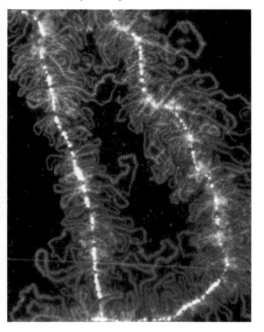

◀ Strands of your DNA like these will one day be tested to predict your chance of getting diseases—eliminating the guesswork for doctors.

The A-T-G-Cs of Biochips

To understand how biochips work, it helps to know a few DNA basics. DNA typically exists in a spiraling pair of complementary strands—the famed double helix—in which As form bonds with Ts, and Gs with Cs. These strands are programmed to reunite with their partner when they are separated, or—and here's the key for biochips—to bond with any other strand of DNA exactly like that partner.

So, if a biochip is going to be used to test for Alzheimer's, for example, segments of DNA containing the Alzheimer's defect are separated and placed on a chip as a probe. Similarly, strands of the patient's DNA are separated, placed in a solution, then washed over the biochip. Only strands with the Alzheimer's defect will bind with the DNA probe. The verdict is in as soon as the chip is analyzed: If the probe has made any matches, the patient has a seven-fold risk of developing Alzheimer's (and knowing this could greatly facilitate the diagnosis of the condition).

And here, at least in theory, is the revolutionary advantage of biochips over earlier screening methods: The entire process—from taking a sample to completing the analysis—will one day be done in a doctor's office in a matter of minutes. Because thousands of DNA probes can be attached to a single chip, it might be possible to screen for thousands of potential problems simultaneously.

Biochips also allow unparalleled diagnostic precision. In February 2000, Stanford University medical researchers used DNA chips to show that a lymphoma previously identified as a single type of cancer was in fact two genetically different diseases. The finding was particularly significant because each of those two cancers requires a different treatment. Biochips offer, for the first time, the possibility of easy, quick, and relatively inexpensive testing to determine the kind of treatment to which a particular disease may respond best.

Another exciting aspect of biochips is that they have the potential to help diagnose not only genetic disorders, but also any illness—or any infectious agent—that carries a distinct genetic marker.

In one of the clearest examples of how extensive the use of biochips could become, researchers announced in October 2000 that they had developed an optical fiber sensor armed with a biochip capable of detecting salmonella and E. coli in meat samples—right in the processing plant. The bacteria's DNA gave them away in about an hour, without any outside lab work. Normal testing for these bacteria can take days.

With news like this breaking every day, it's clear that virtually any troublemaker with a DNA signature will soon be a target for biochips.

WHAT DOES IT MEAN TO YOU?

Researchers are developing better and faster ways to analyze genes. In the future look for:

■ Glass or plastic chips embedded with DNA that can be used to test people for responses to certain drugs, allowing doctors to determine which treatments will be effective—before they prescribe a new medication.

■ Chips that identify antibiotic-resistant strains of tuberculosis, allowing doctors to better target drug therapies.

■ Chips designed to detect genetic mutations linked to breast cancer, Alzheimer's, and other diseases, facilitating early diagnosis.

■ Chips that identify multiple strains of life-threatening infectious diseases, including hepatitis and HIV.

6

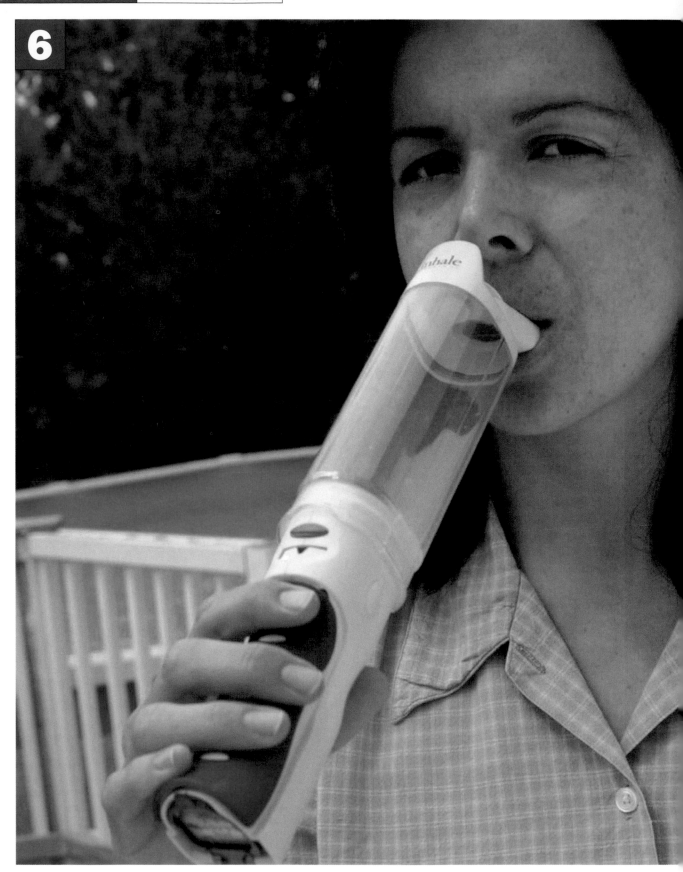

Better Ways to Take Your Medicine

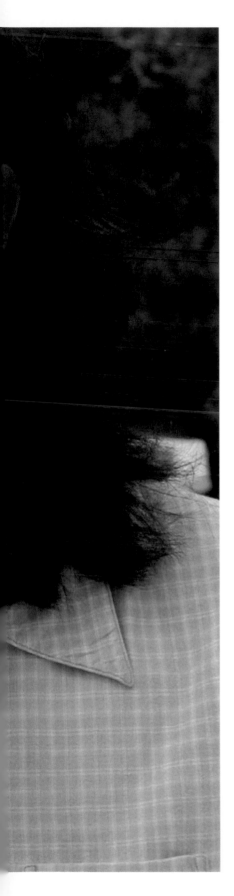

Here: an alcohol swab, a vial, a syringe, a needle, a sting of pain, and a handful of biohazardous waste. There: a compact inhaler, a tilt of the head, and a discreet puff. In both cases, insulin is successfully delivered. In 2001, researchers made significant progress getting from here to there.

Modern medicine is well regarded for developing new drugs, but in many respects the ways we get them into our bodies would be quite familiar to the physicians of ancient Egypt. However, it's become quite clear in recent years that a drug is only as good as its mode of transportation, and scientists are now devising innovative techniques to deliver medications to all parts of the body more easily, effectively, and safely.

By targeting potent drugs—those designed to kill cancer cells, for example—to specific tissues, some of these new drug delivery systems will help reduce debilitating side effects. Others will serve as internal pharmacists, releasing precise doses of medication at preset times. Still others will prevent a drug from

◀ BREATHE EASY
Soon diabetics may be able to get their insulin from an inhaler instead of a needle.

breaking down as it travels through the body to its intended destination.

Dozens of creative drug delivery systems are now in various stages of development. Here are a few noteworthy innovations.

No Need for Needles?

For anyone with insulin-dependent diabetes, injections are a fact of life, if not a way of life—first thing in the morning, before every meal, last thing before bed. But it won't be long before the needles that bear insulin—and many other drugs that must now be injected—join leeches in the archives of medical history. Taking their place will be powders and pills, and sprays and solutions, making the administration of these drugs less painful, less cumbersome, and, at the very least, less anxiety-provoking for the people who need them.

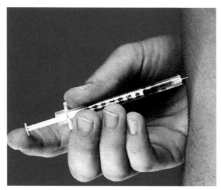

Insulin inhalers were the hot topic in 2001, with a number of biotechnology companies announcing successful clinical trials. That's not surprising: Breathing a drug directly into the lungs is effective as well as non-invasive. The drug, in the form of tiny particles, reaches the lung's millions of bronchioles (small airways) almost immediately. The drug particles easily pass through the walls of the alveoli (tiny air sacs) located at the ends of the bronchioles and are rapidly absorbed into the bloodstream.

Three insulin inhalers were tested in 2001; one of them may be available in 2002 or 2003 if its manufacturer, Inhale Therapeutics, can address concerns about possible side effects. Researchers are also conducting ongoing studies of inhaled versions of human growth hormone, used to treat children with restricted growth and adults with pituitary gland deficiencies, and the multiple sclerosis drug Avonex; both of these drugs are currently available only by injection.

Protein Pills

Powders and sprays are certainly an improvement over needles, but why can't we just pack these chemicals into a pill and down them with a glass of water? Because when they're swallowed, protein drugs such as insulin are digested in the gastrointestinal tract and never reach their target.

▲ **Injections may become a thing of the past for people who take drugs such as insulin, human growth hormone, and heparin.**

It won't be long before the needles that bear insulin—and many other drugs that must now be injected—join leeches in the archives of medical history. Taking their place will be powders and pills, sprays and solutions.

Researchers have come up with scores of possible solutions to the problem, many of which sound like the stuff of science fiction. Encase the drug in a biodegradable shell. Attach it to molecules of vitamin B_{12}, which will escort it intact through the stomach's acidic environment. Lock it behind porous "molecular fences" that open when the drug reaches its destination. This last method, developed by Emisphere Technologies, Inc., led the pack in 2001. Researchers at the Tarrytown, New York, biopharmaceutical company used it to develop insulin capsules that, in initial clinical trials, appear to be safe and effective. Emisphere is also a leader in de-

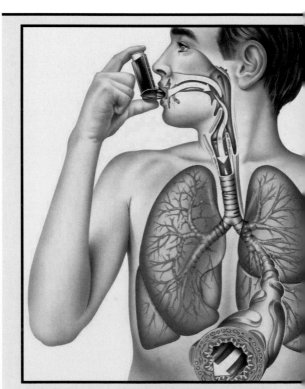

Inhalers deliver drugs deep into the lungs, through the bronchioles to the alveoli, where they are rapidly absorbed into the bloodstream.

veloping oral versions of parathyroid hormone for treating osteoporosis, and heparin, a commonly used blood thinner currently administered intravenously or by injection. Other drugs that may be fit to be swallowed in the next few years include factor VIII (used to prevent bleeding in hemophiliacs), erythropoietin (used to prevent anemia and thereby help avoid the need for blood transfusions), and human growth hormone.

Only Skin Deep

Another new way to take your medicine is through the skin. Typically, drugs that are absorbed through the skin come in transdermal patches—think nicotine patches, hormone replacement patches, and the more recent contraceptive patch (see page 203). Most are designed to offer a constant delivery of medication through the skin, avoiding the side effects that some oral drugs can have on the gastrointestinal tract and liver. Some newer patches can deliver individual doses or vary the dosage with the time of day. Patches also virtually eliminate the problem of missed doses. But for large molecules like insulin and other proteins, as well as for new synthetic biotechnology drugs and the medicines in

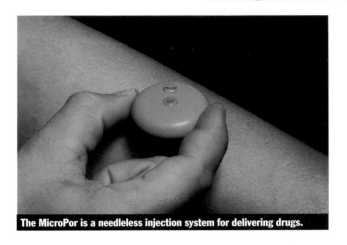

The MicroPor is a needleless injection system for delivering drugs.

vaccines, conventional patches are useless because the drug molecules are simply too large to pass through the skin's protective outer layer. Although skin has pores, it is not porous. In fact, one of the skin's primary functions is to act as a barrier, preventing fluid from getting out while blocking germs from getting in.

Now there are new ways to sneak past this body armor. A number of devices are in development that use either electric current or ultrasound to allow large molecules to penetrate the skin. In the ultrasound method, a device is placed on the skin that emits ultrasonic (very high frequency) sound waves. They cause natural air pockets in the skin to vibrate and the fatty tissues in the skin to become disorganized, allowing drug molecules to pass through the skin and into the bloodstream. A company called Sontra Medical of Cambridge, Massachusetts is currently studying the use of ultrasound to deliver insulin to type 1 diabetics.

A new device called the MicroPor, made by the Altea Development Corporation, is already successfully delivering insulin. Like the ultrasound method, it also creates hundreds of microscopic "pores" in the skin, but it uses a brief burst of electric current to accomplish this. The electrical current is sent to a tiny circuit board, which radiates heat from hundreds of miniscule points for a few milliseconds at a time. The heat vaporizes certain molecules in the paper-thin outer layer of dead skin, creating hundreds of holes no wider than a human hair. The heat is applied for one thousandth of a second, and because it targets only dead skin and does not penetrate to the nerve endings or living tissues below, it is painless. Once the pores are established, an opening in the drug reservoir located above the circuit board allows the medication to migrate through the skin.

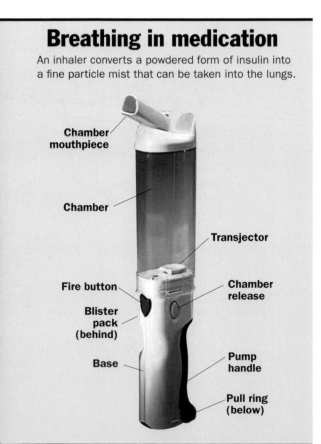

Breathing in medication

An inhaler converts a powdered form of insulin into a fine particle mist that can be taken into the lungs.

Chamber mouthpiece

Chamber

Transjector

Fire button

Chamber release

Blister pack (behind)

Base

Pump handle

Pull ring (below)

The device is currently in phase I trials. It could be used for constant dosing, drug-on-demand dosing, or a combination of both. For example, a constant dose of a painkiller such as morphine could be administered continuously, but the patient would be able to augment the dose by applying another short pulse of electric current if the level of pain increased, as often happens with cancer or after surgery. Likewise, a constant level of insulin could be used for diabetes, with an on-demand increase at mealtimes. MicroPor might also be used to deliver drugs used for chronic illnesses, such as interferon for hepatitis and parathyroid hormone for osteoporosis, or for new or existing vaccines.

Special Delivery

Many important drugs have a fatal flaw: Because they don't dissolve in water, they can't be absorbed into the bloodstream—and therefore they are of little or no help to patients.

"Some 40 percent of new drugs now being discovered are insoluble, lipid-like chemicals," says Dr. Joseph Robinson, Ph.D., a professor at the University of Wisconsin School of Pharmacy and an expert on drug delivery. "But unless a drug can be made to dissolve in water—the main component of blood—it won't have any therapeutic effect."

About ten years ago, researchers conjured up a novel way to make these fat-soluble drugs usable. They packaged them inside tiny synthetic spheres called polymeric micelles. A fat-soluble drug can dissolve in the micelle's fatty inner core, which is surrounded by a water-soluble outer shell that allows the micelle to be absorbed into the bloodstream and the drug to take effect.

It has taken some time, but one of the first drugs to benefit from micelle treatment will be taxol, an important drug for treating breast and ovarian cancer. "To make it more soluble, taxol was first marketed as an emulsion—a mixture of taxol, a fat known as cremophor, and water," says Robinson. "But the cremophor made the emulsion so toxic that taxol sometimes killed the patient. Some other approach was clearly needed."

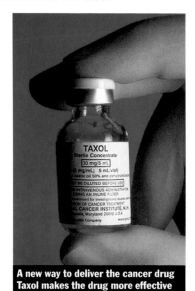

A new way to deliver the cancer drug Taxol makes the drug more effective with fewer side effects.

Doctors are beginning to recognize the importance of a new field called chronotherapeutics, an approach that synchronizes drug therapy with the rhythms of the body.

The polymeric micelle version of taxol, which should soon receive approval from the U.S. Food and Drug Administration (FDA)—phase II trials began in 2001—is a major breakthrough. The drug's solubility in water is increased by a factor of a thousand, making it far more effective than the older version. And with taxol no longer in an emulsion, it's virtually nontoxic.

In the near future, micelles will also help deliver drugs straight to their intended destination, thanks to molecules protruding from their outer shells that will help them bind to particular target cells. They could, for instance, deliver toxins to cancer cells without harming nearby healthy cells. In preliminary research at the University of Tokyo, micelles successfully delivered the chemotherapy drug doxorubicin to solid tumors.

Timing Is Everything

Diseases have their witching hours. Rheumatoid arthritis, heart attack, and stroke tend to prowl the morning; ulcers, asthma, and high cholesterol often get worse at night. Accordingly, doctors are beginning to recognize the importance of a new field called chronotherapeutics (time-related treatment), an approach that synchronizes drug therapy with the rhythms of the body. Practitioners of chronotherapy would advise administering extra doses of certain drugs—antihypertensives (high blood pressure drugs) and anti-clotting drugs, for example—during the morning hours, and others at specific times throughout the day.

The goals of chronotherapy may soon be furthered by a special microchip that takes the concept of time-release to a whole new level. The brainchild of Robert Langer, Ph.D., a professor of chemical and biomedical engineering at the Massachusetts Institute of Technology, the chip stores up to a thousand drugs (or doses) in tiny reservoirs and releases them at pre-programmed times and in particular doses. The dime-size chip, which would be swallowed or implanted under the skin, could also deliver the drugs upon receiving an external signal.

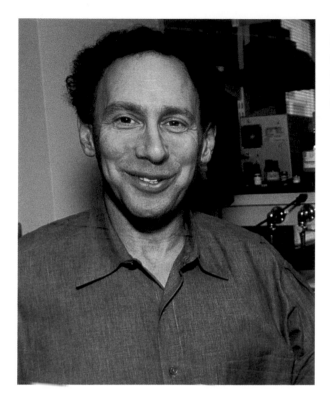

◄ Robert Langer, Ph.D., invented a microchip that stores up to a thousand drugs in resevoirs and releases them at specific times in specific doses.

Langer and his colleagues unveiled the chip in 1999; in 2001 they demonstrated that it could, in fact, release a drug in a controlled manner. It can be programmed to read its host and determine how much of a drug to deliver and when. The microchip could be used for a wide range of medications, including those for cardiac problems, cancer treatment, pain relief, and infertility. In theory, a patient could have the chip implanted and forget about taking their medication for weeks, months, or even years at a stretch.

Drugs That Stick Around

Here and there on the human body lie the so-called mucosal regions—the mucous membranes that line the gastrointestinal tract, the eyelids, the nostrils, and the vagina, for example. These areas have very efficient self-cleansing mechanisms, but that makes it difficult to get drugs to linger there for any length of time. Medications in the mouth are washed away by saliva in four to five minutes, while drugs placed in the vagina are effectively cleared within an hour. But new delivery systems are keeping these drugs in their place. Called bioadhesives, they adhere to mucous membranes for long periods of time, slowly releasing medications all the while.

Bioadhesives can deliver drugs to mucosal areas for up to several days. A conventional drug placed in the eye will be washed away in 90 seconds, for example, but a bioadhesive will keep a drug in the eye for 12 to 15 hours.

Bioadhesives come in various forms, including creams, suppositories, gels, patches, and liquids that solidify once they're in place. In addition to treating eye problems (including glaucoma and infection), bioadhesives can have other local uses, including treating sexually transmitted diseases. Replens, a gel for treating vaginal dryness, remains active for four days after being administered. Crinone, another vaginal gel, delivers progesterone for a variety of conditions, such as endometriosis and female infertility. Other bioadhesive drugs will reach the market in the next few years.

Back to the Future

Most of these technologies are still in the experimental stage and have yet to pass the test of time. But the drugs of the future require special handling, and researchers are rising to the challenge, dressing them in plastic coats, rolling them into padded spheres and onto patches, and storing them on microchips, so that one day the sting of an injection and even the struggle to remember to take your pills might seem quaintly ancient.

WHAT DOES IT MEAN TO YOU?

Drug delivery systems are still playing catch-up with the drugs themselves, but exciting progress is being made that will allow protein-based drugs to be delivered without needles, cancer drugs to hit their targets with less harm to healthy cells, and more. Here are some advances to watch for.

■ Instead of injections, the millions of people who suffer from diabetes will be able to choose from an array of pills, sprays, and inhalers to get the insulin they need every day.

■ Pills and sprays will replace injections for numerous other conditions, including osteoporosis, growth disorders, anemia, and multiple sclerosis.

■ Specially formulated drugs will be able to home in on malignant tumors, thus reducing some of the trauma of cancer therapy.

■ Advances in time-release technology will deliver the right dose of heart, cancer, pain, or other medicine at the right time.

■ Bioadhesive formulations that adhere to mucous membranes will be used to administer hormones and fertility medications and to treat sexually transmitted diseases and gastrointestinal problems.

7

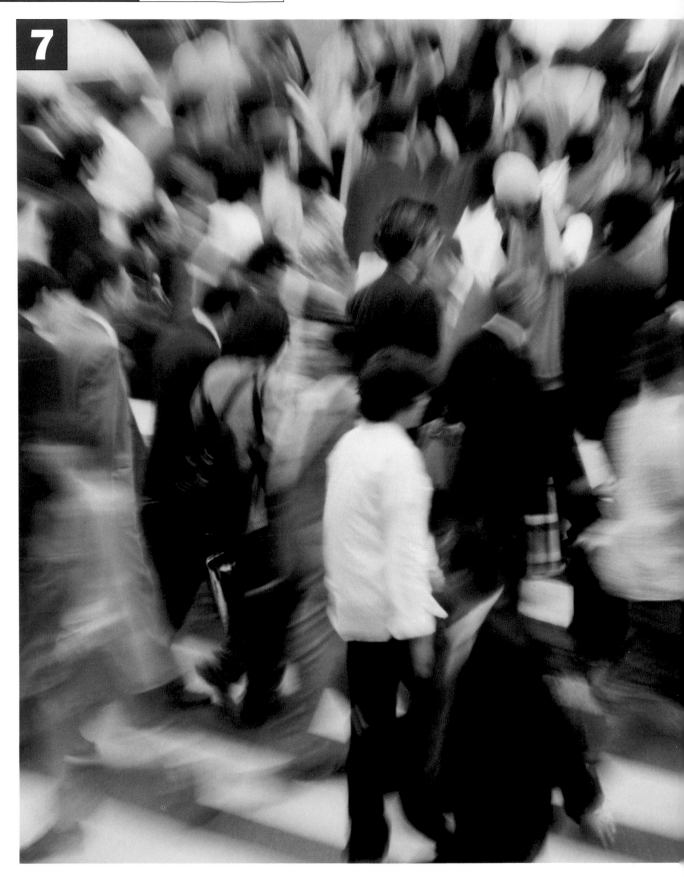

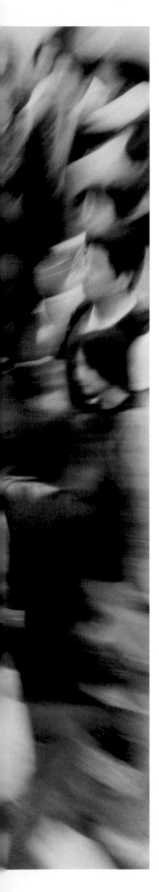

Drugs Get Personal

Two children with leukemia receive the same medication; one child goes into remission, the other dies. After abdominal surgery, two people are given codeine to relieve their pain. It soothes one, but has absolutely no effect on the other. Two patients with high cholesterol are following identical exercise, diet, and drug plans. One's cholesterol level drops, the other's continues to climb.

What's going on here? In recent years, scientists have begun to answer to that question. In 2001, they ventured to bring together the most exciting achievements in genetic testing and the most recent successes in the genetic engineering of drugs, all for the purpose of making sure you get the very best—and the most personal—medical care possible.

What's Good for the Masses

When you go to the doctor with a certain set of symptoms, or when you've been diagnosed with a specific disease, the medication you're likely to be given is one that passed clinical trials—that is, one that worked for a large number of people. The problem is that you can't always count on it working for *you*. Indeed, it's estimated that hundreds of thousands of people are hospitalized every year because of adverse reactions to properly prescribed medicines—and many thousands of those people die.

This happens not because the drug is inherently dangerous, or because the doctor was negligent, or because you took it with food when you were told to take it on an empty stomach. Many factors affect how you respond to a medication, including your age, the severity of your disorder, what you eat, and other drugs you may be taking. But more than any of these, your reaction to a drug is destined by the very stuff that determines who you are: your genes.

Since the 1950s, researchers have known that there is a genetic basis to an individual's response to drugs. But with the completion of the sequencing of the human genome in 2001, scientists at biotech companies, drug companies, and academic institutions are beginning to augment the "one size fits all" philosophy of drug treatment with the more tantalizing "this size fits you" approach.

Whether you call it by its fancy name— pharmacogenomics—or by its friendlier appellation, personalized medicine, it's an enticing vision. Imagine knowing the quirks in your own genome—and then being able to predict how a given medication will affect you. Imagine your doctor prescribing drugs that have been chosen to suit your unique body chemistry. Imagine being treated like the individual you are.

◄ **ONE IN A MILLION Many drugs affect individuals differently. That's why doctors may soon prescribe drugs based on your genetic profile.**

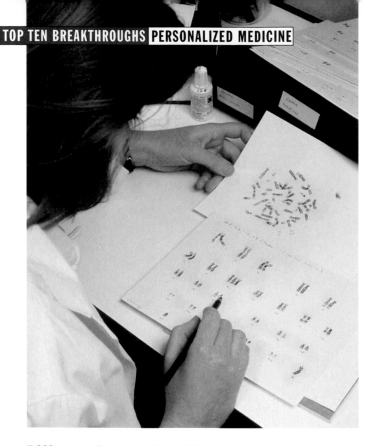

◀ A document of the full complement of chromosomes, called a karyotype, is checked for abnormalities by a cytogeneticist. Knowing whether your genes differ from what's normal will allow your doctor to choose a drug treatment that will work for you.

Different Strokes for Different Folks

Why is the medicine that's so great for Tom such a disaster for Harry? When a drug enters a person's body, the genes direct its action. For one thing, genes regulate the amount of a drug that is rendered inert before it even goes to work. Harry, for example, might be genetically inclined to convert 70 percent of a given dose of a drug to an inactive state, leaving less than a third to do the job. Given the same dose of the same medicine, Tom's genes might carry instructions to inactivate only 1 percent.

Once a drug reaches its destination, the genes are still in charge, determining how sensitive the target, or drug receptor, is going to be. Tom's genetic makeup may be such that he'll respond positively—he'll metabolize a therapeutic amount of the drug in a therapeutic amount of time. In other words, the drug will work. Harry, however, may be genetically disposed to metabolize either so little that the drug is useless, or so much that it becomes toxic.

Sometimes other mechanisms cause the trouble. For example, some five percent of the population has a genetic defect that makes it difficult to eliminate the antidepressant Prozac from the body. This means that the drug accumulates, making it more likely that this group will suffer troubling side effects like insomnia and dips in sexual energy. Even

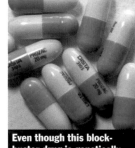

Even though this blockbuster drug is genetically unsuitable for 1 in 20 people, it still racks up sales of over two and a half billion U.S. dollars a year.

killing pain isn't simple: About 20 million Americans (8 percent of whites, 6 percent of blacks, and 1 percent of Asians) lack the liver enzyme that converts codeine to its active form, morphine. These people will still be hurting regardless of how much codeine they take.

Delivering the Goods

So much for Tom and Harry. Here's a sampling of what researchers and clinicians are doing to put pharmacogenomics to work for the rest of us.

■ Each year, some 2,400 American children and adolescents are struck with a kind of blood cancer called acute lymphoblastic leukemia. These patients are routinely given the drug 6-mercaptopurine, which often saves their lives. However, between 10 and 15 percent of these children have a genetic mutation that causes them to metabolize 6-mercaptopurine either too quickly or too slowly. The former don't benefit from the standard dose, while the latter can accumulate lethal levels of the drug. Researchers at St. Jude Children's Research Hospital in Memphis, Tennessee, developed a genetic test that identifies the abnormality and for several years they have been screening children before the drug is administered, enabling physicians to give the child just the right amount.

■ The three most common treatments for asthma do not provide consistent relief, and desperate sufferers often wheeze their way from one to another. Researchers at the University of Cincinnati College of Medicine reported in late 2000 that the effectiveness of one asthma medication, albuterol, depends on a combination of genetic factors. In 2001 scientists at Brigham and Women's Hospital in Boston and elsewhere continued the search for additional genetic explanations for the various reactions to this asthma drug and others. If they are successful, people with asthma could be genetically screened and then prescribed the medication that would work best for them.

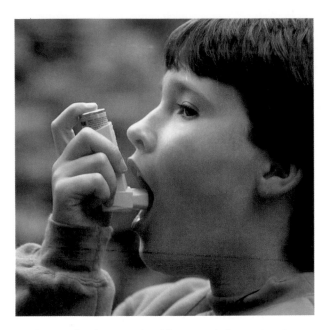

■ Currently, doctors play hit-or-miss with cholesterol medications. It is believed, though, that at least one cholesterol-lowering drug, pravastatin (brand name Pravachol), may be more effective in improving blood cholesterol numbers in people who have a specific genetic variation. In April 2001, the biotech firm Genaissance Pharmaceuticals of New Haven, Connecticut, announced the launch of a clinical trial to analyze subjects' genes to determine which cholesterol-lowering drug would serve them best. The study could also perhaps lead to subtle but significant chemical adjustments to the drugs themselves, making them even more effective.

▲ Researchers have identified 12 genes that determine how well asthma patients respond to albuterol, a drug used to prevent or control acute asthmatic attacks.

Drug Resistance

Like many genetic landscapes, the field of pharmacogenomics is littered with questions that need to be addressed. For starters: When you finally have your own gene profile, should your employer and your insurance company have it, too? When a gene pattern is ethnically linked—and some are—what do we need to do to avoid racial stereotyping? Will doctors be liable if they don't consider a person's genetic information when prescribing a drug?

Not surprisingly, some of the other thorny issues are economic. Is it worth the enormous expense to genotype many individuals in order to design a drug for only a few? Consider oral contraceptives: Birth control pills increase the risk of venous thrombosis (blood clots) among women who have a genetic abnormality called factor V. But is preventing problems for these women worth the cost of testing every woman to see if she carries the defect? Ask a relative of someone who has died of venous thrombosis or pulmonary embolism (a blood clot that has traveled to the lungs) and you'll get one answer; ask the contraceptive's manufacturer and you could well get a different one.

Indeed, the response of the pharmaceutical industry is integral to the future of personalized medicine. Historically, drug companies have depended on a few blockbuster drugs (think Prozac or Claritin) to keep their profits up; personalized medicine could be perceived as being fundamentally disruptive to that method of doing business. Jurgen Drews, chairman of Genaissance and a former head of global research at Hoffmann–La Roche, claims the pharmaceutical firms are afraid of discovering genes that expose "the limitations of their drugs," which could eventually diminish sales. Still, a few pharmaceutical companies have embraced pharmacogenomics—in some cases by acquiring a biotech company or two.

There are many players in the personalized medicine game—researchers, pharmaceutical giants, and patient advocacy groups, to name but a few. These forces are all combining to bring medical treatment to a new level, where personalized medicine means much more than a pharmacist who remembers your name or a doctor with a friendly bedside manner. In this era of custom jeans and sneakers, what could be more important than the development of tailor-made medicine—treatment for the unique person you are?

WHAT DOES IT MEAN TO YOU?

Widespread applications are years away, but pharmacogenomics promises mind-boggling benefits. Here are just a few:

■ Based on your genetic profile, your doctor will know which medication will be most effective for you and whether a particular drug might have toxic side effects.

■ Physicians will be armed with both genetically targeted drugs and detailed information about which diseases you're likely to develop. This will allow them to intervene with preventive medications well in advance of symptoms—so tumors won't ever form, arteries won't clog, bones won't grow brittle, and aging brain cells won't die.

■ Instead of focusing only on medications with mass appeal, pharmaceutical companies could begin to develop drugs to treat disorders that affect smaller numbers of people.

■ Promising drugs that were withdrawn because of unacceptable side effects may be reintroduced for use by people who have genetic immunity to the risks.

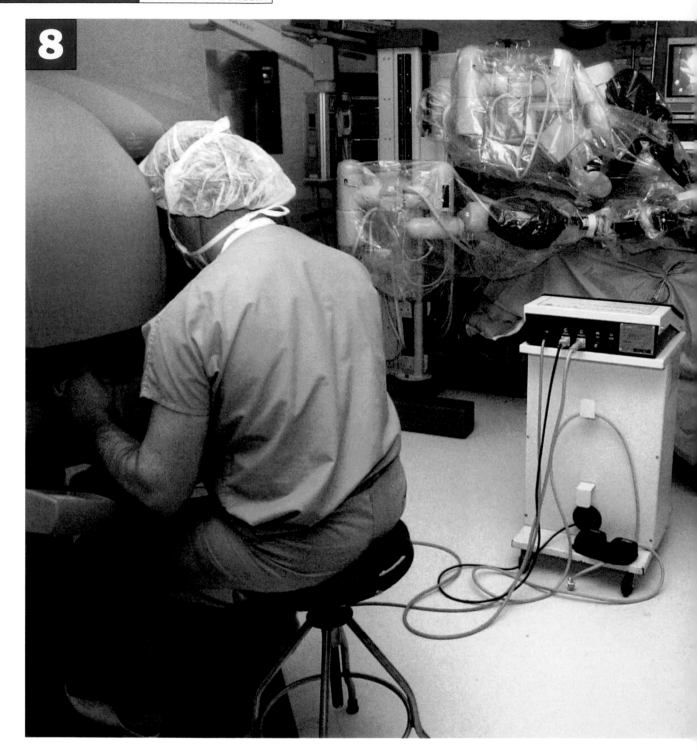

Robots Join the

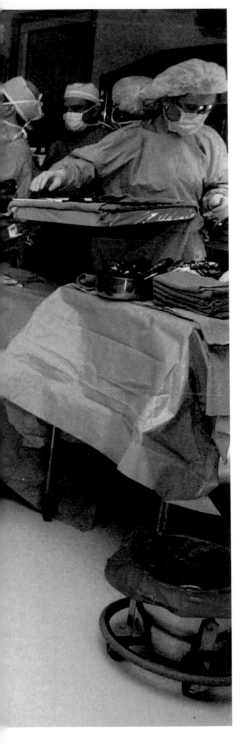

◀ Andrew Boyarsky, M.D., of Robert Wood Johnson University Hospital in New Brunswick, New Jersey, seated left, uses the da Vinci Surgical System to perform a gallbladder operation from about 10 feet away.

I f you ever end up under the knife, what qualities will you want in your surgeon? Nerves of steel? An inhumanly steady hand? Laser precision? Chances are getting better and better that you'll find just what you're looking for. In the year 2001, your operation could well have been performed by a robot.

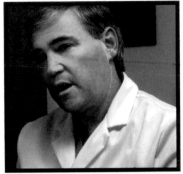

Douglas Boyd, M.D.
"For the first time in 200 years there's a tool in the surgeon's hands that makes the surgeon a better surgeon."

"This is going to make a revolution," says Douglas Boyd, M.D., a surgeon at the London Health Science Centre in Ontario, Canada. In September 1999, Boyd and his colleagues made history: Using the Zeus Robotic Surgical System, they performed a coronary artery bypass operation without stopping the patient's heart.

The following year, the U.S. Food and Drug Administration gave its approval to Zeus's rival, the da Vinci Surgical System, for several types of noncardiac surgery. Both systems are now in clinical trials throughout the United States for cardiac and other procedures. And in Europe, the da Vinci and Zeus systems are already approved for full surgical use in several countries.

Robots are catching on, says Boyd, simply because they can do some things better than people can.

From the moment a Neolithic shaman first sliced into a patient with a stone scalpel up until just a few years ago, surgery has been a matter of educated guesswork. Until they peeled back the layers of flesh, sawed through bone, and pushed aside the intervening organs, surgeons couldn't be sure of what they'd find. A tumor might be larger than they expected—or not there at all. An additional—or different—organ might be afflicted. And there was always a chance the surgery would do more harm than good.

That situation has steadily improved in recent decades. Refined imaging techniques such as magnetic resonance imaging and computed tomography allow surgeons to see within the body before cutting into it. And endoscopes—narrow, lighted viewing tubes often

Surgical Team

fitted with tiny surgical instruments— let doctors enter the body through nickel-sized incisions. But, inevitably, even these tools run up against the limits of human dexterity.

Robots to the Rescue

Imagine picking a lock with only one hand; it's difficult work. Now imagine trying to pick that same lock when it's concealed behind a maze of organs and tissue using the tip of a long, thin instrument. This is just one of the challenges facing surgeons when they perform minimally invasive or "keyhole" surgery.

Keyhole surgery requires a surgeon to manipulate the surgical tool—tipped with a knife, needle holder, or other implement—through small holes while watching the entire process on a TV monitor, earning them the nickname "Nintendo surgeons." Not only is the tool used—an endoscope—long, it

Having a robotic interface between the surgeon and the tip of the endoscope restores the surgeon's dexterity, allows for precise control, and opens up new surgical options.

is also flexible, critically limiting both a surgeon's dexterity and the range of movements available.

How do robots outperform humans? Having a robotic interface between the surgeon and the tip of the endoscope restores the surgeon's dexterity, allows for precise control, and opens up an array of new surgical options. Using robots also creates a more sterile operating environment, reducing the chances of infection. It is far easier to thoroughly clean metal than to scrub germs off hands. Plus, robots don't need to wear masks—they never sneeze.

The use of robots can even reduce the invasiveness of certain surgeries. Consider conventional cardiac surgery: First surgeons must make an incision the length of the patient's chest. Then they split

Long distance surgery

Doctors no longer make house calls, but telesurgery may allow them to operate from afar with the help of robots. In September 2001, surgeons in New York made history by performing a gallbladder operation on a patient in France by remote control, paving the way for other long-distance surgeries.

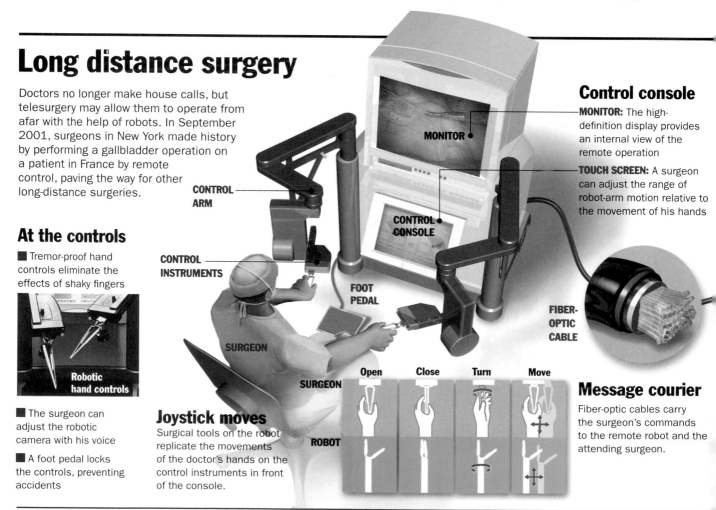

At the controls

■ Tremor-proof hand controls eliminate the effects of shaky fingers

Robotic hand controls

■ The surgeon can adjust the robotic camera with his voice

■ A foot pedal locks the controls, preventing accidents

CONTROL ARM

CONTROL INSTRUMENTS

SURGEON

Joystick moves
Surgical tools on the robot replicate the movements of the doctor's hands on the control instruments in front of the console.

MONITOR

CONTROL CONSOLE

FOOT PEDAL

SURGEON

ROBOT

Open   Close   Turn   Move

Control console
MONITOR: The high-definition display provides an internal view of the remote operation

TOUCH SCREEN: A surgeon can adjust the range of robot-arm motion relative to the movement of his hands

FIBER-OPTIC CABLE

Message courier
Fiber-optic cables carry the surgeon's commands to the remote robot and the attending surgeon.

open the ribs to lay bare the heart, stop it from beating, and transfer its function to a heart-lung machine. Only after all that can the heart itself be worked on. After undergoing this massive trauma, patients typically spend a week recovering in the hospital and cannot fully resume physical activity for about four months.

In contrast, Zeus's miniature hands enter the patient through three small holes, each about the diameter of your little finger, and slip between two ribs. The heart continues to beat on its own while tiny metal pincers cut and stitch blood vessels, sometimes passing needles a dozen times through arteries no wider than a pencil lead. The patient can walk the same day and fully recovers within a month, says Reiza Rayman, M.D., Boyd's colleague at the London Centre.

Several technological advances make the work of these surgical robots possible. Instead of standing over the patient and moving instruments with their own hands, the doctors sit at a console like that of a video game, watching digital images and moving joysticks that control the computer's arms electronically. Some robots will respond to simple voice commands as well, a useful option when both of the surgeon's hands are occupied. And the computer can magnify or reduce motions: A 1-inch thrust on the joystick can become a 1-mm movement within the patient. Or a 90-degree twist can become a 180-degree turn. It's as if the surgeon had shrunk to a tiny size and crawled inside the patient.

It almost looks that way to the surgeon, too. Binocular viewing devices, in which each eye has its own tiny video screen, give the surgeon the crucial depth perception lacking in most endoscopic surgery. And the computers can magnify the images within the body more powerfully than the loupes surgeons traditionally wear for open-heart surgery.

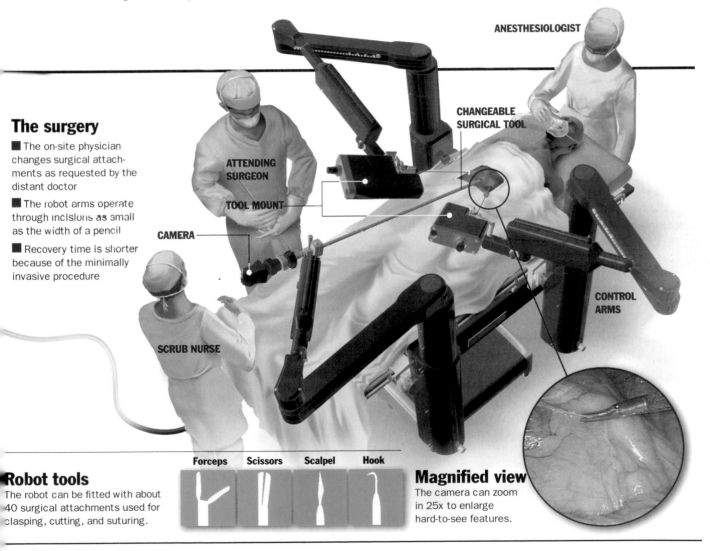

ANESTHESIOLOGIST

CHANGEABLE
SURGICAL TOOL

The surgery
■ The on-site physician changes surgical attachments as requested by the distant doctor

■ The robot arms operate through incisions as small as the width of a pencil

■ Recovery time is shorter because of the minimally invasive procedure

ATTENDING
SURGEON

TOOL MOUNT

CAMERA

SCRUB NURSE

CONTROL
ARMS

Robot tools
The robot can be fitted with about 40 surgical attachments used for clasping, cutting, and suturing.

Forceps   Scissors   Scalpel   Hook

Magnified view
The camera can zoom in 25x to enlarge hard-to-see features.

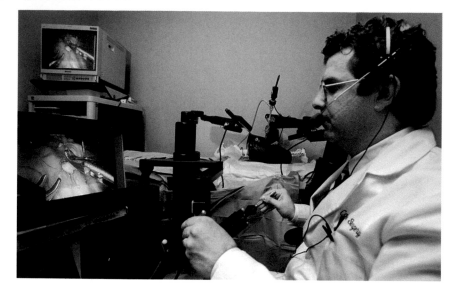

◀ **Robert Lazzara, M.D.,
in Seattle, Washington,
practices a coronary artery
bypass on a model chest
using the Zeus Robotic
Surgical System.**

Surgeons using robots even look different. Sitting 10 feet away from the person on the operating table, they need no gloves or gown (although a scrubbed and gowned team that includes the anesthesiologist is tableside).

Remote Control

Operating a robot's arms through tiny holes, surgeons around the world are repairing heart valves, fallopian tubes, and blood vessels and removing diseased kidneys, prostates, bowel sections, and spleens—all procedures that historically required large incisions. Next, surgeons hope to operate on fetuses within the womb.

Because surgical robots are expensive—about $1 million each—these procedures are more costly than conventional surgery. But factor in the increased productivity of patients who can return to the workplace faster, says Robert Michler, M.D., of Ohio State University, and the operations may already be paying for themselves.

The availability of robots also means that surgeons who presently cannot perform some of the more difficult keyhole surgeries (such as stomach stapling for obesity) may be able to do so now. This could save hospitals the cost of referring patients to the more expensive specialist centers for these types of operations.

Robots may also be capable of coming to the aid of patients far from an operating room. In the late 1990s, U.S. military surgeons conducted an experiment to see if armored robots could operate on soldiers at the front lines while doctors operated the robots from bunkers miles away. "We demonstrated that we could do it," says Richard M. Satava, M.D.,

a Yale University professor and advisor to the U.S. military. There are limitations, of course. In his experiments, Satava's robots didn't work well when they were more than 30 miles from the surgeon. "As you get more distant, the time it takes the signal to get to the scalpel becomes too great," he says. "The surgeon can't compensate for his movements—he might cut the wrong thing." Although the military's work did not come to fruition, the technology that was developed paved the way for today's modern robotic systems.

As of September 7, 2001, a major barrier to long-distance surgery was broken. On that day, a remote gallbladder removal was performed from New York on a patient in France—a distance of nearly 4,000 miles—using the Zeus Robotic Surgical System. The transatlantic surgery was made possible by a fiber-optic link developed by France

WHAT DOES IT MEAN TO YOU?

Surgeons can maneuver robotic arms through nickel-sized holes to perform operations that would otherwise require huge incisions. So far, robots can be used to:
■ Repair or replace damaged heart valves and bypass clogged arteries without breaking the breastbone or stopping the heart.
■ Remove diseased kidneys, prostates, bowel sections, and spleens.
■ Repair fallopian tubes that are blocked or have been tied, giving a woman the possibility of bearing children.
■ Widen the outlet from the stomach to the intestines (pyloroplasty) when they are too narrow, allowing the normal passage of the products of digestion.
■ Remove blood clots and insert catheters in clogged blood vessels.
■ Remove kidney stones.
   Next up, surgeons hope to perform robot-assisted operations on fetuses without removing the fetus from the mother's uterus.

Telecom that allowed signals to arrive with an average delay of only 150 milliseconds. The patient experienced no complications and was released from the hospital two days later. The success of the telesurgery will likely pave the way for other long-range operations performed on patients in different parts of the world.

If robots are so proficient (at least when they're close at hand), why not let them do the surgery on their own? Something like that already happens in thousands of eye doctors' offices around the world. If you're nearsighted, a robot may help you get rid of your glasses. First, a corneal topography machine will collect data about your eye. Using this information, a computer will then direct a laser to sculpt your cornea for better vision while the ophthalmologist stands by as overseer.

Computer-controlled instruments are now used for some stages of standard hip-replacement operations as well, and other kinds of bone surgery may offer opportunities for computer-guided robots.

The Limits of Robotic Surgery

Satava thinks that will be about as far as robots go on their own for a long while; unlike most body parts, Satava notes, corneas and bones don't change shape from one minute to the next. As brilliant as computers are at predictable tasks, they're relatively stupid when it comes to, say, identifying the arteries in a beating heart. "Our computer has almost the same smarts as a lizard," says Satava. "And you don't see too many lizards doing surgery."

Even when computers "learn" to recognize human innards—which would require that they think 10 billion times faster than they do now—it's likely that human surgeons will keep a close eye on them. After all, no one else will ever care as much about saving a human being's life as another human being. "It's like flying a plane," says Andrew Iwach, M.D., an ophthalmologist, who operates eye-sculpting lasers at the University of California, San Francisco. "The computer does everything now. But you still want a pilot up there watching."

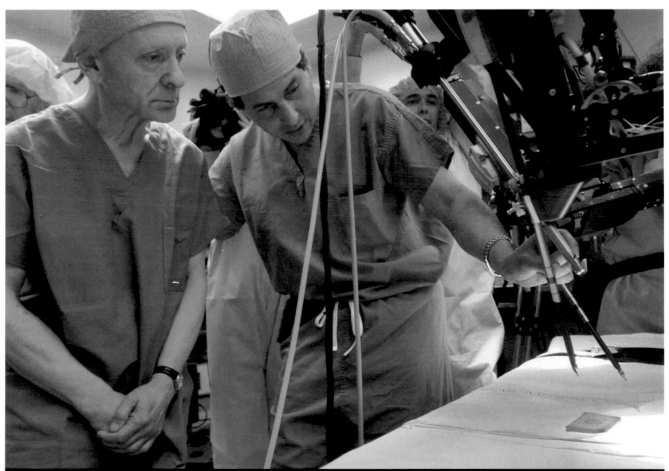

Hani Shennib, M.D., right, of Beth Israel Medical Center, in New York, shows cardiac patient Eugene Bem the robotic device, part of the da Vinci Surgical System, that Bem's surgeon will use to perform his coronary artery bypass.

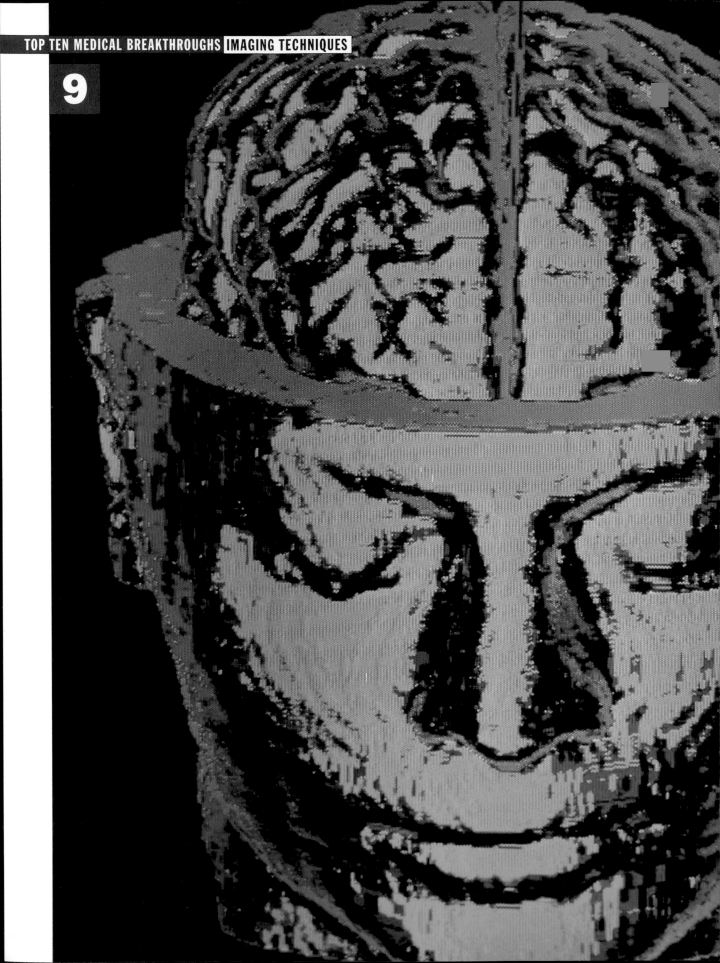

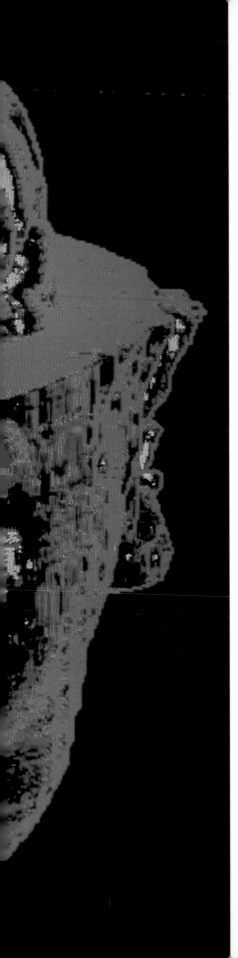

New Views Furnish Lifesaving Clues

Adoctor "flies" through the tunnel of your large intestine, steering around bumps and folds with a computer mouse, zooming in on suspect spots— and you're not even there. You've gone home. Better yet, the equipment for this inspection never entered your body: You were spared the invasion of the viewing tube, the sedation, and the apprehension that prevent many of us from even thinking about undergoing lifesaving tests such as colonoscopy.

Three-dimensional voyages through a live body were once nothing more than fantasy. But now they're real, and virtual colonoscopy and other cutting-edge techniques are being offered by an increasing number of hospitals and medical centers. Physicians using the newest high-speed scanners and computer software can travel, in effect, through just about any part of the body—from bones to

◄ **FANTASTIC VOYAGE**
New imaging techniques such as 3-D CT scanning offer doctors incredible views inside the body.

brain or from colon to windpipe—without touching it. They can study it as a 3-D image, revisit questionable spots that a computer has tagged, store digital images, and transmit them to colleagues near and far.

The new wave of virtual-reality exams isn't the only rich payoff from the past year's advances in medical imaging. Doctors can now monitor processes such as blood flow and even cell chemistry in real time, see immediately whether chemotherapy is helping a cancer patient, make better-informed decisions about treating stroke, and improve their ability to get a head start on diseases such as breast cancer. The rest of us can expect new screening exams that may be just as thorough yet quicker, more comfortable, and perhaps less expensive.

Teaching an Old CAT New Tricks

More than 106 years have passed since the German physicist Wilhelm Roentgen first showed the world what he saw through living skin and flesh—an X ray of the hand of his wife, Bertha. Roentgen's two-dimensional photo of Bertha's bones looks almost like a cave drawing today compared with the increasingly clear and detailed images produced by his modern radiology successors.

At every step along the way, a new technology appears and is soon transformed itself. Magnetic resonance imaging (MRI) gave exquisite images of the brain but didn't seem likely at first to be useful for the heart or other organs that move; now, MRI can clearly show a beating heart or a fetus in the womb. Computed tomog-

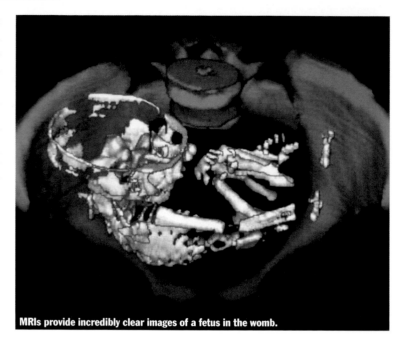

MRIs provide incredibly clear images of a fetus in the womb.

raphy (CAT or CT scanning) started in 1972 as a superb way to show crisp details of any organ in pictures that were, for all their crispness, flat; now, as leaps in speed and detector design give it new power, CT is opening new dimensions for diagnosis and treatment.

Spiral CT, also called helical CT, uses an X-ray tube that rotates continuously while the table carries the patient through the device's center.

Conventional CT remains a diagnostic workhorse. The scanner is a doughnut-shaped X-ray tube that takes cross-sectional pictures of a patient who is moved intermittently on a table though the center of the tube. The X-rays pass through the patient and are picked up by a series of detectors. The data that is acquired is then fed through a computer and the results are displayed on a screen as a series of two-dimensional slices. Details of the body appear layer by layer, much as you see the structure of a tomato when you cut it into thin slices and lay them side by side. In the early 1990s a refinement appeared: Spiral CT, also called helical CT, uses an X-ray tube that rotates continuously while the table carries the patient through the device's cen-

Using MRI, doctors can look closely at the structure of the heart and aorta.

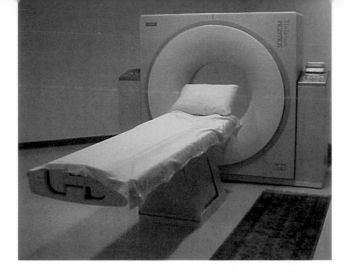

ter. In this way the beam traces a continuous spiral path through the patient. Spiral CT outshines the older technology in several ways:

Speed: Patients love it because it works much faster. Instead of having to hold your breath over and over while the scanner takes pictures and readjusts, you hold your breath once, motor on through, and you're done with it.

▲ In spiral CT scanning, the scanner rotates continuously while the table carries a patient through the device.

Image quality: Here's where spiral CT opens up virtual-reality viewing. As it takes pictures from every angle, it records huge amounts of information about the volume and density of organs and anything in them, such as a tumor. With this volumetric data acquisition, as it's called, computers and software can stack slices in any plane. In other words, spiral CT is ideal for creating virtual 3-D images of the body.

Accuracy: Because all the data is acquired in one breath-holding session, doctors are not faced with picture variation caused by patients breathing differently in each individual picture, as in standard CT.

And now, if there is such a thing as *more* ideal, we have the latest upgrade: multidetector CT, an ultrafast scanner. This new-generation scanner captures even larger amounts of data and works even faster, generating up to a thousand or more slices per scan. There are so many images generated that radiologists need to be equipped with powerful computer workstations and 3-D imaging software in order to best view them.

Multidetector or not, there is plenty a spiral CT can accomplish. You can start at a surface view of the body, then strip away skin, muscles, and overlying organs until you arrive at the place you want to study. Orthopedic surgeons can use 3-D images of complex bone fractures to plan reconstruction. Specialists in every area can get accurate pictures of possible cancers, blood vessel problems, obstructions … you name it. The technique also takes the pain out of tests on practically any part of the body, including arteries and veins, the head and neck, the chest, and the abdomen.

Easier Exams Get Good Grades

That brings us back to colonoscopy, the examination that most of us want to skip even though we know that it saves lives. About 60,000 people die of colorectal cancer every year in the United States. Medical experts figure that many of these people could be saved by early detection of precancerous polyps and tumors. The most thorough screening exam is conventional fiber-optic colonoscopy, but, by some estimates, more than half the people it would help most—everyone over 50 and anyone with a family history of colon cancer—avoid it because they dread taking the exam.

In conventional colonoscopy, a gastroenterologist inserts a long, flexible tube through the rectum and gently pushes it along the entire length of the colon—a distance of five to six feet. The tube contains fiber optics attached to a video monitor and sometimes a camera, plus a wire loop at its tip to lop off any polyps the doctor finds. Pre-exam instructions always mention the possibility—very slight, but still jarring—that the doctor might accidentally perforate your bowel. Before the test you clean out the bowel by fasting and taking a laxative and an enema. The test itself requires intravenous sedatives, so you will need someone to take you home after the procedure.

Virtual colonoscopy—or to use its formal name, three-dimensional CT colography—is easier on the nerves and the body.

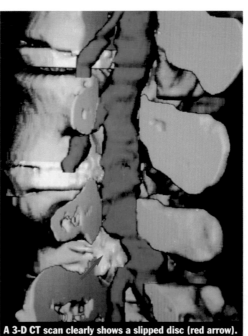

A 3-D CT scan clearly shows a slipped disc (red arrow).

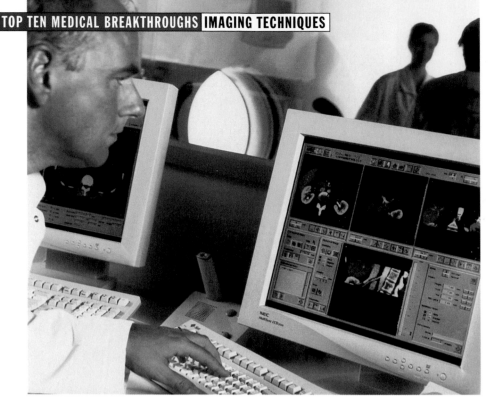

◄ Virtual colonoscopy offers a simpler, faster, and less invasive view of the colon.

al models of colonoscopy in a near dead heat.

At Boston University, researchers tried the virtual exam on 100 volunteers and found it 80 to 90 percent as accurate as the gold-standard conventional exam in detecting polyps larger than 5 mm in diameter (the width of a drinking straw). Polyps smaller than 5 mm generally aren't considered to be a cancer threat. Besides, "Fifty percent of adults older than 50 have at least one polyp, but most of them are smaller than 5 mm or are … not premalignant," said Joseph Ferrucci, M.D., chair of radiology at Boston University, at an American Roentgen Ray Society meeting in May 2001. "It's therapeutic overkill to remove meaningless growths."

A 300-patient study at the Veterans Affairs Medical Center in San Francisco showed that virtual colonoscopy was 90 percent accurate in detecting polyps 10 mm or larger, the threshold for high potential of developing into cancer; it identified all those patients found to have cancer during standard screening. Of note, however, this study included a mix of people without symptoms and those who had symptoms or were at high risk for colon cancer. Whether virtual colonoscopy will have such a high rate of detection in those who are at low risk and have no symptoms will be determined by further studies on this particular group.

If more and larger studies confirm previous results, virtual colonoscopy could gain converts among gastroenterologists and radiologists, many of whom are concerned about the risks of exposing large groups of low- or no-risk people to X rays—a risk that needs to be balanced by clear-cut diagnostic benefits. But patients might not flock to it until it also features virtual bowel preparation. Who will rid us of those laxatives and enemas? Maybe the researchers at Harvard

The only invasion is a little rubber tube, the diameter of a straw, that goes in an inch or two so that the doctor can inflate the colon with air, like a bicycle inner tube. You still have to prepare your colon beforehand (fasting, laxative, enema) —a big annoyance, no doubt about it—and the inflation is sometimes uncomfortable, but no

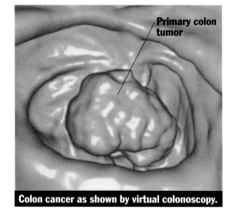

Primary colon tumor

Colon cancer as shown by virtual colonoscopy.

six-foot fiber optic scope, no sedatives. You simply hold your breath for half a minute on a scanning table while the CT scanner clicks. Then you get up, pass wind, and go on your way with no need for help.

How does virtual colonoscopy rank as a diagnostic tool? Most gastroenterologists have their doubts. "Promising, but Not Ready for Widespread Use," the *New England Journal of Medicine* titled a November 1999 editorial. Even so, the author of the editorial, John H. Bond, M.D., of the Minneapolis Veterans Affairs Medical Center, wrote, "Virtual colonoscopy has come a long way in a short time, and its future appears bright." In fact, several carefully controlled studies show the virtual and convention-

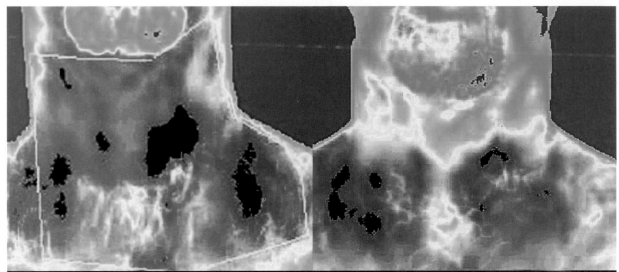

Dynamic infrared imaging helps doctors monitor the effects of cancer treatment. Here, a lymphoma patient before (left) and after treatment.

who have tried a technique called digital stool subtraction. Aiming to let a computer take the place of Colyte, the usual pre-exam laxative, they asked 10 patients to drink a diluted iodine contrast solution. Stool in the colon took up the iodine, which showed up clearly in CT scans. The stool could then be "erased" digitally, just as moviemakers wipe out unwanted backgrounds. Another team at the Mayo Clinic used barium tablets toward the same end.

Watching the Body at Work

Today's imaging techniques are doing more than making procedures easier and providing better internal views of the body. They can also reveal physiological processes—blood flow, for instance, and even the activity of cells—as they occur in living tissue. Functional imaging, as this technology is often called, may turn out to be useful for both diagnosis and prognosis.

One example is dynamic infrared imaging, which was originally developed by NASA to find distant galaxies and spot missile launches for Ronald Reagan's "Star Wars" program. Omni-Corder Technologies licensed the sensor and packaged it in a device called BioScanIR for another use: to spy on cancerous cells and help with studies of cancer treatment. The BioScanIR system can rapidly measure changes in the movement of tiny amounts of infrared light (photons), which are equivalent to temperature variations of less than nine one-thousandths of a degree centigrade, so it can track events that slower, less sensitive thermography tools don't register. For

example, immediately after chemotherapy, it can pick up tiny changes in blood flow patterns from malignant cells, allowing doctors to tell whether the chemo is working.

In 2000 and 2001, researchers at the Dana-Farber Cancer Institute, a Harvard affiliate in Boston, used the BioScanIR system—along with MRI, positron emission tomography (PET), and CT scans—to help judge the effectiveness of

Today's imaging techniques can also reveal physiological proceses—blood flow, for instance, and even the activity of cells—as they occur in living tissues.

new, sharply targeted cancer drugs such as Gleevec, which made news early in 2001 with its success against leukemia and a rare form of abdominal cancer. Dana-Farber wanted BioScanIR because "current technologies to monitor the effects of cancer treatment might miss important biological and clinical effects, especially of newer treatment strategies," said George Demetri, M.D., lead researcher in the Gleevec trials. "People are very excited by the idea that the newer cancer drugs are smarter and more gentle, but they are also occasionally more subtle in terms of their activities." In other words, it can be hard to know when they are working. By providing information that was not available to

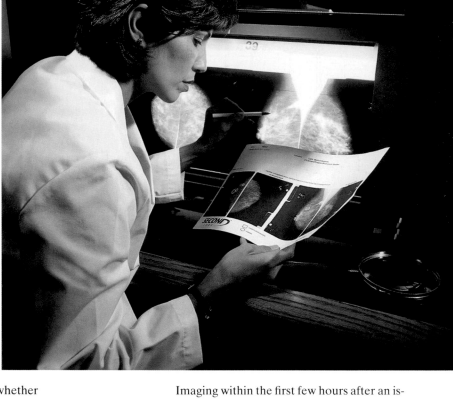

► **CAD technology is designed to assist radiologists with the diagnosis of breast cancer by drawing their attention to suspicious areas.**

researchers until now, the latest heat-measurement method offers doctors a new way to spy on cancer.

Another functional-imaging technique is contributing to better decisions in treating strokes. It has a ponderous name: diffusion-weighted magnetic resonance imaging (DWMRI). When added to the usual stroke assessment tests, this variation on the standard MRI provides a quick, accurate estimate of how a patient is doing.

Standard MRI lines up protons in the body's cells with a strong magnetic field, knocks them out of line with pulses of radio waves, and records the signals they give off as they swing back into place. It provides excellent 3-D images, but those pictures don't tell whether damage to the brain is old or new. The distinction is important because with ischemic strokes (the type caused by blood clots), the sooner you get clot-busting drugs, the better your chances of recovery. DWMRI clears up the picture by analyzing the movement of water molecules in brain tissue. When a stroke kills brain cells, it restricts normal water movement. A bright area on the scan just minutes after a stroke says the stroke has just happened; the bigger the bright area, the worse the stroke is.

A bright area on the scan just minutes after a stroke says the stroke has just happened.

Imaging within the first few hours after an ischemic stroke, combined with ordinary observation, provides an accurate measure of a patient's chances for recovery, researchers from the National Institutes of Health reported in the June 30, 2001, issue of the British journal *The Lancet.* And it helps physicians weigh treatment options. "If we are considering a therapy that might have some risks, and we know that the

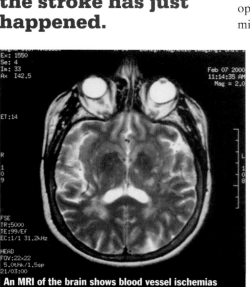

An MRI of the brain shows blood vessel ischemias (strokes), one of which is indicated by an arrow.

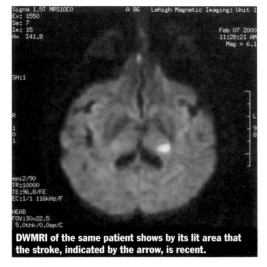

DWMRI of the same patient shows by its lit area that the stroke, indicated by the arrow, is recent.

chance of recovery is high even if we do nothing, we would be less inclined to proceed with that treatment," said Steven Warach, M.D., Ph.D., of the National Institute of Neurological Disorders and Stroke. "But if the chance of recovery is low, we could try more experimental therapies that carry some risk."

A Sum Greater Than Its Parts

While some imaging technologies are advancing on separate tracks, others occasionally converge, with powerful results.

In the diagnosis of breast cancer, for example, two advanced techniques may soon merge to make tumor detection easier and more accurate. The first, mammography assisted by computer-aided detection (CAD), creates a digital image from a mammogram X ray and scans it, marking suspicious areas. This extra electronic eye helps the radiologist detect problems that might have been missed by a conventional mammogram (see also page 97).

The second technique, digital mammography, produces an image that appears on a high-resolution screen within seconds. This is a big improvement over traditional mammograms, which take time to develop. Moreover, digital mammograms allow for easy examination of the entire breast, despite varying tissue density, and they can be stored and transferred electronically for quick access. Will they turn out to make a clear-cut difference for patients? We won't know the answer to that until 2004 at the earliest.

The first major study comparing the real-life results of standard and digital mammography began recruiting women in July 2001. Funded by the National Cancer Institute and run by Johns Hopkins University, it will enroll 49,500 women in the United States and Canada who have no symptoms of breast cancer, give each of them both exams, and follow them for 15 months to gauge which type of exam produces the more accurate diagnosis. Early results from a separate study of 15,000 women, funded by the Department of Defense, give digital mammography a slight edge in diagnosis over the standard mammography technique.

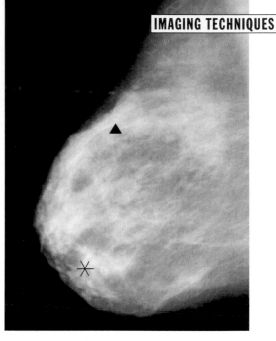

▶ **CAD marks suspicious areas on the digitized mammogram film.**

Tomorrow's Promise

Virtual CT, functional imaging, electronic storage and retrieval of images: These and other nascent imaging techniques are leading us toward noninvasive or less invasive diagnosis and treatment of disease. With each passing year, imaging advances are enabling doctors to probe the body's nooks and crannies ever more precisely, astounding us with jaw-dropping pictures of our inner selves and fulfilling the promise of simpler, less painful, and more successful health care for all patients.

WHAT DOES IT MEAN TO YOU?

Imaging is no longer just a tool for detecting and diagnosing disease. It is becoming an important instrument in the treatment, prognosis, and even prevention of disease. Though high costs curb patient access to some of the new technologies at present, costs may come down as the methods move from breakthrough to mainstream. Here are just a few of the benefits you can expect to see—if not now, then someday soon.

■ **Detecting disease earlier:** CT scanning, for example, plays a significant role in detecting blood vessel disease that can lead to stroke or kidney failure.

■ **Eliminating invasive diagnostic procedures:** Magnetic resonance imaging (MRI) is becoming valuable as a fast, noninvasive tool for diagnosing coronary artery disease and other heart problems.

■ **Making diagnosis safer:** Because it depends on a magnetic field instead of potentially harmful radiation to produce images, MRI is considered safer than X-ray–based technologies such as CT for diagnosing disorders of the reproductive system, pelvis, and bladder.

■ **Targeting treatment:** CT scans can be used to aim radiation at tumors. Up-and-coming brain imaging technologies may help physicians avoid critical areas during the course of performing brain surgery.

10

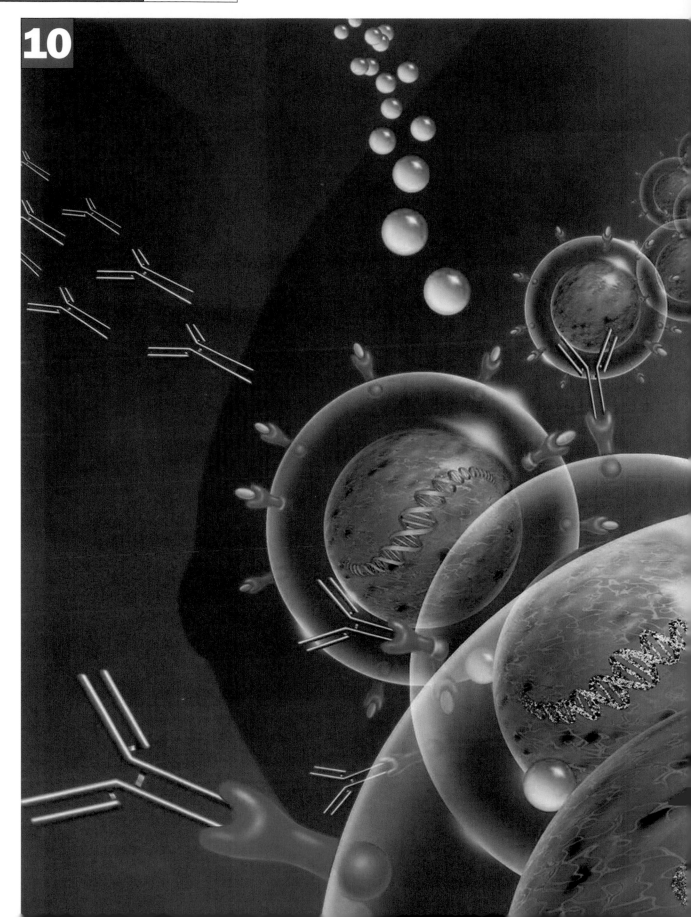

Vaccines: The Next Generation

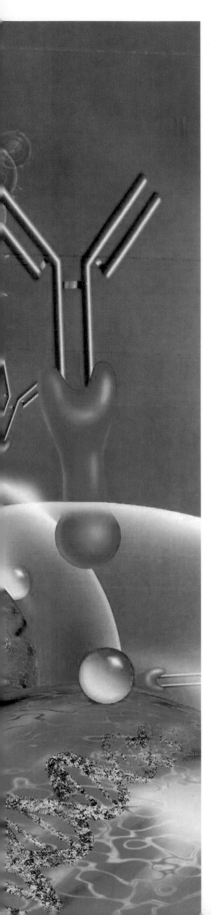

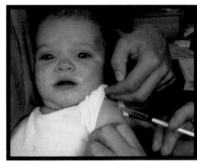

▲ **CRUEL TO BE KIND** Today's vaccines can protect baby from measles and mumps; tomorrow's vaccines take aim at hepatitis, AIDS, and even cancer.

◄ The breast cancer vaccine Herceptin (the Y-shaped molecules) binds to receptor sites on tumor cells, blocking cell proliferation. The vaccine plus chemotherapy (the green spheres), which damages the cell's DNA, deals a deadly one-two punch.

Defeating disease before it can gain a foothold: That has been the goal of every vaccine created since Edward Jenner gave the first modern one to 8-year-old James Phipps 205 years ago. That revolutionary vaccine for smallpox, the scourge of its time, was derived from a dairymaid's cowpox sores. With it, Jenner founded immunology as a science. Now medical researchers are targeting some of the 21st century's worst scourges—from AIDS to diabetes and even cancer—with brand-new approaches that are changing the very meaning of immunization.

Traditional vaccines use a weakened or killed form of the germ you want to stop; they cause just enough of an infection to prompt the immune system to create antibodies—the defensive troops that tag and attack invading organisms—specific to that germ. Should the body ever encounter the live, full-strength form of the invader, these antibodies stall or destroy it. New generations of vaccines—including several that showed promising test results in the past year—are safer, and they may prove effective against diseases that traditional vaccines haven't been able to stop, such as malaria and even AIDS. They are made from snippets of the germ's own DNA containing instructions for producing a specific protein: the antibody for that germ. (Antibodies are one of the half-dozen major kinds of protein. The DNA in a cell determines which proteins the cell will make.) With these vaccines, you aren't exposed to the whole germ—just its DNA. As a result, you avoid the small risk of infection that still comes with some traditional vaccines.

DNA vaccines may also prove more powerful than the older kinds, in the sense that they stimulate cells to keep producing antibodies for a long time, unlike vaccines that require repeated injections to maintain immunity. And vaccines for many different diseases can be combined in a single inoculation. By contrast, a full course of childhood immunizations in the United States requires as many as 18 visits to a doctor or clinic. And DNA vaccines don't need the careful refrigeration that older vaccines must have. They can be stored, dried or in solution, under almost any conditions, so they can be used easily in remote areas of the world.

New Techniques, New Targets

That's the origin of some big news. Because the DNA in these new vaccines can be chosen to produce antibodies that will attack just about any type of offending cell, they are not limited to targeting invaders from the outside—infectious organisms like the ones that cause smallpox, polio, measles, AIDS, herpes, and tuberculosis. Indeed, some of the most exciting developments of the past year emerged from vaccines aimed at problems that arise when the body's own systems go awry—for instance, diabetes that occurs when the body destroys its own insulin-producing cells, or cancer that occurs when cell division runs amok.

In June 2001, researchers at the University of North Carolina announced a successful test in mice of an experimental vaccine against type 1 diabetes, the kind that typically strikes young people and requires daily insulin shots. It occurs when the immune system produces too many killer cells called TH-1, which destroy insulin-producing cells in the pancreas. The vaccine works by stimulating the immune system to produce more of a cell type called TH-2, which, in healthy people, keeps the number of TH-1 cells in check.

That announcement came on the heels of a successful vaccine trial targeting rheumatoid arthritis, another disease in which the immune system attacks healthy tissues. The vaccine, tested in rats in Haifa, Israel, is based on a gene that produces the kind of protein responsible for the inflammatory process that causes pain and swelling in arthritic joints. This vaccine stimulated the rats' immune systems to produce antibodies against the protein.

For both vaccines, researchers warn that human trials may still be a few years away. But, bolstered by their recent successes, scientists can talk hopefully about using vaccines to prevent some forms of diabetes, rheumatoid arthritis, and other autoimmune disorders such as multiple sclerosis.

Keeping AIDS and Cancer at Bay

The two biggest recent headline grabbers, though, have been experiments that raise the possibility of immunization against AIDS and certain cancers.

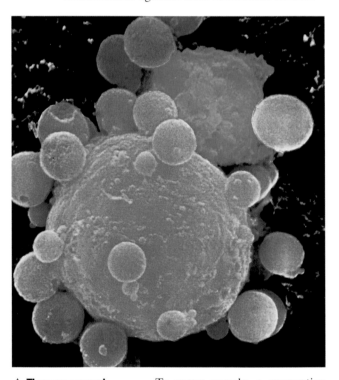

▲ **There are several approaches to making a cancer vaccine. One involves stimulating the body's own killer T-cells (in orange) to move in and kill the cancer cell.**

To many people, a preventive vaccine is the holy grail of AIDS research—perhaps the best hope for fighting the disease. "Preventive" may be too strong a word: Such a vaccine wouldn't stop HIV (the virus that causes AIDS) from entering the body. But it could make it possible to control infections and keep them from causing full-blown AIDS. That's how many flu vaccines work.

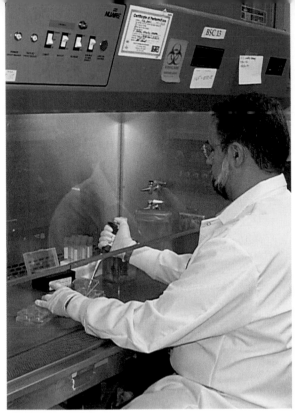

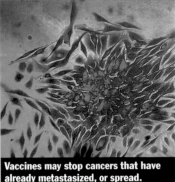

Vaccines may stop cancers that have already metastasized, or spread.

Optimism about an AIDS vaccine was fueled in 2001 by the first phase III (the final stage before FDA approval) clinical trials in North America of a human HIV vaccine, dubbed AIDSVAX. Made of a synthetic viral protein, it stimulates production of HIV antibodies. If found to be effective, AIDSVAX could be on the fast track for U.S. Food and Drug Administration approval. Other trials involve vaccines based on harmless viruses or bacteria containing a few HIV genes; still others use DNA fragments from the virus or shards of the virus protein.

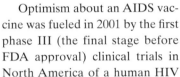

▲ Researchers at Therion Biologics are conducting groundbreaking cancer vaccine studies.

Another encouraging report came from recent animal trials of vaccines against a virus similar to HIV: Simian Immunodeficiency Virus (SIV), which infects rhesus monkeys. In a trial conducted by Harvard Medical School and the drug company Merck, vaccines made of pieces of virus DNA plus a chemical to boost the immune system created strong immune responses against the virus. None of the vaccinated animals developed SIV during the experiment. Unvaccinated monkeys got sick.

Recent trials with cancer vaccines have also brought encouragement. The goal of the vaccines is not to prevent cancer but to prevent a treated cancer from recurring or augment standard cancer treatments by coaxing the immune system to stop cancer cells from spreading.

The problem with developing a cancer vaccine has been finding ways to enable the immune system to recognize cancer cells as foreign. Cancer cells produce unique proteins, but they are so similar to the protein markers of normal cells that the immune system usually ignores them. The challenge, then, is to fine-tune the identification process so that immune cells will detect the minor variations in the proteins and then attack. That's where DNA-based vaccines hold the greatest promise. By identifying cancers at the genetic level, they may make precision targeting of cancer cells possible.

In May 2001, Therion Biologics announced success in trials of a vaccine-based therapy for patients with cancers that had already metastasized, or spread beyond their original site. Scientists have lauded the effort, and so has the government. The National Cancer Institute has partnered with Therion, believing this and other therapeutic vaccines the company is developing have great potential.

Two centuries ago, Edward Jenner found little support for his vaccine. That didn't stop other doctors around the world from observing that it worked and, on May 8, 1980, the World Health Organization declared that smallpox had been eradicated. Today, as discoveries in one field of medicine smooth the path for breakthroughs in others, there is every reason to expect rapid progress on vaccines that could one day make deaths from cancer, AIDS, and other ailments a thing of the past.

WHAT DOES IT MEAN TO YOU?

Several forms of cancer and other disorders—including AIDS, rheumatoid arthritis, and multiple sclerosis—are among the health problems for which researchers are actively seeking vaccines. Also on the hit list:

■ **Alzheimer's Disease.** Mice treated with an experimental vaccine had fewer of the brain-destroying plaques associated with Alzheimer's disease than the mice that were not treated with the vaccine. (See also pages 74–76.)

■ **Type 1 Diabetes.** As well as experimenting with vaccines designed to stimulate the immune system to protect insulin-producing cells, researchers are giving insulin itself to healthy individuals with a family history of type 1 diabetes. The hope is that the insulin will somehow prevent or reduce the body's destruction of insulin-producing cells.

■ **Hepatitis B.** One newly developed vaccine, based on the DNA of hepatitis B, conferred full immunity on volunteers in a clinical study who had failed to respond to standard vaccines.

ADVANCES

Nearly every part of your body, from your brain to your toes, stands to benefit from this year's medical breakthroughs. They are arranged here by 11 major categories for easy look-up.

72 BRAIN AND NERVOUS SYSTEM

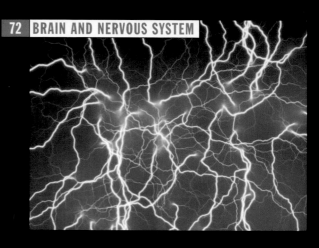

132 EYES AND EARS

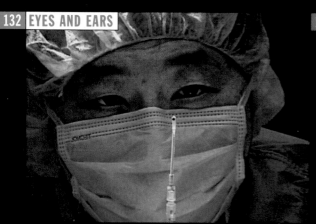

144 HEART AND CIRCULATORY SYSTEM

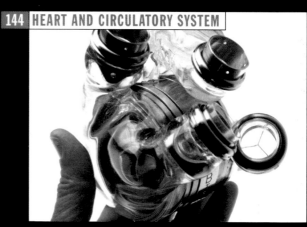

196 REPRODUCTIVE AND SEXUAL HEALTH

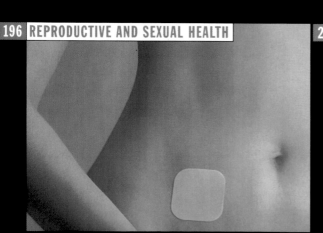

210 RESPIRATORY SYSTEM

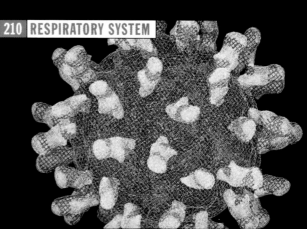

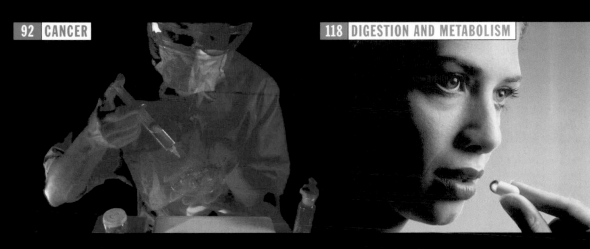

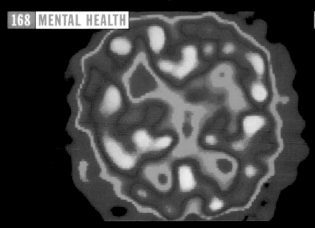

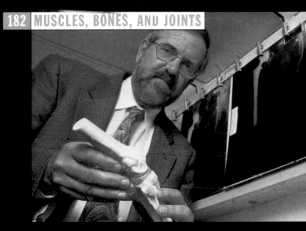

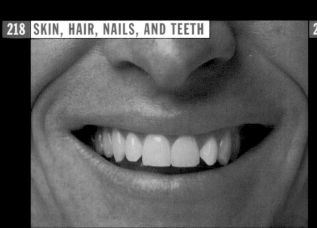

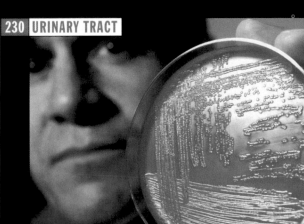

The amazing human brain is finally yielding up some of its secrets, and people with conditions as diverse as epilepsy, insomnia, and multiple sclerosis are going to benefit. For instance, scientists used to think we were born with all the brain cells we'd ever have—and that once these cells were dead, they were gone forever. But, in the past 10 years, we learned that new brain cells do form as we age. And in the year 2000, we found that these newly acquired brain cells quickly become involved in forming new memories. This may prove to be exciting news for people who have sustained damage from stroke and other diseases. With some high-tech genetic manipulation, it turns out that spinal nerves can regenerate, too—lending hope to people with spinal cord injury. And soon you may be able to head off a migraine by sticking a patch, impregnated with a local anesthetic, on your forehead. What could be simpler?

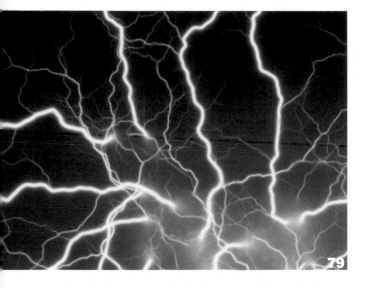

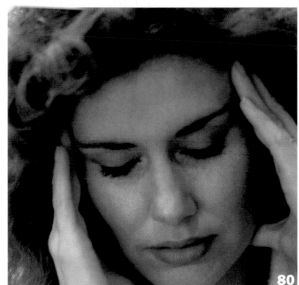

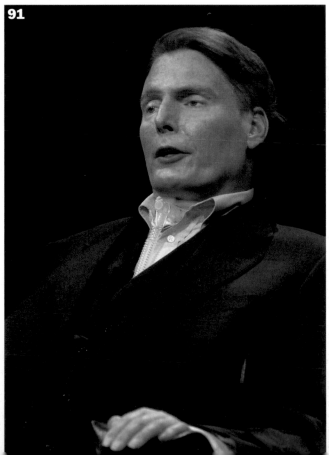

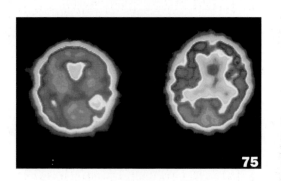

Progress in Prevention

A Vaccine to Protect Against Alzheimer's?

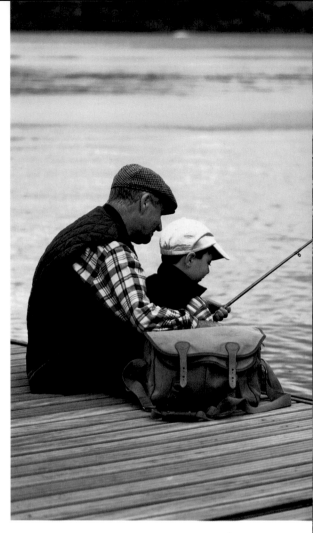

If preventing or delaying the onset of Alzheimer's were as simple as getting an annual shot, few people would balk at the sight of the needle. In December 2000, two separate research teams reported exciting progress in the quest for a vaccine against Alzheimer's, a disease that affects memory, thought, language, and reasoning.

The vaccine passed the first stage of clinical trials after being tested in more than 100 people.

Mice in these experiments swam through a maze until they learned the location of an underwater platform. A simple task for mice with all their mental faculties—but not so simple for those that have been genetically programmed to develop an Alzheimer's-like disease. Vaccinated mice, though, performed better than those that weren't vaccinated, and in one of the studies, they did as well or nearly as well as normal mice.

How it works. Researchers aren't certain why the vaccine worked. But they know that the mice treated with

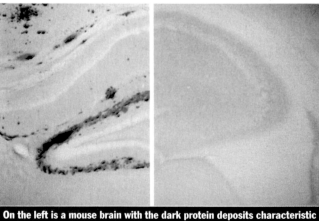

On the left is a mouse brain with the dark protein deposits characteristic of Alzheimer's disease. On the right is the brain of a mouse that was treated with an experimental Alzheimer's vaccine.

the vaccine had fewer brain plaques—clumps of protein that accumulate on nerve cells of Alzheimer's patients. It's possible that the vaccine reduced new plaque formation or removed old plaque. It may also have somehow protected the nerve cells from the harmful effects of the plaque.

Diagnostic Advance

Brain Scans Show Telltale Signs of Early Alzheimer's

Researchers have identified many promising strategies for preventing Alzheimer's disease. But until recently, there's been no way to know whether such therapies will work without following patients over the many years it takes the disease to develop. An imaging technique called positron emission tomography (PET), which provides a detailed look at the inner workings of the brain, may be just the thing medical investigators need to monitor the effects of preventive measures in the earliest, presymptomatic stages of the disease.

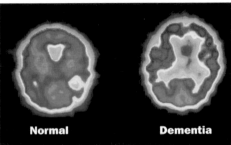

Normal   **Dementia**

PET scans of the brain are being tested as a way to check for the brain changes of Alzheimer's in people at risk for the disease.

Using PET scans, researchers at Good Samaritan Regional Medical Center in Phoenix, Arizona, found lower-than-normal levels of sugar metabolism—reflecting reduced activity—throughout the brains of healthy people who are at increased genetic risk of Alzheimer's. Armed with this insight,

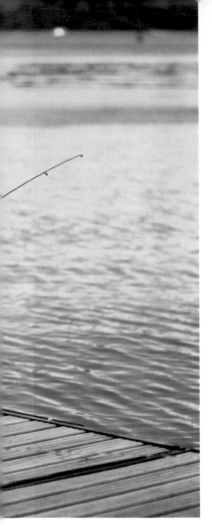

▲ **HOPE ON THE HORIZON**
Ten percent of people over age 65 suffer from Alzheimer's. Now scientists are one step closer to a vaccine that can protect your senior years by preventing or delaying the debilitating disease.

Availability. In July 2001 it was announced that the vaccine had passed the first stage of clinical trials after being tested in more than 100 patients with mild to moderate Alzheimer's. It proved to be well tolerated, and no safety concerns were evident. Now it will be tested in approximately 375 people in the United States and Europe. This study is expected to take approximately two years. A commercially available vaccine is still many years away.

STAY TUNED FOR...

Anti-inflammatories for Alzheimer's

Many small studies have suggested that anti-inflammatory drugs, commonly used to treat arthritis, may slow or halt the progression of Alzheimer's. Researchers at four medical centers in the United States are now in the process of recruiting 2,625 healthy people over age 70 with family histories of the disease for the Alzheimer's Disease Anti-inflammatory Prevention Trial (ADAPT). In this study, one-third of patients will take the anti-inflammatory drug naproxen every day; one-third will take a different anti-inflammatory, celecoxib (brand name Celebrex), daily; and the remaining one-third will take a placebo. All patients will be evaluated for signs of thinking and memory problems three times in the first year of the trial and twice a year thereafter, for a maximum of seven years.

The technique is likely to speed the quest for treatments that stop or slow the progression of Alzheimer's.

these investigators were able to track the progression of Alzheimer's-related brain changes long before behavioral symptoms such as memory lapses and irritability emerged. Their findings are very similar to ones noted in May 2000 by UCLA researchers for an older group of genetically at-risk people who had reported minor memory complaints. The imaging technique is likely to speed the quest for treatments that stop or slow the progression of Alzheimer's.

How it works. Several minutes before the PET scan is done, the patient inhales or is injected with a radioactive tracer. During the test, the patient lies still, with his or her head positioned beneath the arch of the scanner. The computer tracks how fast the tracer deteriorates to calculate activity—in this case, sugar metabolism—within the brain.

By using PET scanning in high-risk patients (people with a certain gene that accounts for about half of all Alzheimer's cases), the Arizona researchers say that the time needed to evaluate new treatments could be significantly reduced because researchers would not need to wait the many years it normally takes for symptoms to develop and treatment effects to be seen.

Availability. The use of PET scans to monitor brain function in patients at risk for Alzheimer's disease is still experimental. Although some doctors may order these scans to help diagnose the condition, Medicare and other health insurers don't cover the scans for this purpose. If you carry the Alzheimer's gene and you enter a clinical trial of a treatment to delay the onset of the disease, periodic PET scans may be part of the study.

FAST FACTS
18 MILLION Number of people worldwide with Alzheimer's **40** Earliest age at which Alzheimer's may become apparent **10** Percentage of people over 65 with Alzheimer's disease

Diagnostic Advance

New Test May Put ADHD Controversy to Rest

Estimates of the number of schoolchildren with attention deficit-hyperactivity disorder (ADHD) in the United States vary widely, from 1 percent in some studies to 20 percent in others. Adding to the confusion, the diagnosis is almost unheard of in France and several other countries. What's the reason for this lack of agreement? So far, no precise way has been found to test for ADHD in children — or in adults, for that matter.

Doctors base their diagnoses on observations of behavior, reports from teachers and family members, and results of psychological tests. Without a surefire diagnostic test, there's a concern that hundreds of thousands of children may be needlessly medicated for misdiagnosed ADHD. A new test may soon put those fears to rest.

The test—which uses an imaging technique called single-photon emission computed tomography (SPECT) together with a new diagnostic agent called Altropane—indirectly measures levels of dopamine, a brain chemical involved in regulating attention and inhibiting impulses. People with ADHD have lower levels of this chemical.

How it works. Given in an injection before the scan, Altropane—marked with a radioactive "flag" so that it shows up on SPECT scans—"hitches a ride" with proteins called dopamine transporters, which are present in higher levels in

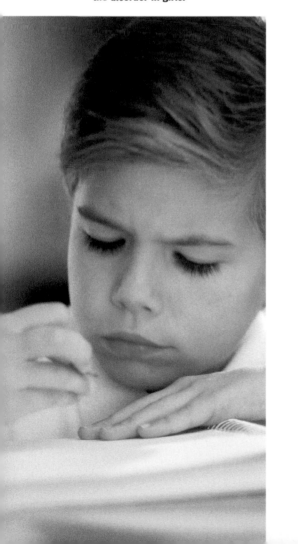

▼ More boys than girls are affected by ADHD, but part of this difference may be due to a failure to recognize the disorder in girls.

Mixed-up messages

Dopamine, a neurotransmitter, carries messages across the gap between nerve cells (called the synapse) and plays a critical role in several disorders such as ADHD, Parkinson's disease, and schizophrenia. People with ADHD have lower levels of dopamine in the brain.

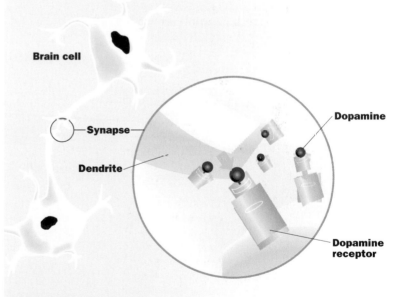

Brain cell

Synapse

Dendrite

Dopamine

Dopamine receptor

[**FAST FACTS**
3–5 Most reliable estimate of the percentage of school-age children with ADHD **75–91** Percent chance that if one of a pair of identical twins has ADHD, the other twin will **1 MILLION** Number of American children who take prescription medications for hyperactivity **3 BILLION** Estimated expenditures of U.S. school districts on managing students with ADHD]

people with ADHD. (It is thought that higher concentrations of dopamine transporters lead to lower dopamine levels by making dopamine less available for the brain to use.) Dense concentrations of Altropane on SPECT images may be the chemical marker of ADHD that researchers have long been seeking.

Availability. Early in 2001, Altropane completed the second phase of testing needed for market approval by the U.S. Food and Drug Administration, with successful results. The Altropane-SPECT test will not be available for a few years, however, because further studies are needed to validate its use.

STAY TUNED FOR...

Safer ADHD Drugs
The pipeline for ADHD medications is certainly not empty. Tomoxetine is a promising newcomer without the stimulant effects of widely used ADHD drugs, which can make the patient feel "wired." Recent clinical trials found it almost as effective as methylphenidate hydrochloride (Ritalin), the standard treatment. Results from the final phase of clinical trials are expected this year, meaning the drug could become available as soon as early 2002. Two other non-stimulant drugs are also under development but are at earlier stages of testing.

RESEARCH ROUNDUP

■ **BRAIN WAVE CLUES TO ADHD.** Psychologists at the University of Virginia School of Medicine in Charlottesville have developed a test for ADHD based on research done on fighter jet pilots at the National Aeronautics and Space Administration (NASA) in the United States. The test measures brain waves in children as they shift from task to task. Normally, brain-wave patterns remain steady when we change activities, but in children with ADHD, they become chaotic. This brain-wave disruption may be a unique feature of ADHD—one that could help doctors diagnose the disease. Further research examining brain-wave patterns in children with ADHD is now under way. The goal is to confirm the results of an early preliminary study.

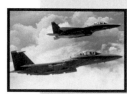

Diagnostic Advance
Better Seizure Prediction on the Horizon

An epileptic seizure is something like an electrical storm—both are characterized by chaotic power surges that may leave damage in their wake. But while you can usually see a storm coming, seizures often strike out of the blue. This unpredictability is a major threat to people with uncontrolled epilepsy and a cause of disability and mortality. In the future, however, there may be better ways to predict them, thanks to recent work by a team of international researchers who devised a new way to analyze scalp electroencephalograms (EEGs), tracings of the electrical changes in the brain.

▶ Sometimes compared to lightning storms, epileptic seizures involve electrical disturbances in the brain.

How it works. As reported in the January 20, 2001, issue of *The Lancet*, researchers in France used continuous scalp EEG recordings and video monitoring for 18 patients with temporal lobe epilepsy to capture the half-hour to 1-hour period before seizures. After reviewing the recordings, the researchers could identify electrical changes that foretold the seizure at least 7 minutes in advance. In the past, this type of electrical change could only be noted on EEG monitoring that was done from electrodes implanted within the brain (intracranial monitoring). Five patients in this study underwent intracranial as well as scalp EEG monitoring, and the electrical changes shown by each method corresponded well.

Availability. At this point, continuous scalp EEG monitoring is not designed for patient use, but the recent findings are a big step toward a monitoring system that a patient might one day be able to use at home as an early warning device, allowing treat-

▶ EEGs allow researchers to measure electrical changes in the brain and may one day be a useful tool for predicting seizures.

ment intervention such as the administration of an anticonvulsant drug, electrical stimulation, and mental or behavioral countermeasures. First, further testing of larger groups of people over a longer period are needed to verify and fully understand these new findings.

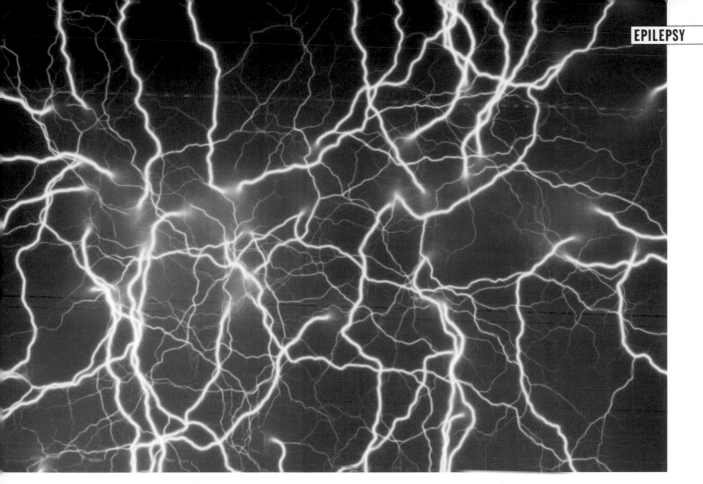

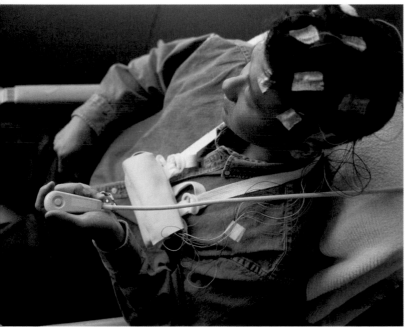

RESEARCH ROUNDUP

■ **EPILEPSY IN CHILDREN.** Why do children with newly diagnosed seizure disorders often have behavioral problems? Until this year, conventional wisdom held that acting out with defiant or destructive behavior was a sign of poor adjustment to the condition. However, a study in the January 2001 issue of *Pediatrics* showed that one-third of children actually displayed problem behavior during the 6 months before their first recognized seizures. Does this mean that behavior problems and seizures are part of the same neurological picture? Or are children with undiagnosed epilepsy distressed because they don't feel quite right but don't know why? In either case, researchers stress disruptive behavior is often overlooked as an early sign of epilepsy.

FAST FACTS
80 Number of times per second that brain cells normally fire **500** Number of times per second that brain cells fire during a seizure **1.2** Percentage of people who have had at least one seizure **40** Number of different types of epilepsy **80** Percentage of people with epilepsy who can control their disorder with medications or surgery

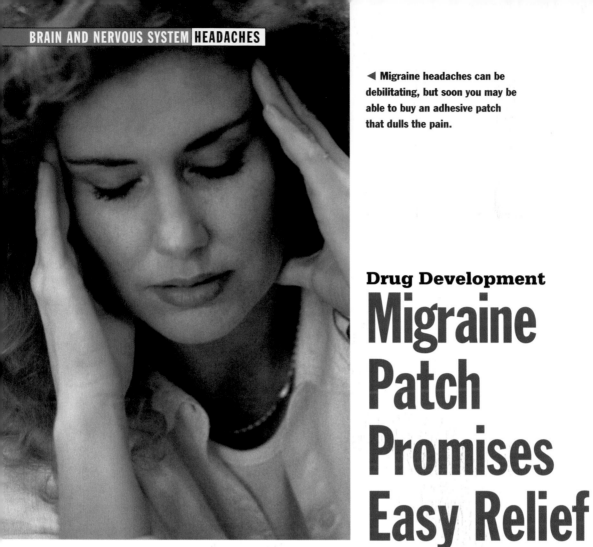

◄ Migraine headaches can be debilitating, but soon you may be able to buy an adhesive patch that dulls the pain.

Drug Development

Migraine Patch Promises Easy Relief

If you don't head a migraine off at the pass by taking oral or injected medication at the first inkling of pain, you may be in agony for hours, and even days in the worst-case scenario. But nausea and vomiting may occur with migraine attacks, so it's often a challenge to keep medication down. Not everyone has the intestinal fortitude to self-administer a shot, either—and injectable migraine drugs are usually reserved for those who have severe attacks.

Soon, however, it may be possible to stave off a migraine simply by placing a clear, thin, adhesive patch, impregnated with the local anesthetic lidocaine, on your forehead. In a trial reported at the March 2001 meeting of the American Society for Clinical Pharmacology and Therapeutics, every one of 40 migraine patients reported a reduction in pain

Doctors foresee using the patch on its own or in combination with other types of treatment.

almost immediately after applying the patch. After two hours, seven of these patients were pain free. After eight hours, the participants said their pain had decreased by an average of 30 percent. The only side effect, experienced by just a few patients, was a slight tingling or burning sensation at the patch site.

How it works. Exactly how lidocaine works for migraines is unclear. Theoretically, it numbs one of a pair of nerves that carries sensations to the mouth, teeth, face, and nasal cavities. Previous studies have shown limited success with lidocaine delivered via nasal spray, and applying it to the forehead may be an even better approach.

Availability. Further clinical tests of a lidocaine patch with the brand name EpiCept are currently under way. Doctors foresee using the patch on its own or in combination with other types of treatment. Since lidocaine is already widely used as a topical anesthetic, quick approval by the U.S. Food and Drug Administration is expected.

Drug Development

New Drug Halts Migraines with Fewer Side Effects

Stopping a migraine headache in its tracks is the goal of drugs called triptans. Unfortunately, the side effects of these drugs, especially chest pain, can make some people reluctant to use them. Now there's a new triptan that offers highly effective pain relief with little or no chest pain. This is important to the millions of people who suffer from migraines (10 to 15 percent of all Americans and Europeans), which the World Health Organization recently called a "major disabling condition."

A study published in the *Archives of Neurology* in June 2001 found that the drug almotriptan (brand name Axert) was as effective as sumitriptan (brand name Imitrex), the gold standard of triptans, but was better tolerated. As a result, patients may be more likely to take their medication as soon as the symptoms of migraine appear, notes Egilius Spierings, M.D., of Harvard Medical School, the principal investigator of the drug trials. This is critical, since migraine drugs are most effective when taken during the earliest stages of the attack.

How it works. Although the medical profession still can't agree on the exact cause of migraine, a leading theory holds that swelling of blood vessels in the brain are to blame. Triptans appear to reduce this swelling by increasing the level of serotonin (a chemical messenger) in the brain. They also may interrupt the transmission of pain signals within the brain and block the release of pain-causing substances from nerve endings.

A cautionary note: All triptans have the potential to cause sudden spasms of a blood vessel and cannot be used by people with heart disease.

Availability. Almotriptan, approved by the Food and Drug Administration in May 2001, is now available by prescription from your doctor. An added bonus: the new drug is cheaper than other triptans.

The root of migraines

New research shows that migraines may occur when abnormally sensitive brain cells fire electrical pulses in a wave that ripples through the brain, ending in the brainstem, where pain centers are located. Interruption of this wave could stop the pain of migraine.

Pain centers

Brainstem

When brain cells transmit pulses...

...blood flow is increased, inflaming blood vessels.

Inflamed blood vessel

RESEARCH ROUNDUP

■ **NO GLUTEN, NO HEADACHES.** "An ounce of prevention" is often a wise approach, even to headaches. A small, preliminary study reported in the February 13, 2001, issue of the Journal *Neurology* found that removing gluten (a protein in wheat and other grains) from the diet of 10 people with a known gluten sensitivity led to fewer or no headaches in 9 of the subjects. One person refused to go on the gluten-free diet. All 10 of the patients had complained of occasional headaches and had shown abnormal findings on magnetic resonance imaging of the brain. The gluten-free diet also relieved their symptoms of poor muscle coordination and unsteadiness.

FAST FACTS
45 MILLION Number of Americans who have chronic headaches
70 Percentage of headache sufferers who are women **72** Number of hours a migraine attack can last

Diagnostic Advance

Pinpointing the Cause of Memory Loss

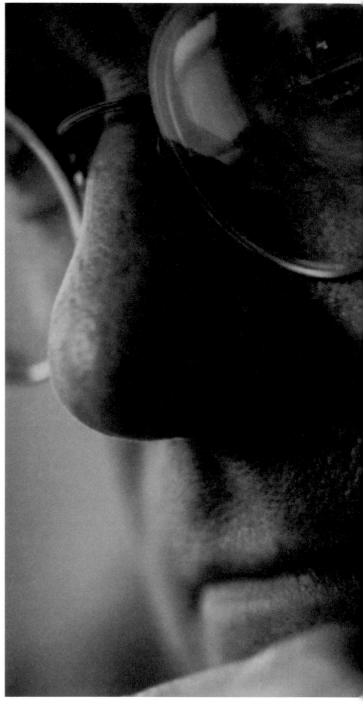

Soon doctors may have a way to determine the cause of memory loss early, so they can start people on appropriate treatment before permanent damage occurs. A new imaging technique called high-resolution magnetic resonance imaging (MRI) is allowing them to see changes and track nerve activity in the hippocampus, a structure deep in the brain that is central to learning. In the December 2000 issue of *Neuron*, researchers from Columbia University College of Physicians & Surgeons in New York City reported their success in using high-resolution MRI in mice to identify abnormal activity in the hippocampus, even before there was irreversible structural damage.

How it works. High-resolution MRI is a variation of functional MRI, which takes thousands of still images a fraction of a second apart to show changes in brain activity while a person is doing a specific task. But the result shown with functional MRI is akin to a photograph of someone running: You can see a large, general pattern of movement, but you lose the fine details. The new high-resolution MRI, on the other hand, analyzes MRI signals over longer periods, providing clearer images of a particular region of the brain, such as the hippocampus. Precise identification of the part of the hippocampus affected in a person with memory problems could provide researchers with important clues to the underlying cause.

Availability. High-resolution MRI is generally available only in academic research facilities. However, standard MRI equipment could be used for high-resolution MRI because taking high-resolution images requires no special equipment. What's different is the way the images are processed — which could be done at a central location equipped with the necessary technology. Countries with national health programs typically license only enough MRI facilities to serve people in a relatively large area, so the technique may not be adopted as quickly outside of the United States.

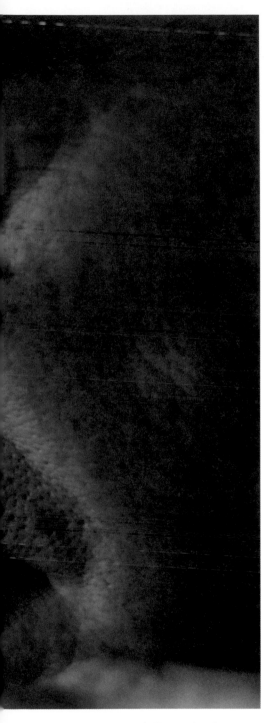

▲ Memory loss is not uncommon in older adults. Now researchers are looking deep in the brain to find out why.

Nutrition Tip
Potatoes for Breakfast?

In a small study of older adults, researchers at the University of Toronto found that a breakfast of carbohydrates such as potatoes or barley increased participants' performance on memory tests. Reporting in the March 2001 issue of *Neurobiology of Learning and Memory*, they explained that a diet lacking in carbohydrates reduces the brain's supply of glucose (blood sugar). This hinders the synthesis of acetylcholine, a messenger chemical that helps brain cells communicate with one another. The researchers also found that rats fed high-fat diets scored lower on tests of learning and memory than rats fed a standard diet. A high-fat diet impedes the metabolism of glucose and may promote resistance to insulin, a protein that controls blood sugar. One more reason to pass up the bacon and eggs.

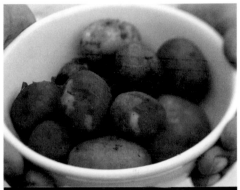

New research shows that eating a breakfast rich in complex carbohydrates — for example, one including potatoes — may boost memory.

RESEARCH ROUNDUP

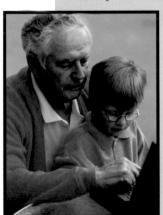

■ **OLD BRAINS, NEW MEMORIES.** For decades, scientists have believed that new brain cells cannot develop later in life. Fortunately, they were wrong. Not only do our brains continue to produce new brain cells as we age, but a study published in the March 15, 2001, issue of the journal *Nature* found that newly generated neurons (nerve cells) quickly become involved in the formation of new memories. This means we have been drastically underestimating the regenerative powers of brains that have been damaged by stroke or by other diseases.

In an earlier study, the same researchers also showed that when it comes to the new brain cells, it's a case of "use it or lose it." They found that new cells in the adult rat brain die within weeks of their "birth." But putting the brain to work with learning exercises improved their survival rate. Another reason to continue learning new skills throughout life.

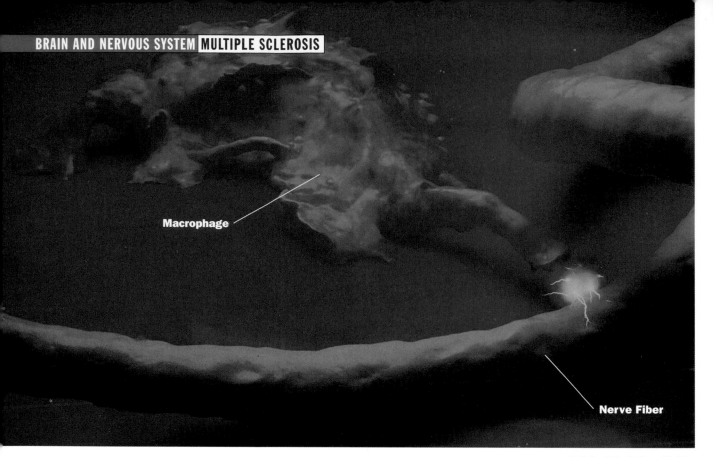

Macrophage

Nerve Fiber

Drug Development
First-Ever Therapy for Severe, Progressive Form of MS

▲ Scientists believe that in some people, macrophages and other white blood cells attack nerve fibers, causing symptoms of multiple sclerosis. A drug can stop these attacks.

Multiple sclerosis (MS) follows several different patterns of progression. Until recently there was no treatment for patients with the secondary progressive type of MS, a stage of advancing deterioration that usually begins after years of relapsing-remitting MS, the most common form of the disease. Now there is a drug that can help these patients—one already used to treat prostate cancer and leukemia.

How it works. MS is an autoimmune disease, which means the immune system responds to some part of the body as if it were a dangerous invader. A drug called mitoxantrone (brand name Novantrone) reins in the immune system by suppressing white blood cells known as T cells, B cells, and macrophages. Scientists believe it's these cells that mistakenly attack the body, targeting the fatty coating around nerve fibers (called the myelin sheath) and destroying it. This makes it more difficult for the nerve cells

> **Until recently there was no treatment for patients with the secondary progressive type of MS.**

to transmit electrical impulses. In clinical trials, mitoxantrone delayed the first relapse of symptoms requiring treatment and also succeeded in delaying MS progression in patients with secondary progressive or progressive relapsing disease.

Availability. In October 2000, the U.S. Food and Drug Administration approved mitoxantrone for secondary progressive MS, as well as for worsening relapsing forms of MS. Patients take mitoxantrone by intravenous infusion once every three months. Those with a history of serious heart problems, liver disease, or certain blood disorders should not use mitoxantrone, nor should women who are pregnant, trying to become pregnant, or breastfeeding. In fact, because of the drug's potential to damage the heart, patients are limited to 8 to 12 doses over two to three years. Also, blood samples need to be taken before each dose is given to check blood counts and liver function.

Drug Development
Smarter MS Treatment Spares the Immune System

Common sense would tell you that it's good to know your friends from your enemies. But the immune system of people with multiple sclerosis (MS) lacks this ability. That's why it attacks a key structure of the nervous system—the protective covering around nerve fibers, called the myelin sheath—leading to damage that slows or blocks nerve signals.

The current approach to treating MS and other autoimmune diseases, using powerful immune-suppressing drugs that increase the risk of infections and other illnesses, is something like wielding a baseball bat to swat a mosquito on your knee: You'll smash the bug, but you may wind up with a broken kneecap. By contrast, an experimental MS treatment called antigen specific immunotherapy targets only the immune system's T cells, leaving the rest of the immune system intact. In February 2001, a report in the *Journal of Immunology* described successful experiments using this therapy in monkeys with an MS-like disease. Before long, it could be tested against MS and other autoimmune diseases in humans.

How it works. Exposure to small amounts of the protein that makes up the myelin sheath primes T cells to attack the myelin. However, large amounts of the protein have just the opposite effect: They cause the T cells to self-destruct. None of the monkeys given large doses of myelin protein developed MS-like symptoms. Although the monkeys had some myelin damage (which showed up on magnetic resonance imaging scans), it was far less severe than the damage seen in groups that did not receive this type of treatment.

Availability. More trials in animals are planned, and the company that developed the myelin protein used for treatment, Alexion Pharmaceuticals, has applied for a permit to proceed with testing on people. Even if the therapy turns out to be safe, many years of study will still be needed before it becomes widely available.

How multiple sclerosis interferes with nerve signals

Nerve cells are connected by fibers, some of which have a protective covering called the myelin sheath. In multiple sclerosis, T cells attack the myelin sheath, making it harder for nerve cells to transmit electrical impulses.

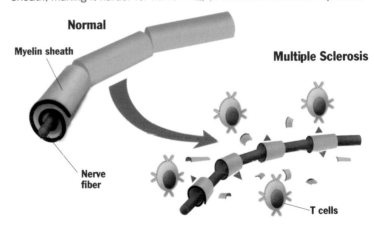

Normal

Myelin sheath

Multiple Sclerosis

Nerve fiber

T cells

RESEARCH ROUNDUP

■ **A DRUG TO STAVE OFF MS?** According to a recent study at the State University of New York School of Medicine at Buffalo, an existing drug used to slow the progression of MS may actually ward off MS in people with early signs of the disorder. The drug, interferon beta-1a (brand name Avonex), is currently part of the standard treatment for MS once a pattern of symptoms and progression is established.

The study, reported in the September 28, 2000, issue of the *New England Journal of Medicine*, compared the effects of Avonex injections with placebo (non-treatment) injections in 383 men and women who had experienced at least one sign of MS and whose brain scans showed typical MS brain lesions (areas where myelin has been damaged). During three years of treatment, people in the group receiving Avonex were significantly less likely than people in the placebo group to suffer a second episode of myelin damage. The treated group also had fewer and slower-growing MS lesions. Because Avonex worked so well, the researchers stopped the study early to offer the drug to people in the placebo group. Whether Avonex can ward off MS indefinitely remains to be seen.

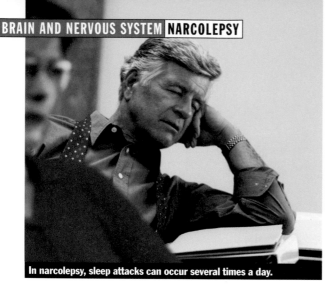

In narcolepsy, sleep attacks can occur several times a day.

Key Finding

Researchers Find Chemical Clue to Narcolepsy

Insomniacs might wish they could fall asleep at the drop of a hat, but people with narcolepsy—uncontrollable daytime sleep attacks that often occur at inopportune times—would probably do anything to stay awake. In 2000, two separate teams of researchers uncovered an important clue about what makes narcoleptics conk out without warning. The key is a brain cell that secretes chemical messengers called hypocretin peptides. People with narcolepsy have up to 95 percent fewer of these cells than do people with normal sleep patterns.

Researchers also found that people with narcolepsy have a type of brain inflammation that has been linked to brain cell degeneration. This deterioration may explain the loss of hypocretin peptides. But what causes it? Genetics, autoimmune factors, or environmental or biological toxins—either individually or in combination— could all play a role.

Pinpointing a cause of narcolepsy could one day also help millions of more people than the relatively small number of individuals who have the disorder: If scientists knew the location of the master sleep switch, researchers could also devise better treatments for the opposite problem—insomnia.

High-Tech Help

Reversing Parkinson's with Gene Therapy

Gene therapy experiments have successfully reversed changes that occur in the brains of monkeys with a disease that closely resembles Parkinson's. The therapy also relieved the tremors, muscle stiffness, and other motor symptoms that are characteristic of the disease. The experiments were conducted at Rush-Presbyterian-St. Luke's Medical Center in Chicago and

RESEARCH ROUNDUP

■ **BLAME IT ON YOUR GENES.** Researchers at Duke University Medical Center, leading a team of researchers from 13 different sites, identified a genetic mutation that appears to be connected to both early- and late-onset Parkinson's disease. A few years ago, Japanese researchers found that a mutation of this Parkin gene was responsible for a disorder similar to Parkinson's that strikes young people. Now the Duke researchers and their colleagues have found another mutation on the Parkin gene by studying over 800 people in more than 175 families affected with Parkinson's disease. The mutation makes the Parkin gene the second one to be implicated in Parkinson's and the first to be linked with the late-onset form of the disease. No blood test for Parkinson's exists yet, but these discoveries are first steps in that direction.

The gene therapy totally prevented the brain cell degeneration associated with Parkinson's disease. The monkeys who didn't receive it became severely impaired.

Lausanne University Medical School in Switzerland and published in the October 27, 2000, issue of the journal *Science*.

How it works. Researchers used a modified virus to deliver a gene into the brains of monkeys. This gene is responsible for the production of a nerve-cell growth factor that strengthens and protects brain cells that normally die as Parkinson's progresses. The growth factor, called GDNF, or glial-derived neurotrophic factor, also increases production of dopamine, a brain chemical largely responsible for normal movement.

After undergoing the gene therapy, one group of old monkeys with early Parkinson's-like disease showed a dramatic increase in the production of dopamine. A second young group of monkeys was first given a chemical that induces the disease; this caused poor performance on a hand-reach test. Some of these monkeys then received gene therapy a week later, and their performance on the test returned almost to normal. In addition, the gene therapy in this group totally prevented the brain cell degeneration associated with Parkinson's disease. The monkeys who didn't receive it became severely impaired.

Availability. These results suggest that a long-term, non-toxic approach to forestalling progression of the disease in newly diagnosed Parkinson's patients may be possible. Clinical testing of the viral delivery system for GDNF should begin in Switzerland and the United States in less than five years, following review by the U.S. Food and Drug Administration.

How the gene therapy works

Parkinson's is caused by the death of dopamine-producing cells in the brain. Researchers reversed it in monkeys by inserting a gene that protects these cells.

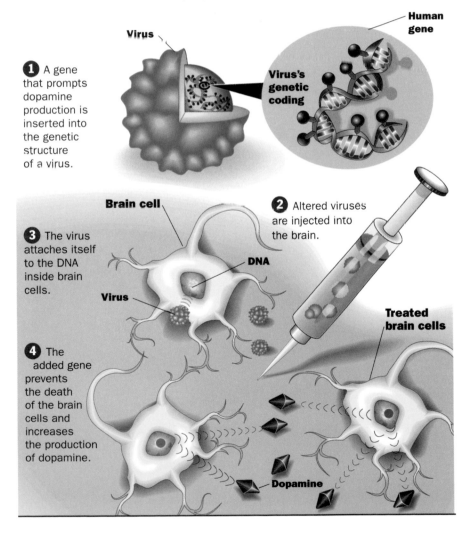

Virus

Human gene

Virus's genetic coding

1 A gene that prompts dopamine production is inserted into the genetic structure of a virus.

Brain cell

2 Altered viruses are injected into the brain.

DNA

3 The virus attaches itself to the DNA inside brain cells.

Virus

Treated brain cells

4 The added gene prevents the death of the brain cells and increases the production of dopamine.

Dopamine

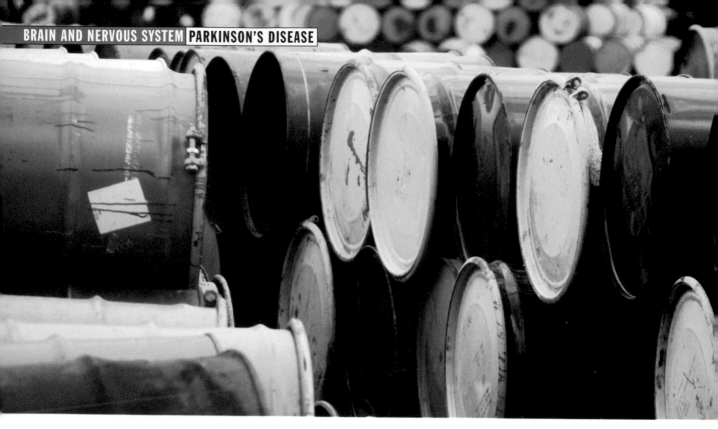

Key Finding
Parkinson's Patients: Like the Canary in the Coal Mine?

Several recent studies have linked Parkinson's disease to environmental toxins—in particular, pesticides, herbicides, solvents, and manganese. Researchers caution that exposure to toxins is unlikely to be the only cause of Parkinson's. Rather, some people who develop the disease may have an inborn susceptibility to develop it as a reaction to toxins and other, unknown, factors.

Pesticides and herbicides. Within the past year, two separate animal studies have implicated pesticides and herbicides as causal factors in the development of Parkinson's. In one study, rats exposed to rotenone, a common chemical used to kill garden pests, developed Parkinson's-like symptoms. Another study suggested that combination chemicals can be particularly damaging. Mice injected with the herbicide paraquat and the fungicide maneb had symptoms similar to those of Parkinson's and showed damage in the same brain area that is abnormal in humans with Parkinson's. The authors of the latter study recommend that safety standards for these substances be reevaluated. Currently, paraquat and maneb are used in combination throughout the United States.

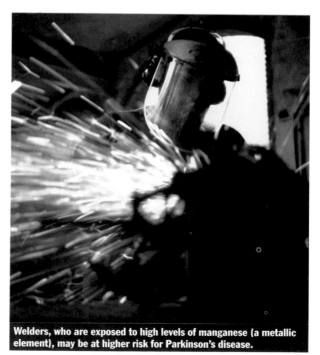

Welders, who are exposed to high levels of manganese (a metallic element), may be at higher risk for Parkinson's disease.

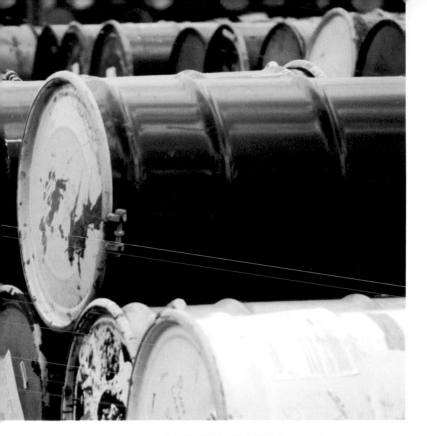

▲ **CHEMICAL CULPRITS Exposure to toxins such as pesticides and solvents may contribute to the development of Parkinson's disease.**

Solvents. A study of 1,000 Italians found that workers in the plastics, petroleum, rubber, and paint industries, all of which involve on-the-job exposure to solvents, developed Parkinson's disease at an earlier age and had more severe symptoms than other Parkinson's patients with different types of occupations.

Manganese. Another study, published in *Neurology* in January 2001, found that welders who were exposed to heavy doses of manganese developed Parkinson's disease an average of 15 years earlier than the typical age of onset. And scientists at the University of California, Santa Cruz, showed that animals exposed to low levels of manganese experienced an accelerated version of Parkinson's. Both reports are particularly worrisome given that manganese is being used increasingly in industrial processes and that a gasoline additive containing manganese (MMT) has been approved for use in the United States.

FAST FACTS
1.2 MILLION Number of people in the United States and Canada living with Parkinson's disease **50,000** Number of people in the United States diagnosed with Parkinson's each year **60** Average age of Parkinson's onset **5–10** Estimated percentage of people under 40 who have Parkinson's

Diagnostic Advance
Is Sleep Apnea Causing Your Snoring?

Imagine gasping for breath up to hundreds of times each night. That's what it's like for people with sleep apnea. In this condition, tissues in the back of the throat temporarily block the passage of air, forcing the person to awaken. Besides the obvious disruption of sleep, apnea has also recently been linked to cardiovascular problems, such as high blood pressure, heart attack, and stroke. So being able to diagnose the condition is all the more pressing. Yet only one out of 10 people with sleep apnea is actually diagnosed with the disorder.

Up until now, the only way to diagnose sleep apnea was to spend the night in a sleep laboratory, the cost of which ranges from $1,100 to $4,000. Now a low-cost, reliable screening device recently approved by the U.S. Food and Drug Administration helps identify which people really need to make that trip to the sleep lab.

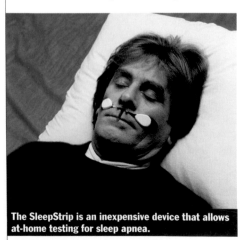

The SleepStrip is an inexpensive device that allows at-home testing for sleep apnea.

How it works. Developed at the Sleep Research Laboratory of the Technion-Israel Institute of Technology in Israel, the SleepStrip allows one-night, at-home testing for sleep apnea. Patients fasten a 4-inch (10-cm) -long plastic strip to the upper lip before going to sleep. Powered by an eight-hour battery, the device contains temperature sensors that record when breathing stops. In the morning, the patient removes the strip and takes it to the doctor, who reads the results on a built-in display.

Availability. The SleepStrip is available in the United States and parts of Europe by prescription.

RESEARCH ROUNDUP

■ **YOUR GAIN, YOUR LOSS.** It's not exactly news that extra weight adds to your risk of snoring and sleep apnea. But specific numbers reported in the *Journal of the American Medical Association* in December 20, 2000, show just how strong the link between apnea and obesity really is. Researchers at the University of Wisconsin Medical School found that a 10 percent weight gain over a four-year period resulted in a six-fold increase in the likelihood of developing sleep-related breathing problems. People who already had sleep apnea got 30 percent worse after a 10 percent weight gain. The extra fat not only blocks the airways, but softens the tissues in the back of the throat, contributing to the problem.

■ **HRT FOR APNEA.** As if the decision about hormone replacement therapy (HRT) weren't already complex enough, women approaching menopause have one more factor to consider. A study of 1,000 women between ages 20 and 100 showed that postmenopausal women had higher rates of sleep apnea than those of premenopausal women. But undergoing HRT evened the score. Preventing apnea may be more important than you'd think: Recent findings indicate that sleep-related breathing problems may trigger high blood pressure. In fact, HRT's protection against apnea may partly account for its benefits to the heart.

High-Tech Help
New Hope at Last for Spinal Cord Injury

I f it worked in dogs, it may work in humans. That's the hope of researchers at the Center for Paralysis Research at Purdue University, in Indiana, who successfully repaired damaged spinal cords in dogs with natural injuries, allowing a few of them to walk again. The researchers used an implanatable device called an oscillating field stimulator to bathe injured nerve cells with weak electrical fields mimicking those that regenerate tissue naturally in the body.

How it works. About the size of two joined lipstick cases, the device has six electrodes radiating out from it. They produce electrical fields that act on growth-promoting receptors on the damaged nerves, causing them to move to the ends of the nerves, thereby allowing the outward expansion of nerve fibers. Because nerve fibers grow toward a negative electrical charge, the field reverses periodically to allow regrowth on both sides of the injury. This device has promoted rapid nerve regeneration in laboratory animals and recovery from paraplegia (paralysis of the legs) in dogs.

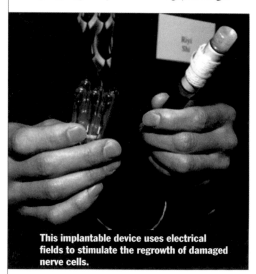

► The actor Christopher Reeve, who was paralyzed in 1995 from an injury to his spinal cord, has been recognized by the Society for Neuroscience for his efforts to promote research into treatment for spinal cord injury.

This implantable device uses electrical fields to stimulate the regrowth of damaged nerve cells.

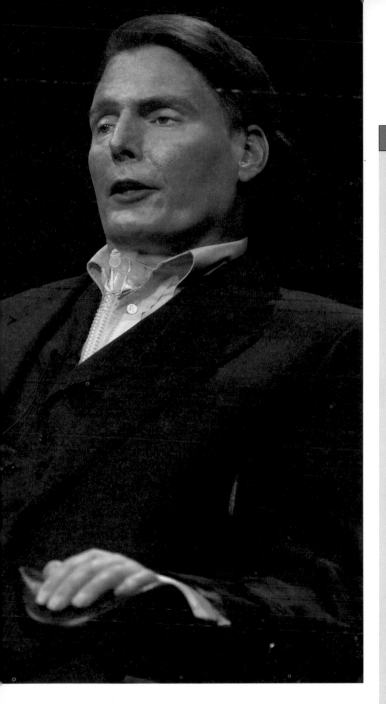

RESEARCH ROUNDUP

■ **STEM CELL TRANSPLANTS FOR PARALYSIS.** Scientists at the Society for Neuroscience meeting in November 2000 reported on a procedure that helped paralyzed rodents recover some movement. Working with rodents with complete paralysis of the hind limbs, these investigators transplanted neural stem cells (immature cells with the potential to become any kind of cell) into the animals' spinal fluid. The stem cells traveled up and down the spinal cord, with a small percentage transforming into neurons (nerve cells). The result? Hind leg movement improved in 12 of 18 rodents. Some had slight movement; some even took steps. Long-term animal trials are needed before human studies can begin.

■ **SPONTANEOUS RECOVERY FROM SPINAL INJURY.** Tree branches sprout after pruning. Miraculously, similar regrowth of spinal nerves can happen after a spinal cord injury, as reported in the *Proceedings of the National Academy of Sciences (USA)* on March 13, 2001. Despite the loss of all but 3 percent of the spinal nerve fibers in a part of the spinal cord that controls movement of the paws and

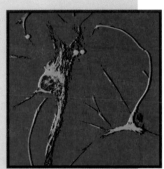

Animal studies have shown that damaged nerves can grow again.

feet, rats gradually recovered movement in these limbs and within a month were no different than rats that had not been injured. The small number of intact nerve fibers had sprouted new connections and increased contact with other cells by more than 300 percent. This phenomenon helps explain the spontaneous recovery of motor function that happens with about 40 percent of humans after spinal cord injury. The next step the researchers will take is to see what effect nerve growth factors (proteins that stimulate nerve growth) may have on encouraging nerve fiber regrowth.

Availability. The U.S. Food and Drug Administration has approved the testing of the technique in humans, and trials began in April 2001 at the Indiana University School of Medicine. At first, the device is being implanted in only 10 people no more than 18 days after a spinal injury. Researchers want to know, among other things, whether the device used will have any negative effects. If no safety concerns arise, the trial will be expanded to include more people. Ideally, the researchers hope to duplicate in humans the promising results that have already been seen in restoring feeling and some function in animals. The goal is an increase in the quality of life of those paralyzed, according to Richard Borgens, M.D., the director of the Center for Paralysis.

FAST FACTS
82 Percentage of spinal cord injuries occurring in males **44** Percentage of spinal cord injuries caused by motor vehicle accidents **7,600-10,000** Number of new spinal cord injuries occurring in the United States each year

CANCER

We're still years away from being able to say there is a cure for cancer—and in fact, some researchers are loath to mention the word "cure." Nevertheless, this has been an exciting time for cancer patients and researchers alike. Gleevec, the first of a brand-new class of cancer drugs, has been compared to a stealth missile or sniper's bullet in the precision of its attack on leukemia, and similar weapons against other cancers may be just around the corner. Another new high-tech family of drugs called monoclonal antibodies may change the face of treatment and the survival rates for many people—those with colon cancer and lung cancer among others. And with vaccines in the pipeline for cervical cancer and prostate cancer and new imaging techniques leading to more accurate diagnosis of breast cancer, this cutting-edge area of research is hurtling forward at breakneck speed.

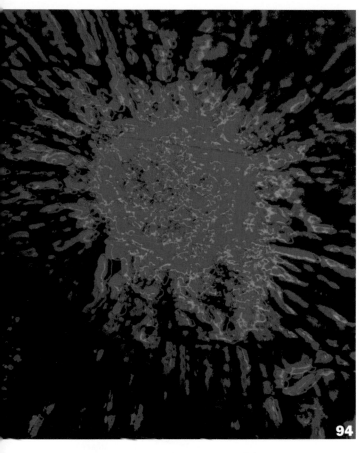

94

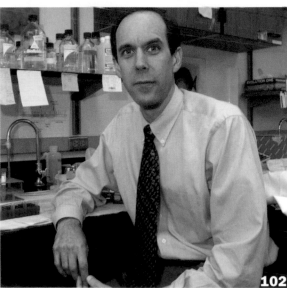

102

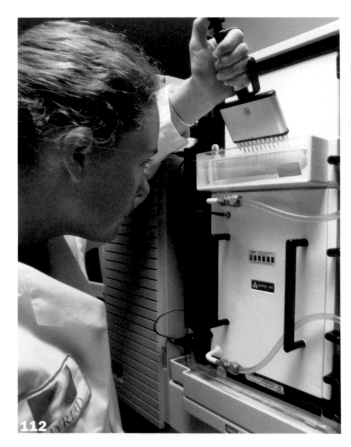

112

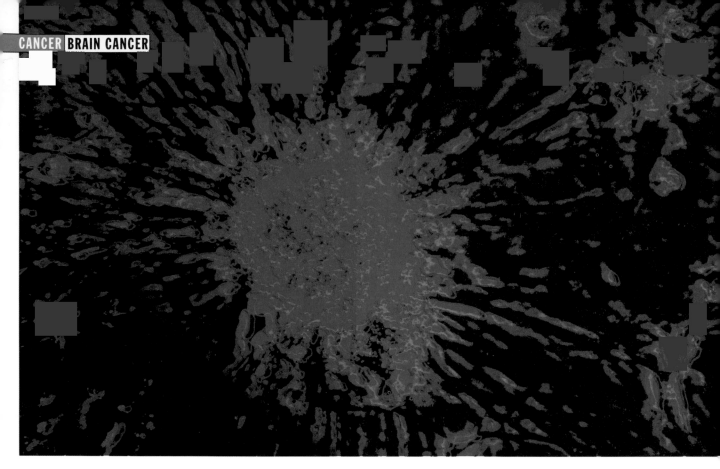

Progress in Prevention
New Vaccine Targets Aggressive Form of Brain Cancer

▲ A vaccine made from cancer cells offers new hope to people with glioma, a deadly type of brain tumor.

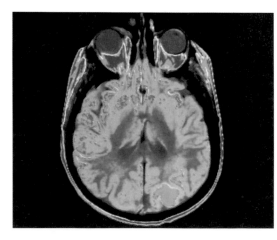

► Cancer cells can be identified by an MRI brain scan.

An aggressive type of brain tumor called a glioma carries a veritable death sentence: People diagnosed with this type of cancer generally have less than a year to live. But a newly developed vaccine that engages the immune system may be able to prolong their lives.

Scientists at the Maxine Dunitz Neurological Institute at Cedars-Sinai Medical Center in Los Angeles have had preliminary success with a vaccine called a dendritic cell vaccine. It doesn't cure the cancer, but it does provoke the immune system to wage a much stronger battle against the stubborn disease. The survival rates of the patients in the study improved from an average

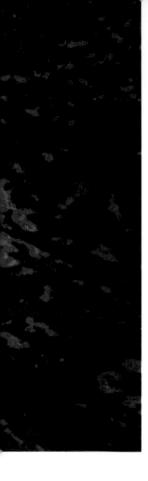

of 257 days to 455 days. "Although this first study was conducted with a small number of patients, the results greatly exceeded our expectations," wrote Keith L. Black, M.D., in a Cedars-Sinai Medical Center statement.

How it works. Researchers created the vaccine by removing cancer cells from the tumor and mixing them with dendritic cells, a type of cell found in the bloodstream that helps identify targets to be attacked. Normally, the body can't distinguish between cancer cells and regular cells, so the dendritic cells are an essential component of the vaccine. The nine patients who were injected with the vaccine all showed activation of tumor-specific white blood cells called T-cells. In other words, their immune system began to identify, target, and kill cancerous cells. No serious adverse reactions were noted.

Availability. Following the positive results of this Phase I trial, Phase II trials are under way to further the understanding of how the vaccine works and confirm its effect on survival.

FAST FACTS

17,200 Estimated number of malignant tumors of the brain or spinal cord that will be diagnosed in the United States during 2001
13,100 Estimated number of people in the United States who will die from these conditions in 2001 **BLOOD-BRAIN BARRIER** The nearly impermeable brain blood vessels, which prevent certain substances—including anti-cancer drugs—in the blood from entering the brain, making it more difficult to treat brain tumors

Key Finding
Secrets to Chemotherapy Success

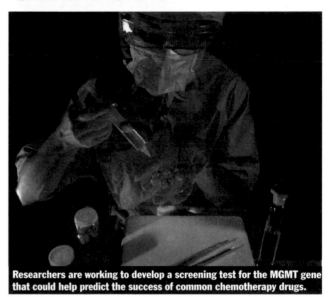

Researchers are working to develop a screening test for the MGMT gene that could help predict the success of common chemotherapy drugs.

Why do some patients respond well to chemotherapy, while others don't? Recent studies in people with a type of brain cancer called glioma filled in a critical piece of the puzzle. In one of the studies, reported in the November 9, 2000, issue of the *New England Journal of Medicine*, researchers discovered that a common chemotherapy drug worked best in people with a certain alteration of a gene called MGMT (methylguanine-DNA methyltransferase), known as the DNA repair gene.

In healthy cells, MGMT helps prevent DNA damage that causes cancer. In cancerous cells, it protects the cell from destruction by certain chemotherapy chemicals—bad news for people undergoing chemotherapy. But in some people, the gene is altered in such a way that it is turned off—good news for those individuals receiving alkylating agents, the most common type of chemotherapy drug.

Of the 47 patients in the study, 40 percent tested positive for the alteration. Of these patients, 64 percent had a better survival rate, showing complete or partial response to the chemotherapy drug used to treat their cancer. Only 4 percent of those who tested negative for the alteration had a similar

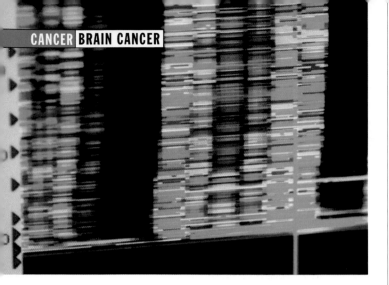

▲ By looking at differences in patients' DNA, researchers are beginning to understand why chemotherapy shrinks the brain tumors of some people and not others.

response. Identifying which patients have an altered MGMT gene would help predict who may do well on alkylating agents and who might need a different type of drug.

More exhaustive study is needed before screening for the gene alteration can be recommended for patients. In the meantime, an international biotechnology company, Virco Lab Inc., has bought the licensing rights for the development of an MGMT screening test. They plan to market the test to doctors to help them target which type of chemotherapy drugs would be best for their patients. Virco is also working to develop a drug that will switch off the gene in those patients in whom it is still active so that they too can benefit from the standard drugs.

RESEARCH ROUNDUP

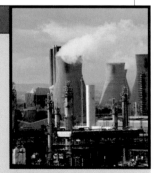

A new study links brain tumors in children with exposure to the toxins released by petrochemical plants.

■ **BRAIN CANCER CULPRIT.** "What caused my cancer?" is an often-repeated question, and it is rare that a doctor can provide an accurate answer. But there are exceptions. Lung cancer, for instance, can often be attributed to smoking. And sometimes investigations of "cancer clusters" (geographic areas with higher-than-normal rates of certain cancers) reveal environmental causes. A recent study in Taiwan, funded by the National Institutes of Health and the Brain Tumor Society, has found such a link.

Ninety-two new cases of brain tumors in children under age 19 were found in the villages located less than 3 kilometers from four large petrochemical industrial complexes (PICs), which produce fuel, among other chemical products. Up to 10 times more hydrocarbons (compounds containing hydrogen and carbon) and other toxic substances are released there than in industrialized communities in the United States. Though the actual number of cancer cases in the study was relatively small, the increased rates within 1 kilometer of the PICs were considered significant.

Diagnostic Advance
Ductal Lavage: A Pap Test for the Breast?

What if there were a way to detect abnormal cells in the breast long before a lump could be felt or even seen on a mammogram? In women at high risk for breast cancer, a new technique called ductal lavage could help doctors find atypical cells in the breast—which can indicate an increased risk for breast cancer.

Just as the Pap test dramatically lowered the death rate from cervical cancer during the second half of the last century, ductal lavage could potentially lower the death rate for breast cancer. However, unlike the Pap test, this method is designed only for women who have been determined to be at high risk for breast cancer (defined as having a personal history of breast cancer; a mother, daughter, or sister with breast cancer or two or more other close relatives with breast cancer; or evidence of a genetic change that increases susceptibility to breast cancer).

Final results of a clinical trial presented at the 23rd Annual San Antonio Breast Cancer Symposium at the end of 2000 found atypical cells in 23.5 percent (90 women) of 383 high-risk women who had ductal lavage and malignant cells in 0.5 percent (2 women)—cells that would have gone unnoticed without the new technique. It should be stressed, however, that ductal lavage has not yet been tested enough to determine its accuracy in identifying cancerous cells and is primarily intended to detect atypical cells.

How it works. Ductal lavage is based on the fact that most breast cancers originate in the breast's milk ducts. Performed under local anesthesia in either a doctor's office or an outpatient clinic, it involves two steps. First, a suction cup, much like a breast pump, draws any existing fluid from the milk ducts. Because such fluid can be a danger signal, this step identifies which ducts may need further examination. Then, saline is inserted through a tiny catheter into the suspect ducts to "rinse" the ducts and collect cells for examination. ("Lavage" is the French word for "rinse.") The cells are then sent to a lab for analysis under a microscope to determine whether they are normal or abnormal.

Availability. The devices used for ductal lavage have been cleared for marketing in the United States, and several breast cancer centers around the country already offer the screening technique. If you know you are at high risk for breast cancer, speak to your doctor about whether you are a candidate for ductal lavage, which can be used in addition to mammography and physical examination.

▼ In ductal lavage, cells are collected from a milk duct in the breast through a tiny catheter. If any suspicious cells are found, a woman may be at increased risk for breast cancer.

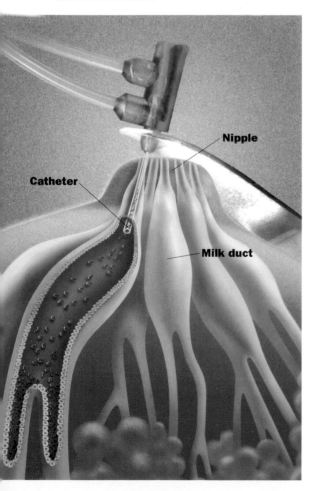

Catheter

Nipple

Milk duct

Diagnostic Advance
Computer-Assisted Mammograms Detect More Breast Cancers

Computers can help us in so many areas of our lives—including our health. Now they're helping make mammograms more accurate, possibly saving lives in the process.

How it works. After a regular mammogram is taken, computer-aided detection (CAD) creates a digital version of the image, then scans it, marking any suspicious areas. Think of it like running a manuscript through a spellchecker: CAD helps radiologists catch any potential problems they didn't see with their own eyes.

In a study of 12,860 women presented at the annual meeting of the Radiological Society of North America in November 2000, the computer-assisted technique detected 20 percent more breast cancers than radiologists did on their own. But CAD was not perfect: It also missed some cancers that only the radiologists noticed.

Availability. The only FDA-approved CAD system is R2 Technology's Imagechecker, which costs $200,000 and can add $15 or more to the cost of mammography. Larger trials are needed to demonstrate its cost-effectiveness.

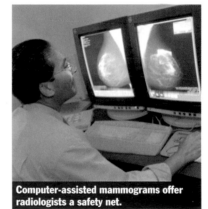

Computer-assisted mammograms offer radiologists a safety net.

CAD is currently available in about 100 centers in the United States. But researchers remind us that the overall accuracy rate for the gold standard, mammography, is 85 to 90 percent without CAD, so women need not feel that their mammogram is not accurate without the use of this new tool. Good advice is to make sure that your mammograms are read by an experienced radiologist who examines thousands of mammograms a year.

FAST FACTS

182,800 Estimated number of women in the United States who will be diagnosed with invasive breast cancer during 2001
75 Percentage of women diagnosed with breast cancer who are over age 50 **5–10** Percentage of breast cancers that are inherited

Progress in Prevention
Vaccine Could Cripple the Virus that Causes Cervical Cancer

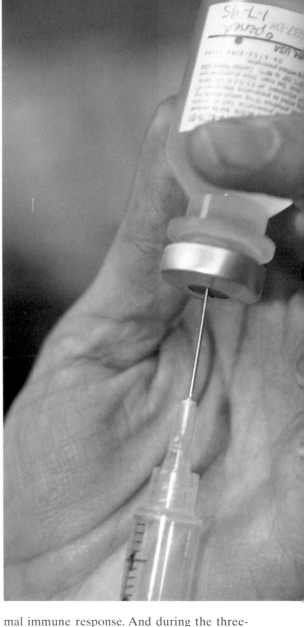

If initial positive results with a vaccine hold up under further scrutiny, deaths from cervical cancer could drop dramatically. Cervical cancer, which grows initially in the lining of the lower part of the uterus, is inextricably connected to human papillomavirus (HPV)—the same virus that causes genital warts. There are more than 100 types of HPV. But recently, the identification of about a dozen high-risk types has led to experimentation with a vaccine that could theoretically protect against 80 percent of cervical cancers.

▶ To prove whether the HPV vaccine actually prevents infection and reduces cancer, researchers will be studying thousands of women in Costa Rica, where the rate of cervical cancer is much higher than that in the United States.

The vaccine was tested in 72 volunteers, who received it over a four-month period. The results were published February 21, 2001, in the *Journal of the National Cancer Institute*.

How it works. Just as a flu vaccine contains parts of influenza viruses, the HPV vaccine was created from HPV proteins, specifically those of HPV-16—one of the high-risk strains, which accounts for more than half of all cervical cancers. During the study, researchers found that in response to the vaccine, the immune systems of inoculated healthy volunteers mounted a defense 40 times stronger than a nor-

The immune systems of inoculated volunteers mounted a defense 40 times stronger than normal.

mal immune response. And during the three-month follow-up period, the worst side effect experienced was a mild irritation at the injection site.

Availability. As always, the early research caveat applies: More study is warranted. And if this vaccine is successful, more vaccines will be needed to fight the other strains of HPV. But these early results are promising—so promising that Novavax, a Columbia, Maryland, drug delivery company, has been awarded a $1 million contract from the National Cancer Institute to manufacture an HPV vaccine. A clinical trial with 20,000 volunteers that will further test the effectiveness of the vaccine began in 2001. Though these are significant steps, the vaccine is still years away from becoming widely available.

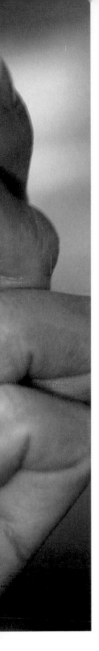

Diagnostic Advance
New Test Helps Clarify Inconclusive Pap Results

For years the Pap test, which involves microscopic examination of cervical cells, has been the gold standard when it comes to screening for cervical abnormalities, including cervical cancer. But the results aren't always clear-cut, and sometimes further tests are needed to clarify what they mean.

When the lab report reads "atypical squamous cells of undetermined significance" (ASCUS), what happens next? That depends on the health care provider. In some cases, the patient will be immediately referred for colposcopy, an exam using an instrument that magnifies the cervix. Any precancerous or cancerous tissue can be removed during the exam. Other doctors might take a "wait and see" approach, ordering a follow-up Pap test for the patient within a few months.

Either tactic can be effective, but neither is perfect. Colposcopy is expensive and uncomfortable. And a repeat Pap test is not infallible; it can miss cellular changes that are early indicators of cancer. But a third type of follow-up test, for the human papillomavirus, or HPV, may be the best answer yet. Why? Because more than 95 percent of cervical cancers are caused by HPV infection.

The HPV test was evaluated, along with the two

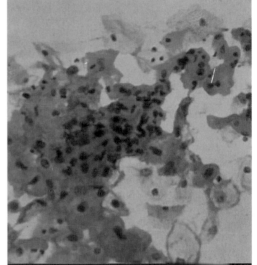

Of the more than 100 types of human papillomavirus (above), more than 30 can be transmitted through sexual contact, and about a dozen have been linked to cervical cancer.

The Pap test is a way of detecting abnormal cells on the cervix (above), which can be an early indication of cervical cancer. Now a new test can help clarify ambiguous Pap results.

existing options, in a comprehensive clinical trial reported in the February 21, 2001, issue of the *Journal of the National Cancer Institute*. The study looked at more than 3,500 women who had received Pap test results of ASCUS and had been given a colposcopy, either after receiving the HPV test or after having a repeat Pap test. About 5 to 10 percent of the women were found to have precancer or cancer on colposcopy; of these, over 96 percent had received a positive HPV test, as opposed to 85 percent having a positive repeat Pap test. In addition, 99.5 percent of women with a negative HPV test were found not to have precancer or cancer.

While a positive HPV test does not mean that precancer or cancer is present, a negative or positive test result in addition to an uncertain Pap finding can lead to a better decision about whether a colposcopy should be scheduled.

Availability. The HPV test is not yet available everywhere, but given its effectiveness, it's likely that it will soon become a standard test given at the same time as the Pap test.

> **FAST FACTS**
> **500,000** Estimated number of new cervical cancer cases worldwide in 2001 **74** Percentage decline of cervical cancer deaths between 1955 and 1992, largely attributed to more widespread use of the Pap test **70 PERCENT** Five-year survival rate for cervical cancer **ALMOST 100 PERCENT** Five-year survival rate for precancerous cervical conditions **2** Number of the most common types of cervical cancer: squamous cell carcinoma and adenocarcinoma

Drug Development
Cancer Vaccine Shows Early Promise

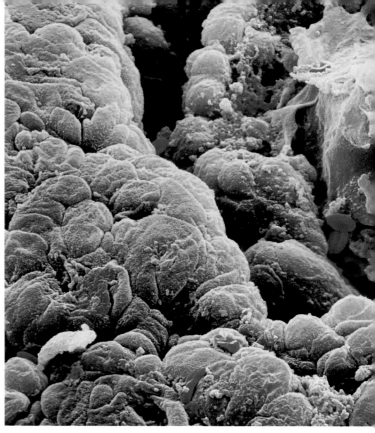

▲ Unlike a healthy colon (right), a cancerous colon (above) contains a multitude of tumors. The tumors are pictured in yellow, blood cells in red, mucus in blue, and bacteria in green.

Researchers at Stanford University in California are optimistic that a vaccine may one day offer another treatment option for cancer patients. In a study presented at the 2001 annual meeting of the American Society of Clinical Oncology, 12 patients with either advanced colorectal or lung cancer were treated with a vaccine made from a specific type of immune system cell (called a dendritic cell) that was removed from the patients. The cells were altered to produce a certain kind of cancer protein commonly found in lung and colorectal cancers. When the altered dendritic cells were injected back into the patients, they induced a powerful immune reaction to the cancer protein in the body, causing the patients' immune systems to attack the tumors.

Two of the patients with advanced colorectal cancer experienced complete remission. One has remained cancer-free for almost a year, but in the other patient, cancer recurred in a different location after 10 months. Two others showed clinical improvement. These results are encouraging because, in the past, cancer vaccines have not been successful against solid tumors (cancer of body tissues other than blood, bone marrow, or the lymphatic system) because these tumors tend not to trigger an immune response in the body.

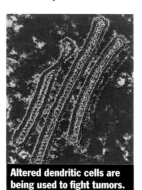

Altered dendritic cells are being used to fight tumors.

Outsmarting cancer cells. The thinking behind using vaccines to treat cancer is straightforward: Once the immune system is exposed to an antigen—a cancer protein—carried by the vaccine, it learns to identify and destroy the antigen. Therefore, the cancer vaccine eventually trains the immune system to recognize and kill antigens found in tumor cells. So far, the treatment has proven to be nontoxic. What is particularly exciting, says one researcher, is that the vaccines can be customized to each patient and his or her particular type of cancer. The vaccine will be tested next in patients with colorectal cancer who are less ill.

RESEARCH ROUNDUP

■ **SPARING CERTAIN PATIENTS FROM CHEMOTHERAPY.** Research is under way to pinpoint which patients might benefit most from chemotherapy after surgery. Although chemotherapy is often given to all patients in an attempt to kill off any cancerous cells that surgery failed to remove, it doesn't help everyone. A new study, published in the *New England Journal of Medicine* on April 19, 2001, examined tissue from the tumors of 460 patients with stage III or high-risk stage II colon cancer. They found that in people with certain molecular markers—characteristics of the tumor tissue—the five-year survival rate after chemotherapy was no better than that without chemotherapy. In other people, chemotherapy boosted their chances of survival. Scientists hope that these markers will provide the critical first step toward individualized cancer treatment based on the molecular characteristics of the person's tumor.

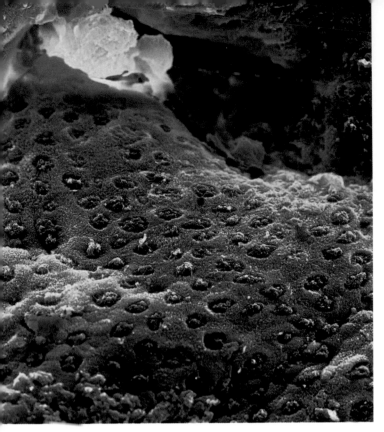

Drug Development
Breast Cancer Drug Approved for Colon Cancer

The first oral drug for treating metastatic colorectal cancer was approved by the U.S. Food and Drug Administration (FDA) in May 2001. Already used to treat breast cancer, capecitabine (brand name Xeloda) is only the second treatment for colon cancer approved by the FDA in the past 40 years.

How it works. When capecitabine enters the body, it reacts with an enzyme that converts it into 5-fluorouracil, or 5-FU, a standard therapy for cancer that has been used for many years. Unlike the typical intravenous cancer treatments, which require a trip to the hospital, this drug can be taken at home, in two daily doses. A 30-week study conducted at the University of Texas showed that patients who took capecitabine survived as long as patients on standard therapy but experienced fewer side effects.

Availability. The FDA approved capecitabine as a breast cancer treatment in 1998, so it is widely available by prescription.

Drug Development
Experimental Drug Gives New Hope to Patients with Advanced Colon Cancer

For patients with advanced colon cancer that no longer responds to chemotherapy, there may be a way to shrink the tumor and prolong life. An experimental drug called IMC-C225 (also known as cetuximab) blocks a protein called epidermal growth factor (EGF) that tumors need in order to grow. The drug may not be able to kill cancer cells outright but it can weaken them enough to allow chemotherapy to finish them off.

Researchers presented their latest findings at the annual meeting of the American Society of Clinical Oncology in May 2001. They gave the drug to 121 patients with advanced colon cancer that was no longer responding to standard chemotherapy treatment. In more than one-fifth of the patients, the tumors shrank by more than 50 percent. Said the study's leader, Leonard Saltz, M.D., of Memorial Sloan-Kettering Cancer Center in New York: "This is a significant result. We have a group of patients who have failed to respond to two other therapies, and now we're getting a 22.5 percent response rate from this new regimen."

How it works. In many tumors, EGF must attach to its EGF receptor (located on a cell's surface) in order for the cell to begin a chain of activities that allow the tumor to grow. IMC-C225 is a monoclonal antibody (a laboratory-produced substance) that binds to the EGF receptor, preventing EGF from linking up to it. Many types of solid tumors have been found to have EGF receptors, including colorectal, head and neck, and pancreatic cancers.

Availability. IMC-C225 is still being tested for colon cancer and several other types, such as cancers of the head, neck, pancreas, and lung. Phase III clinical trials for colorectal cancer patients are scheduled to begin during 2001.

Dr. Leonard Saltz discusses his research on a drug that blocks tumor growth in people with colon cancer.

Drug Development

Breakthrough Leukemia Drug Zeros In on Cause of Cancer

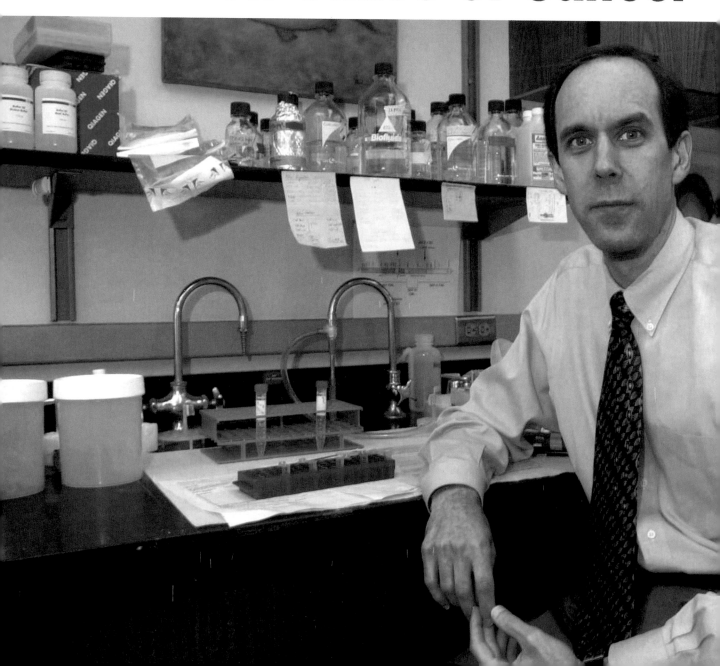

"Paradigm shift" is a phrase that's used judiciously in oncology circles, but it was invoked following the announcement of a revolutionary new anti-cancer drug for chronic myelogenous leukemia (CML), a rare, life-threatening type of leukemia. The drug, imatinib mesylate (brand name Gleevec), was approved by the U.S. Food and Drug Administration (FDA) in record time because of its impressive results in patients during clinical trials. The time it took the drug company, Novartis, to manufacture Gleevec was also cut in half, largely due to an Internet petition signed by thousands of patients clamoring for the drug.

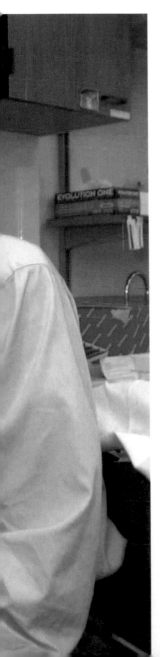

▼ Dr. Brian Druker was part of the team of visionaries who developed Gleevec, a drug that may revolutionize cancer treatment.

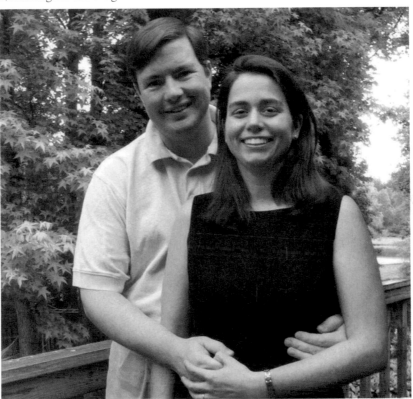

How it works. Gleevec is the first in a new class of drugs — one that represents an entirely fresh approach to treating cancer. These drugs target an abnormal growth-signaling protein that is present in nearly all CML patients and is probably the cause of the disease. By blocking the protein, called BCR-ABL, the drug kills the leukemia cells.

▲ Frank Gibbe, shown with his wife, Elizabeth, participated in a clinical trial for the leukemia drug Gleevec. Gibbe is now cancer-free.

Because Gleevec takes aim directly at the protein molecules that cause the cancer, it leaves healthy cells alone, which sets it apart from most chemotherapy drugs. Although Gleevec does have side effects, such as nausea, diarrhea, swelling, and muscle pain, they are minor compared with those of traditional cancer drugs. Gleevec's triumph over CML is sure to spur the development of similar drugs for other cancers.

Explains Richard Klausner, M.D., director of the National Cancer Institute, "For the first time, cancer researchers now have the necessary tools to probe the molecular anatomy of tumor cells in search of cancer-causing proteins. Gleevec offers proof that

Gleevec is the first in a new class of drugs— one that represents an entirely fresh approach to treating cancer.

"When you feel like you've lost your life, no one can put into words what it feels like to have it back."

molecular targeting works in treating cancer, provided that the target is correctly chosen. The challenge now is to find these targets."

Unlike typical chemotherapy drugs, which are given intravenously, Gleevec is taken orally once a day. Although it is most effective with the first stage of CML, the drug is approved for use with all three stages. In clinical trials it triggered remission in up to 78 percent of patients. In one trial, abnormal cells disappeared from the blood of 53 out of 54 patients. These are impressive results, yet researchers caution that the drug has not been available long enough to evaluate its long-term benefits or risks.

Availability. Gleevec was approved by the FDA in May 2001 for CML. It also appears to work against a second type of cancer known as gastrointestinal stromal tumor (GIST), which is usually incurable if surgery for it fails. It is currently being tested in other cancers as well, including glioma and soft-tissue sarcoma.

PATIENT PROFILE

Surviving CML with Gleevec

At first, he noticed at work that he wasn't quite himself. "I had a lot of fatigue and was making mental mistakes, which was unusual for me," says Philip Russell, a 50-year-old electrical contractor. Then, as a licensed soccer referee, he was trying to train for an upcoming season and found he couldn't run more than a quarter mile. But it wasn't until he noticed one night that the entire left side of his abdomen was as hard as a rock that he knew something was terribly wrong. "Even with the sit-ups I did, my stomach never felt like that," says Russell. "It turned out that my spleen had grown so huge it was collapsing part of one lung."

Blood tests revealed a white blood cell count 28 times the normal level. The diagnosis: chronic myelogenous leukemia (CML). Ironically, Russell had been the executive director of the San Francisco Leukemia Society in 1976. "Back then, everyone died, so when I got this diagnosis, I started 'folding up my tent.' Later, I found out there was more hope than ever."

At first, Russell underwent courses of chemotherapy and interferon, an immune system stimulant. The interferon helped, but not without dire consequences. Russell dropped 30 pounds in the first two months. He was extremely fatigued, lost his appetite, and couldn't do anything athletic. After almost two grueling years on interferon, he was lucky enough to become part of a Stanford, California, clinical trial for Gleevec beginning in March 2001.

With Gleevec he had pain in his hips and legs for about four weeks, but it was nothing compared to the side effects he experienced with interferon. "I call us the Gleevec babies—we have this bright-eyed look—because we not only get to go on living, but we get to feel good doing it," says Russell, whose white blood cell count is now closer to normal. Russell is ecstatic that he will be able to see his two teenagers finish growing up. "When you feel like you've lost your life, no one can put into words what it feels like to have it back," he says. Most days, "the sky is unbelievably blue and the grass unbelievably green. It's like looking down a long hallway at a bright light. The hallway gets longer, but you still see the light. You never forget."

Philip Russell, here with his son, Ben, has a lower white blood cell count thanks to Gleevec.

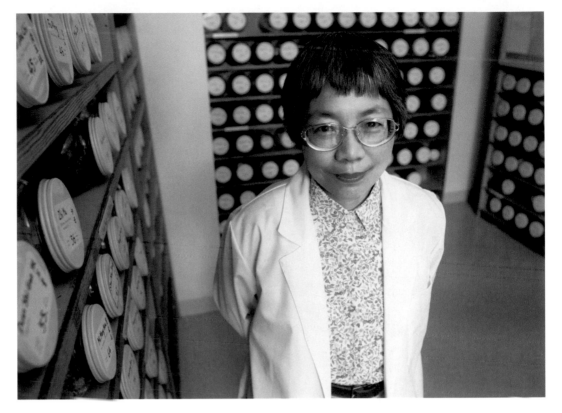

► Traditional Chinese medicine has included arsenic therapy for years. Now Western doctors are using this notorious poison to treat leukemia.

Drug Development
Harnessing a Poison's Powers

What doesn't kill you makes you stronger. This aphorism describes the impressive results of a drug called arsenic trioxide (brand name Trisenox) in treating acute promyelocytic leukemia (APL), a fatal cancer that affects the blood and bone marrow. Used in China for many years, arsenic-based therapy is now approved in the United States for treating leukemia in patients who have not responded to or who have relapsed after standard therapy.

How it works. With APL, a mistake in the cellular DNA prevents otherwise healthy cells from maturing normally. As they continue to reproduce, they take up increasing space in the bone marrow, crowding out normal cells. Arsenic works by forcing the cancer cells to mature and die off rapidly. Then, normal cells can return to the bone marrow to do their job of making blood.

The arsenic course consists of daily injections for up to 60 days. After the bone marrow is cleared of leukemia cells, a second course continues for 25 days, starting three weeks after evidence of remission. One research study published in July 2000 showed remission in 88 percent of patients.

> **Arsenic works by forcing cancer cells to mature and die off rapidly. Then, normal cells can return to the bone marrow.**

Availability. Trisenox was approved by the U.S. Food and Drug Administration in September 2000. Although side effects can be severe, they do not appear to be permanent or irreversible. They include inflammation of heart and lung tissues, changes in cardiac rhythm, abdominal discomfort, nausea, vomiting, headache, fatigue, and skin changes. Studies are being conducted to see if arsenic trioxide may be effective in treating other cancers such as chronic myelogenous leukemia, lymphoma, and cancers of the cervix, bladder, and kidney.

> **FAST FACTS**
> **30,800** Estimated number of new leukemia cases diagnosed in the United States in 2001 **21** Percentage drop in deaths from leukemia in the last 20 years for men and women under age 65 **57** Percentage drop in the death rate during the last 30 years for children with leukemia. Still, in the United States, leukemia causes more deaths in children under 15 than any other disease.

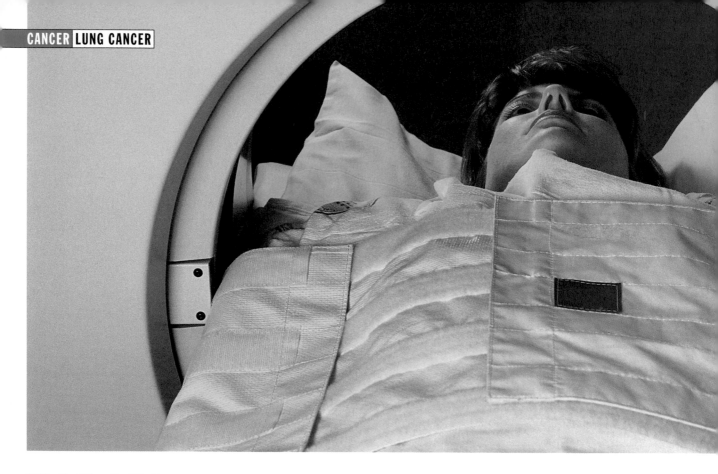

High-Tech Help

PET Scans Help Cancer Patients Get Smarter Treatment

A high-tech radioactive scan may soon become part of the diagnostic workup of a patient with suspected cancer and a routine exam for people suffering from cancer. Although the technology has been available since the 1970s, more and more studies are showing that PET (positron emission tomography) scans help doctors make better and more informed decisions about how to treat their patients.

PET scans are highly sensitive full-body scans that can detect cancer cells that may be left over from cancer treatment, as well as check whether or not a suspicious mass is, in fact, cancerous. The latest study from Queen's Medical Center in Honolulu, reported in the May 1, 2001, issue of the *Journal of Clinical Oncology*, showed that PET scans may help doctors pinpoint the most appropriate drugs and procedures for patients who are diagnosed with lung cancer and other cancers.

In people already being treated for cancer, PET scans can change the treatment direction a doctor might take. For example, in 33 percent of 53 cases studied (mostly lung cancer), ex-pected surgery was canceled after doctors reviewed the scan results. In 15 percent of cases, chemotherapy or radiation was added to the treatment plan. And treatment was canceled in 7 percent of the patients because the PET scan showed that they did not, in fact, have cancer.

How it works. PET scans measure the use of glucose (sugar) in the body's cells. Since cancer cells consume more sugar than normal cells, the scan can identify cancerous cells and detect whether any of them have spread beyond the original tumor location.

Availability. Although the technology has been available for about 30 years, its use was limited to large research universities. Health insurance companies only recently began to cover the cost after major hospitals started buying the machines. Though PET scans are more expensive than CT (computed tomography) scans, researchers suspect that the test is worth the extra cost since it can rule out what could be unnecessary and costly treatment.

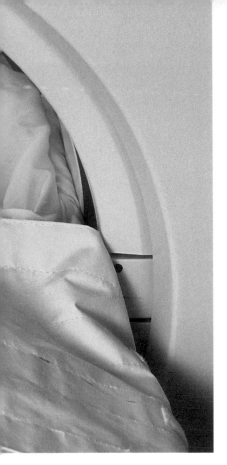

▲ This multimillion-dollar machine can detect cancer cells that other tests might miss, helping doctors make better-informed treatment decisions.

Nutrition Tip
Study Finds That Fish Wards Off Cancer

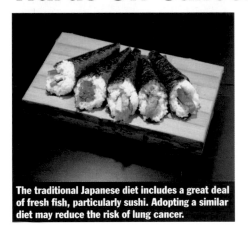

The traditional Japanese diet includes a great deal of fresh fish, particularly sushi. Adopting a similar diet may reduce the risk of lung cancer.

According to a recent study, eating fresh fish—particularly sushi—may protect people from lung cancer. In Japan, lung cancer rates are less than two thirds of those in the United States and the United Kingdom. Dietary factors, such as frequent intake of fish, soybean products, and green tea, have long been thought to be one reason. Until recently, though, research studies have often reported inconclusive or contradictory findings. But a new study, published in the *British Journal of Cancer* in May 2001, finally offers proof.

The researchers examined the diets of over 1,000 Japanese men and women with different types of lung cancer and compared them with more than 4,000 healthy Japanese subjects. The study found that people who ate the most cooked or raw fish were half as likely to develop rare cancers of the lung called adenocarcinomas compared with people who ate less fish.

Fish contains oil made of polyunsaturated fatty acids, and many scientists think that it is this oil that provides the protective effect against cancer. Consumption of dried and salted fish did not seem to provide any protection against lung cancer.

RESEARCH ROUNDUP

■ **A NEW WAY TO SPOT LUNG CANCER BEFORE IT'S TOO LATE.** Detecting cancer in its earliest stages is the ticket to beating it. In the case of lung cancer, early detection is especially important, since by the time most lung cancers are caught, the overall five-year survival rate is only 13 percent.

Unfortunately, chest X rays aren't very helpful when it comes to spotting early lung cancer. And other screening methods aren't sensitive enough to detect the few cancer cells that may be present in blood or sputum (coughed-up fluid). But a new screening test now being studied can. This test, called RT-PCR, is so sensitive that it can detect as few as 10 cancer cells added to two teaspoons of blood or 100 cancer cells in one teaspoon of sputum, according to a study published in the *International Journal of Cancer* on April 1, 2001. Research is continuing on practical applications of these findings.

A new test can detect as few as 10 cancer cells in two teaspoons of blood.

Drug Development

Cancer Drug Takes Aim at Hodgkin's Disease

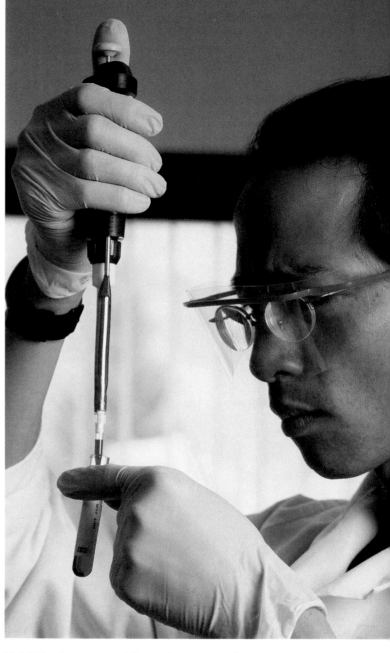

▲ A laboratory-engineered protein is being used to tag cancer cells so the immune system can destroy them.

T rial and error is an age-old scientific precept, and sometimes it pays off, as it did in the case of a new treatment for relapsed Hodgkin's disease, a cancer that occurs mainly in young people. The reward came in the form of a drug currently used to treat cases of relapsed non-Hodgkin's lymphoma (NHL).

Noting that both Hodgkin's disease and NHL are cancers of the lymphatic system—an integral part of the immune system—scientists theorized that the NHL drug rituximab (brand name Rituxan) might work for Hodgkin's, too. And recent U.S. and European trials are already showing promising results.

How it works. Rituximab is a monoclonal antibody—a laboratory-engineered protein that can bind to dangerous cells and "tag" them so that they can be destroyed. The drug is designed to attack B-lymphocytes (one of two main types of lymphatic system cells) by binding to a marker, called CD-20, on the cell's surface. All B-lymphocytes, both the cancerous and the healthy ones, have this marker.

In three separate studies, the majority of patients had partial or complete disappearance of their cancer.

In most people with NHL, the cancer originates in the B-lymphocytes, so killing these cells makes sense. But for Hodgkin's patients, who do not typically have cancerous B-lymphocytes, the use of rituximab was a gamble. The results were lucky: In three separate studies, the majority of patients had partial or complete disappearance of their cancer following this treatment.

Availability. Rituximab is not yet approved for use with Hodgkin's disease although that approval is probably not far off. But future clinical trials are required to confirm its efficacy and any other potential uses.

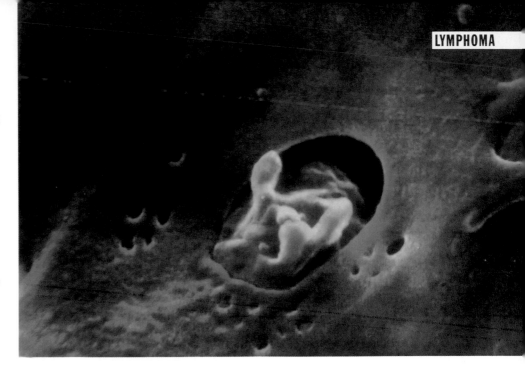

▶ Stem cells, produced in the bone marrow, are the precursors of all blood cells. (Here, a white blood cell migrates from bone marrow.) Removing them before chemotherapy or radiation, then giving them back, can help the patient beat cancer.

Drug Development
Combination Therapy Boosts Survival Rates in Cancer Patients

Increasingly, researchers are looking at combining two or more treatment approaches as a way to dramatically improve survival rates among cancer patients. According to a February 2001 article published in the *Journal of Clinical Oncology,* one such combination is being tried for follicular lymphoma, a type of non-Hodgkin's lymphoma (cancer of the lymph nodes). It involves high doses of either chemotherapy or radiation plus stem cell transplantation—a reintroduction of stem cells retrieved from the patient prior to treatment.

How it works. High-dose chemotherapy or radiation works because it kills more cancer cells than a standard dose would. However, in the process, more healthy cells are killed, too. Among these are the all-important stem cells—cells produced in the bone marrow (the spongy tissue inside the large bones in the body) and responsible for the development of three essential kinds of blood cells. Taking stem cells from the patient prior to chemotherapy or radiation and giving them back afterwards can help restore levels of these blood cells and help the patient survive.

Data recently analyzed from the European Bone Marrow Transplant Lymphoma Registry showed that 77 percent of patients who underwent high-dose therapy and stem cell transplantation had partial or complete disappearance of their cancer three months following treatment. Five years out, half of the patients were still alive, with 30 percent having no relapse.

Availability. Patients with follicular lymphoma can currently explore this treatment option with their doctors.

FAST FACTS
62,300 Estimated number of new lymphoma cases diagnosed in the United States during 2001
54,900 Number of these that are non-Hodgkin's lymphoma
51 PERCENT Five-year survival rate for non-Hodgkin's lymphoma **31 PERCENT** Five-year survival rate for non-Hodgkin's lymphoma between 1960 and 1994
100 PERCENT Increase in the incidence rate (annual new case rate) of non-Hodgkin's lymphoma since the early 1970s

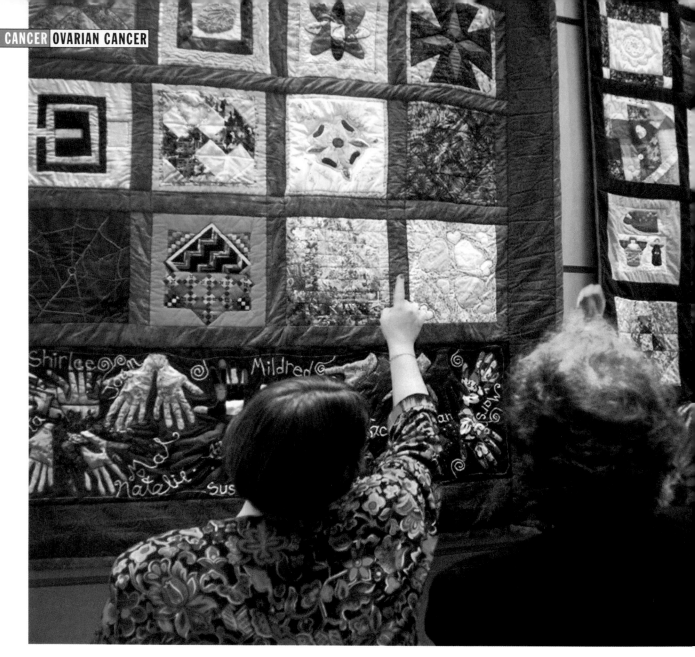

Diagnostic Development

Simple Blood Test May Spot a Silent Killer

It's a classic case of catch-22: Ovarian cancer is highly curable in its early stages, but it remains silent until it has spread beyond the ovary, at which point it's difficult to treat successfully. Ovarian cancer is not only devoid of symptoms early on, it's also difficult to detect. But that may change now that recent genetic advances have paved the way for an ovarian cancer blood test.

How it works. Scientists at Johns Hopkins University recently identified a protein produced by ovarian tumors that prompts the immune system to make antibodies against it. The blood test looks for these antibodies—a sure sign of ovarian cancer. Given that the cure rate for ovarian cancer more than triples if it's caught

Key Finding
Aspirin May Join the Arsenal in the War against Cancer

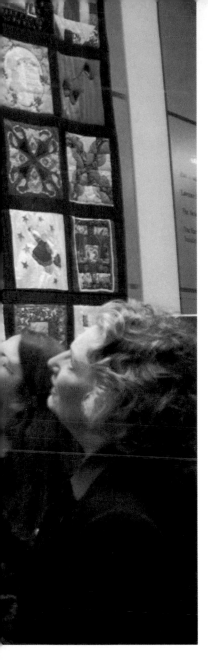

◄ **Women and their families memorialized their battle with ovarian cancer in this quilt, displayed at Beth Israel Medical Center in New York City. A new test may help spot the disease early, when it is more easily cured.**

It's the wonder drug indeed, and now it might even help keep cancer at bay. Evaluating surveys from a long-term study of more than 12,000 women in New York State, researchers found that women who took aspirin at least three times a week for six months or more had up to a 40 percent lower incidence of ovarian cancer originating in the tissue covering the ovary. The results were presented at the 32nd annual meeting of the Society of Gynecologic Oncologists on March 7, 2001.

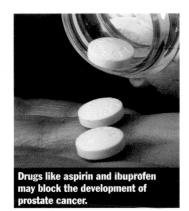

Drugs like aspirin and ibuprofen may block the development of prostate cancer.

Evidence suggests that chronic inflammation—from factors such as ovarian endometriosis or pelvic inflammatory disease—is associated with ovarian cancer. So it would seem reasonable that an anti-inflammatory drug, such as aspirin, might change the course of ovarian cancer.

It may be a little too soon to stock up the medicine cabinet, however. As the researchers admit, a larger study is needed to more thoroughly weigh the benefits of long-term aspirin use against the risks of gastrointestinal bleeding and other serious side effects. And some call the data from this study into question because the questionnaire depended heavily on the long-term memories of the participants. Still, look for more conclusive studies in the near future examining the benefits of aspirin against this and other types of cancer, such as colon cancer. Researchers are currently testing aspirin's ability to prevent polyps from turning cancerous, especially in people with familial polyposis syndromes, inherited forms of colon cancer.

early, a test of this type could significantly improve survival rates, according to a March 27, 2001, report in the *Proceedings of the National Academy of Sciences*.

Availability. Amplistar, Inc. has begun developing the blood test, and the company is optimistic that it will gain approval from the U.S. Food and Drug Administration by 2003. Another blood test for ovarian cancer developed by Atairgin Technologies is currently undergoing a large clinical trial. It tests for LPA, or lysophosphatidic acid, a lipid (fat) found in high quantities in the blood of ovarian cancer patients.

FAST FACTS

95 PERCENT Five-year survival rate for women whose ovarian cancer is diagnosed and treated before the cancer spreads outside the ovary **25** Percentage of ovarian cancers found at an early stage, before spreading beyond the ovary **SYMPTOMS** Pelvic or abdominal pain or bloating, frequent urination, changes in bowel habits, weight loss or gain especially in the abdomen, pain during intercourse, fatigue

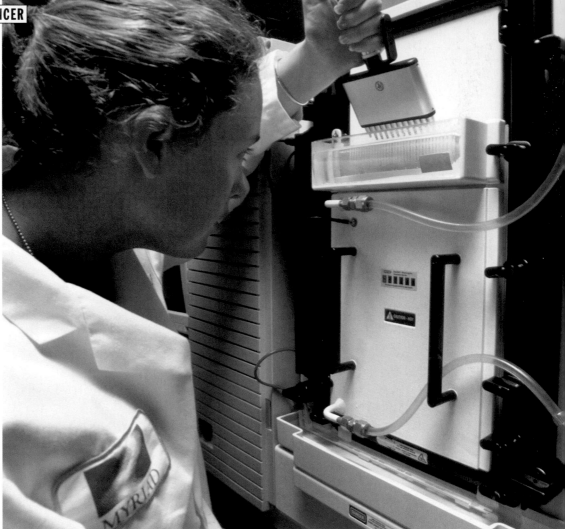

▶ A lab technician at Myriad Genetics performs genetic sequencing. The company has identified genetic abnormalities that increase the risk of prostate cancer.

Progress in Prevention
One Gene, Four Mutations, and 127 Utah Families

Although the average lifetime risk of developing prostate cancer is 5 to 10 percent, men with a father or brother who has the disease run a 20 to 30 percent risk. This year, researchers at Myriad Genetics in Salt Lake City, Utah, identified a group of genetic abnormalities responsible for this increased risk. The culprits: four different mutations (alterations in the sequence of building blocks that make up our genes) in a gene known as hereditary prostate cancer 2 (HPC2), located on chromosome 17.

How it works. Analyzing genetic material from members of 33 Utah families in which prostate cancer rates were up to 10 times higher than expected, the geneticists determined that relatives who developed the disease had some abnormality on chromosome 17. (Chromosomes are the paired coils of genetic material in the nucleus of each cell.) By expanding the study to include 127 high-risk families, they were able to identify four specific variations, two of which are linked to greatly increased risk and two of which

Geneticists identified four different mutations that are linked to an increased risk of prostate cancer.

are linked to moderately increased risk.

Availability. Like the test for the genes that have been linked to breast cancer in some families, a test for HPC2 and other, as yet undiscovered genes that predispose men to prostate cancer could become available in the next decade. Men with family histories of prostate cancer could then be tested when they are in their 20s or 30s, with the goal of taking preventive measures and getting regular checkups if they have inherited high-risk genes.

STAY TUNED FOR...

News on Prostate Cancer Prevention

In 2003, look for results from the Prostate Cancer Prevention Trial, which enrolled 18,000 men in 1993 to test the drug finasteride (brand name Proscar), typically used to treat prostate enlargement, in preventing prostate cancer. Also ongoing is a two-year trial comparing a plant-based, low-fat diet (the Ornish diet) and stress management to conventional treatment in early-stage prostate cancer. By the middle of 2001, 93 of the planned 150 men had entered the study, and first-year data on that group were being analyzed. Final results should be out in 2003.

Scientists have also begun recruiting participants for the Selenium Vitamin E Chemoprevention Trial, which will ultimately follow 32,400 men in a study to determine whether dietary or supplemental antioxidants (substances, such as vitamin E, that prevent cancer-promoting cell damage) lower the risk of prostate cancer.

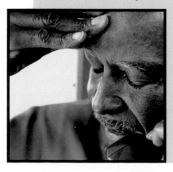

Studies suggest that lifestyle changes, like stress management, may reduce the risk of prostate cancer.

High-Tech Help
Better Seed Mapping Improves Radiation Treatment for Prostate Cancer

Brachytherapy, the placement of radioactive seeds into the prostate to kill cancer cells, is an alternative to surgery and another radiation treatment, called external beam radiation. It's the treatment that Mayor Rudolph Giuliani of New York City chose when he was diagnosed with prostate cancer in 2000.

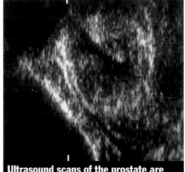

Ultrasound scans of the prostate are used in placing radioactive seeds.

Now, new developments in seeding mean faster and more accurate seed placement. They can also help surgeons place many more seeds in the prostate instead of in surrounding healthy tissue, where the lingering effects of so-called hot spots can include incontinence, a common side effect of brachytherapy.

How it works. Seed mapping, or deciding where to place the seeds based on ultrasound scans, usually takes four to eight hours. But computers being tested at Memorial Sloan-Kettering Cancer Center in New York City promise to cut mapping time to a mere 5 to 15 minutes by rapidly processing ultrasound readings and converting them to images and measurements that immediately guide urologists to tumors. The reduced mapping time means that images can be obtained and seeds can be placed almost simultaneously, making placement even more accurate.

Availability. Computer-assisted seed mapping is currently being evaluated at Memorial Sloan-Kettering Cancer Center and other medical institutions. Ask your doctor when it might be put to use in your hospital.

Drug Development

Aspirin-like Drugs Make Cancerous Prostate Cells Self-Destruct

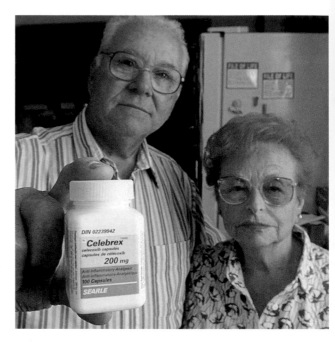

▲ Although most often prescribed for arthritis, drugs like Celebrex may fight prostate cancer.

The painkillers millions of people take every day for headaches and arthritis hold potential as powerful weapons in the fight against prostate cancer, according to the latest research. Although studies of how these medications, called non-steroidal anti-inflammatory drugs, or NSAIDs, could be deployed against prostate cancer are still at the test-tube stage, it is clear that NSAIDs block chemical reactions involved in the progression of the disease.

How it works. Aspirin, ibuprofen, naproxen, and the newer NSAIDs, such as rofecoxib (Vioxx) and celecoxib (Celebrex), halt the formation of substances that promote both inflammation and cancer. These substances, called prostaglandins, are byproducts of a fatty acid—arachidonic acid—found in meat and, in lesser amounts, produced by the body. In test-tube experiments, certain prostaglandins promote the spread of prostate cancer cells and keep them from dying. One experiment found that adding an NSAID-like compound that inhibits a particular prostaglandin to cultures of prostate cancer cells resulted in the cancer cells' death within eight hours.

NSAIDs could be used against cancer within the next decade.

Availability. This research is at an extremely early stage. Although NSAIDs are widely available, no one has yet figured out the best way to harness their cancer-fighting properties. Celecoxib, a relatively new NSAID, has been approved for preventing a particular kind of precancerous growth in the colon, so other NSAIDs could be put to a similar use against prostate cancer within the next decade.

RESEARCH ROUNDUP

■ **PROSTATE CANCER VACCINE.** For men with prostate cancer, a new vaccine has been designed to make the immune system recognize and attack cancer cells. In a preliminary study at the University of California at San Francisco, it was given over two months to patients with advanced prostate cancer. In two-thirds of the patients, it was successful in slowing disease progression. The vaccine is made from a protein found on prostate cells and dendritic cells, specialized cells that tell the immune system to attack particular tissues. Further studies are planned to find the best dosage of the vaccine and to see if it works well in combination with standard prostate cancer treatments. The scientists who developed the vaccine also plan to test it in men with less-advanced cancer.

[
FAST FACTS

75 Percentage of prostate biopsies that are unnecessary **10** Number of years it takes for a small prostate tumor to spread **HIGH-FAT DIET** Possible risk factor for prostate cancer **80** Percentage of men with prostate cancer who are over age 65 **90** Percentage of men with prostate cancer who will die from some other cause
]

High-Tech Help
Early Warning System for Deadliest Skin Cancer

When former U.S. president Bill Clinton was diagnosed with basal cell carcinoma in January 2001, he became one of millions of people who have had skin cancer. Luckily for Clinton, the lesion on his back was easily removed with a "scrape and burn" procedure, but other types of skin cancer aren't quite so curable. As the deadliest form of skin cancer,

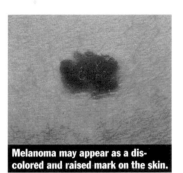
Melanoma may appear as a discolored and raised mark on the skin.

malignant melanoma attracts most of the attention; although it accounts for only 4 percent of all skin cancers, it causes more than 80 percent of skin cancer deaths.

A new digital imaging system that works via a home computer could help people concerned about skin cancer detect changes in their skin—and possibly melanoma—much earlier than was previously possible. Results of a study evaluating the system's effectiveness were presented at the annual meeting of the American Academy of Dermatology in March 2001.

How it works. It's a bit like time-lapse photography: A patient sends two sets of photos taken 6 to 12 months apart to the Western Research Company, which digitizes the images and perfectly aligns them using their DermAlert system. When the photos are displayed on the patient's computer monitor with the DermAlert software, differences become obvious: Any new lesions flash on screen, and lesions that have changed in size pulsate. The system can show lesions as small as 1 mm in diameter and changes of as little as 10 percent in size, and the lesions can then be brought to a dermatologist's attention for diagnosis and treatment. By alerting people to tiny skin changes they otherwise wouldn't notice, the device could greatly improve the rate of early detection.

Availability. The DermAlert system is available from Western Research Company for home use and can be ordered on-line from the company.

FAST FACTS
50 Percentage of all new cancers that are skin cancers **1 MILLION** Estimated number of new cases of skin cancer that will be diagnosed in the United States in 2001 **1** Number of people who die of melanoma each hour

STAY TUNED FOR...

Cancer-Fighting Weeds
A humble folk remedy for warts could be a cure for nonmelanoma skin cancers. The poisonous radium weed (also known as petty spurge, or *Euphorbia peplus*) is commonly found in Australian gardens and along roads. In a pilot study at Mater Adult Hospital in Brisbane, Australia, actinic keratosis (rough, scaly patches that can develop into skin cancer), squamous cell carcinoma, and basal cell carcinoma disappeared in 88 percent of patients after treatment with the plant's active compounds. Additional studies will determine the plant's effectiveness in different formulations against skin cancers that cover more extensive areas of the body.

Using One Disease to Fight Another
A mutant strain of herpes simplex virus called HSV1716 seems to kill melanoma cells without harming the surrounding tissue. A pilot human study published in the February 2001 issue of *The Lancet* involved people with small masses in the soft tissue (tissue that surrounds, connects, or supports the structures and organs of the body, such as muscle, tendon, and fat). Researchers injected these masses with HSV1716. When the masses were removed

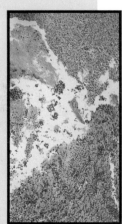
A pilot study showed that a type of herpes virus may kill melanoma cells.

after two sets of injections, dead melanoma cells were found in them, but healthy tissue was not harmed. Future studies will test the effectiveness and toxicity of higher doses of the mutant virus.

Surgical Solution
"Keyhole" Surgery Benefits Testicular Cancer Patients

When it is found early, testicular cancer can almost always be cured by removing the diseased testicle, followed in most cases by radiation or chemotherapy, depending on the type of cancer. Men with the most common types of testicular tumors (nonseminomatous tumors), though, often need additional, painful operations to remove lymph nodes deep in the abdomen. These lymph nodes are the first stop for testicular cancer cells on their way to colonizing other organs.

Now, European urologists have developed a minimally invasive technique for removing these lymph nodes using a fiber-optic viewing instrument, called a laparoscope, that allows the surgeon to view real-time video of the abdominal cavity on a television monitor during the operation.

How it works. The surgeon makes three small incisions in the abdomen and inserts the laparoscope through one of them and tiny surgical instruments to remove the lymph nodes through the others. In a recent French study of 25 patients who underwent laparoscopic lymph node removal, each procedure took about four hours, and the average hospital stay was just over one day.

The standard or "open" operation to remove these lymph nodes may be quicker than the laparoscopic method, but recovery is far more painful and prolonged because the incision goes either from the breastbone to the pubic bone (and through the underlying muscle and fat) or from the left side to the breastbone down to the pelvis. The open method also requires temporary removal of one rib.

Availability. This technique is being pioneered in Europe, but surgeons in other parts of the world are watching it closely and will probably adopt it if further studies show positive results.

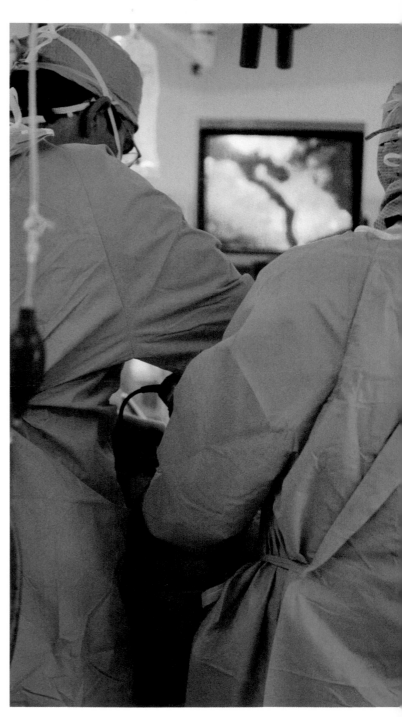

▶ Many men with testicular cancer must have the lymph nodes in the abdomen removed. A new technique allows surgeons to access the abdominal cavity without making a large incision.

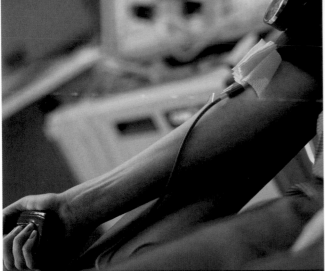

By taking blood in advance and harvesting its stem cells, doctors can protect the immune system from the damaging effects of chemotherapy.

Drug Development
Rebuilding Bone Marrow After Chemotherapy

At least 9 out of 10 patients with advanced testicular cancer can be cured with chemotherapy and surgery. But for men who don't respond to standard doses of chemotherapy, the only option until now was high-dose chemotherapy with powerful drugs that destroy stem cells—blood-making cells found in the bone marrow and bloodstream—followed by bone marrow transplantation to restore these cells.

High-dose chemotherapy itself can be fatal, and bone marrow transplantation lessens the danger. But removing the bone marrow prior to chemotherapy is a painful process, one that involves making several cuts in the skin over the pelvic bone and driving a large needle into the bone at each cut. And marrow transplants from donors can result in graft-versus-host disease, in which the donor marrow attacks the patient's blood cells as if they were a disease or foreign invader.

Now scientists have found a way to make high-dose chemotherapy safer and bone marrow salvage less painful.

The key: transplanting stem cells found in the patient's own bloodstream. Stem cells can be harvested without anesthesia and with less discomfort than bone marrow removal. Also, using a patient's own stem cells (or bone marrow) eliminates the risk of graft-versus-host disease.

In an Indiana University Medical Center study published in the *Journal of Clinical Oncology* in October 2000, 37 out of 65 patients whose cancers had recurred or failed to respond to initial chemotherapy were disease-free after receiving two rounds of high-dose chemotherapy followed by stem-cell transplantation.

How it works. In most cases, the patient's own stem cells are removed from the bloodstream and frozen for later transplantation. Because only small numbers of stem cells normally circulate in the blood, patients usually take medication for several days to stimulate the release of more stem cells. When there are enough circulating stem cells to collect, the patient undergoes a procedure called apheresis, in which all the blood in the body is gradually diverted through a machine that filters out stem cells, then sends the blood back to the body.

One or more cycles (usually consisting of treatments every other day for eight days) follow, after which the stem cells are returned to the body through a catheter placed in the neck or chest. After they are infused, stem cells go automatically to the bone marrow and begin to multiply and mature into healthy blood cells.

Availability. Doctors worldwide are studying stem-cell transplantation with high-dose chemotherapy for the treatment of several types of cancer. The studies in testicular cancer are still very preliminary, though, and to enter one of these studies, you have to have advanced cancer with no other treatment options.

RESEARCH ROUNDUP

■ **TESTICULAR CANCER–INFERTILITY LINK.** Testicular cancer and male infertility have both become more common in the past few decades, and Danish researchers comparing semen samples and health records from 32,000 men say it's probably no coincidence. Over time, men with poor sperm quality and fertility problems were two to three times more likely to develop testicular cancer than men with normal sperm.

A study from the University of Buffalo Department of Social and Preventive Medicine in Buffalo, New York, reached a similar conclusion from a different starting point: Men diagnosed with testicular cancer, along with healthy men from the same neighborhoods, were asked how many children they had. The testicular cancer patients were two-thirds less likely to be fathers and nine times more likely to have been diagnosed as infertile. Researchers think events during fetal development are responsible for both the fertility problems and the increased risk of testicular cancer.

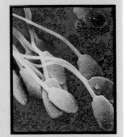

Recent studies suggest that men with poor sperm quality are more likely to develop testicular cancer.

DIGESTION AND METABOLISM

A camera in a pill—the stuff of science fiction? Now it's fact. Instead of undergoing an uncomfortable, invasive procedure to pinpoint the cause of your intestinal trouble, you can swallow a capsule that takes images of your innards to help your doctor diagnose such conditions as inflammatory bowel disease. New drugs on the way may take the guesswork out of treating irritable bowel syndrome by targeting a brain chemical responsible for intestinal spasms. People with diabetes may soon be able to get their insulin from an inhaler or a coated pill instead of a needle. They can already monitor their blood sugar levels by wearing a high-tech "wristwatch" that measures the glucose in their sweat—no drop of blood required. And, for the people who regularly down heartburn pills to keep acid reflux in check, there's a simple new outpatient surgery that can cure the condition for good.

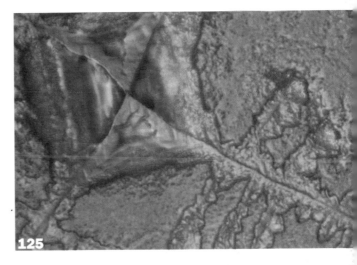

125

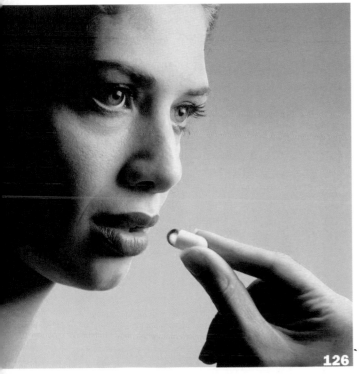

126

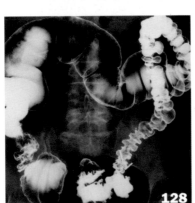

128

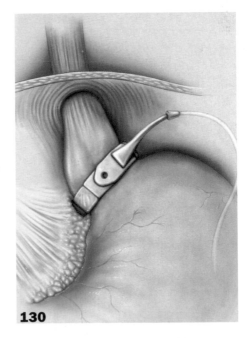

130

High-Tech Help

For Diabetics, an Easier Way to "Watch" Your Blood Sugar

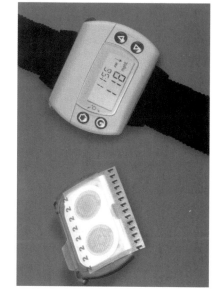

everal times a day, diabetics follow a routine that involves pricking their finger and placing a drop of blood on a test strip to monitor their blood sugar level. Maybe that's why many diabetics check their blood sugar level only twice a day instead of the recommended four to eight times. But in March 2001, the U.S. Food and Drug Administration (FDA) approved a special wristwatch, called GlucoWatch, that offers diabetics an easier and less painful way to manage their condition.

▶ Worn like a wristwatch, the GlucoWatch can help patients track patterns in their blood-sugar levels.

Unlike an earlier device called the MiniMed Continuous Glucose Monitoring System—an implantable sensor that monitors glucose levels every five minutes for up to three days—Gluco-Watch is worn externally. It checks glucose levels up to three times an hour.

How it works. The key to the system is a small pad that fits on the back of the watch. It captures glucose molecules that are drawn from the sweat glands by infinitesimal electrical impulses emitted by the device. GlucoWatch analyzes the sample and calculates your blood sugar level, warning you with a built-in alarm if the reading is too low or too high. It can store three months of data, which can be downloaded to a computer and transmitted to a doctor's office.

GlucoWatch is not foolproof. The FDA warns that it can produce false readings up to 25 percent of the time, especially if the arm is very sweaty or when glucose levels are very low. Consequently, it should be viewed as a supplemental information source that does not completely free a diabetic from daily blood tests.

Availability. GlucoWatch is available through a doctor's office and is approved for people 18 years and over. It is not approved yet for children. Doctors must be trained in its use, and they will advise patients on the number of daily blood tests they must continue to perform.

How GlucoWatch works

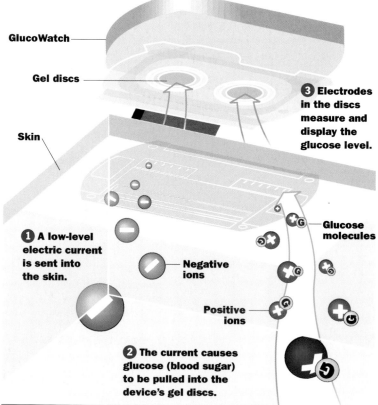

GlucoWatch

Gel discs

Skin

❸ Electrodes in the discs measure and display the glucose level.

Glucose molecules

❶ A low-level electric current is sent into the skin.

Negative ions

Positive ions

❷ The current causes glucose (blood sugar) to be pulled into the device's gel discs.

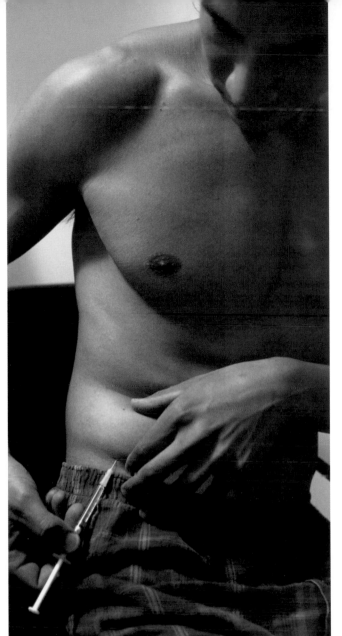

▲ A new sustained-release formulation of insulin means that many diabetics will need only one injection a day, at bedtime.

Drug Development
Human Pincushions No More

Insulin is a necessary medication for many diabetics because it helps nutrients such as blood sugar (glucose) get into the cells of the body's tissues. Insulin is a protein, so it can't be taken in pill form because the body would simply digest it, making it ineffective. In order to reap its benefits, patients have to stop what they're doing several times a day and use a hypodermic syringe to inject themselves with the drug—or at least they did in the past.

Now, diabetics with moderate insulin needs can use a new, once-a-day formulation that's injected at bedtime and is designed to be absorbed slowly into the bloodstream for 24-hour coverage. The drug, L-glargine (brand name Lantus), reached the U.S. market in May 2001.

As a result of its chemical structure, it releases insulin into your body steadily and continuously, reducing the blood sugar spikes that are common with other long-acting types of insulin. And it is effective for a broader range of diabetic patients than any other insulin preparation on the market. Lantus is not a panacea, however. People with type 1 and type 2 diabetes who have more significant insulin needs will still need a rapid-acting insulin at certain times—for example, before eating.

RESEARCH ROUNDUP

■ **CLOSER TO A CURE.** A cure for diabetes is the Holy Grail of research into the disease, and it just might be on the horizon with word that scientists at the University of Alberta in Canada have successfully implanted insulin-producing cells, called islets, into diabetics. The islets have been producing all or much of the insulin needed by the study subjects for two years. Previous attempts have worked for a year at best and in only 8 percent of patients. Follow-up studies using the so-called Edmonton Protocol are now under way at Alberta and research facilities in the United States to confirm the initial, exciting findings of this potential cure for the disease.

■ **PREVENTING STROKE IN DIABETICS.** Exercise can dramatically reduce the chances of developing heart disease or having a stroke caused by diabetes—by as much as 40 percent for women—says a recent Harvard study of 5,125 women with type 2 diabetes. As little as four hours of moderate exercise a week is all it takes.

Progress in Prevention
Stopping Diabetes Before It Starts

Until now, it's been unclear whether changing your diet and getting more exercise can prevent the slide into full-blown diabetes for people at high risk for the disease: those who have developed impaired glucose tolerance, a condition in which blood sugar levels are higher than normal but not yet considered diabetic. Now new research out of Finland—a country with one of the highest incidences of type 2 (non–insulin-dependent) diabetes—proves it.

The results of the three-year Finnish Diabetes Prevention Study were published in the May 3, 2001, issue of the *New England Journal of Medicine*. In the study, one group of overweight people with glucose intolerance received detailed diet and lifestyle counseling seven times a year, along with a free health club membership. Subjects in this group were given personalized advice on how to lose weight, lower their intake of saturated fat to 10 percent of total calories, increase their intake of dietary fiber, and increase their level of physical activity to at least 30 minutes a day. Members of the other group were given general information on the benefits of losing weight, exercising, and healthy eating in the prevention of diabetes, but they didn't get individual attention and met with their health-care team only once a year.

The result? People in the first group had an impressive 58 percent lower incidence of type 2 diabetes, even though weight loss was only marginally different between the two groups.

Findings from a larger, more recent U.S. trial, the Diabetes Prevention Program, support the Finnish results and extend them to a more diverse population.

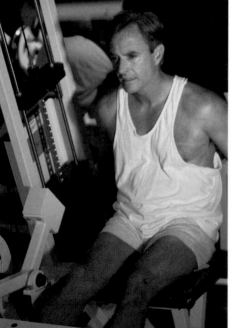

◀ Two new studies show that exercise helps ward off diabetes.

Inhaled Insulin
For both type 1 and type 2 diabetics, easier blood sugar control may soon be a breath away. That's because research has found that getting insulin from an inhaler (like those used by asthmatics) is just as effective as injected insulin. The lungs are an excellent entry point to the bloodstream; in fact, if one takes into account the surface area of all of their air sacs (alveoli), the lungs have a surface area the size of a tennis court! One important caveat is that the inhaled insulin is short acting, so it is useful only for moderate post-meal rises in blood sugar. The approach is also seen by some people

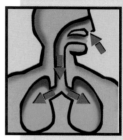

A new form of insulin is delivered by an inhaler and transmitted to the bloodstream through the lungs.

as wasteful because it requires 20 times more insulin than the injection method. And there are concerns among some researchers that when inhaled on a daily basis, insulin, a growth hormone, might cause abnormal growth in the lungs—although studies have found that using inhaled insulin for up to four years does not produce any serious side effects.

Other New Delivery Devices
Several other insulin delivery devices are under development, including a mouth spray that allows the insulin to be absorbed through the cheeks, and pills that pass through the stomach intact and are absorbed through the intestinal wall. There's also an implanted insulin pump currently in use in Europe and awaiting approval from the U.S. Food and Drug Administration. Placed under the abdominal skin, it uses a concentrated form of insulin to mimic the body's own delivery of the hormone.

FAST FACTS
90 Percentage of diabetics who have type 2 (non–insulin-dependent) diabetes **50** Percentage of diabetics who die of coronary artery disease **120 MILLION** Number of people worldwide with diabetes

High-Tech Help
Turning Up the Heat on Heartburn

Instead of taking heartburn drugs for the rest of your life, there's another option: a simple surgery to prevent the backwash of stomach acid into the esophagus that can cause pain and, in rare cases, lead to esophageal cancer. A recent study found that the Stretta procedure provides an effective solution to the problem of severe and chronic heartburn. The study was presented at the annual Digestive Disease Week conference in Atlanta, Georgia, in May 2001.

Sealing the deal. During the Stretta procedure, the physician places an endoscope (a thin, lighted, flexible tube) fitted with needle electrodes down the patient's throat and into the digestive tract. Once it is in position at the junction between the esophagus and the stomach, radiofrequency heat is applied to the area between the esophagus and stomach to create burn-like lesions. When the lesions heal, the scars leave less room for stomach acids to wash back up the esophagus, reducing the frequency of heartburn caused by acid reflux.

Doctors at several U.S. medical centers evaluated 118 long-term sufferers of gastroesophageal reflux disease (GERD)—a condition that produces chronic heartburn—who had undergone the new surgery. A year later, 70 percent reported that they suffered less than they had beforehand, categorizing their symptoms as the same as or less severe than those they experienced while taking medication to control their heartburn. The study results also showed there was less need for costly proton pump inhibitor drugs (such as Prilosec) following the procedure.

It's a cinch. In addition to the Stretta procedure, another endoscopic surgery has been developed called EndoCinch. In this technique, a tiny device at the end of the endoscope places stitches in two different locations near the junction between the esophagus and the stomach to "tighten" that region of the lower esophagus, preventing the stomach contents from flowing back into the esophagus and causing heartburn.

How the Stretta procedure works

In the Stretta procedure, **(1)** the doctor uses an endoscope placed down the patient's throat to deliver radiofrequency heat at the junction of the esophagus and stomach. **(2)** The heat creates thermal lesions (indicated by small white circles). **(3)** When the lesions heal, there is less room for stomach acids to wash back up into the esophagus.

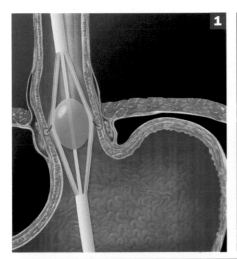
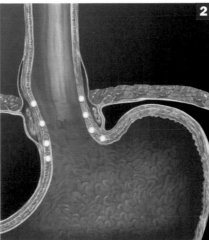
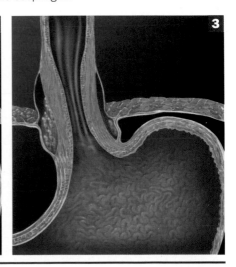

Both are outpatient procedures, done under conscious sedation, and are less invasive than the older techniques of Nissen fundoplication and laparoscopic fundoplication. Patients need less recovery time and don't run the risk of infection common to surgeries that open up the stomach.

Both the Stretta and EndoCinch procedures were given approval by the U.S. Food and Drug Administration in April 2000; they are now becoming more available in the United States and many European countries as more physicians train in their use.

STAY TUNED FOR...

Prilosec at the Drugstore

The FDA may soon allow the proton pump inhibitor omeprazole (brand name Prilosec) to be sold without a prescription. One reason this drug has not yet been approved for over-the-counter (OTC) sale has to do with people's perceptions about how the drug works. While the OTC formulation appears to effectively prevent heartburn, it does not immediately relieve existing heartburn. And although prevention is its aim, it appears that most consumers associate the use of OTC heartburn products with the relief of symptoms. Subject to correct labeling, this medication will be available by 2002. The advantage to consumers: a much lower price.

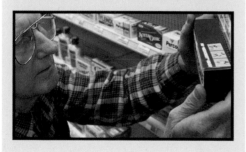

FAST FACTS

50 MILLION Number of bottles of a popular U.S. heartburn remedy manufactured each year **600,000** Number of Americans who go to the emergency room each year with chest pain **100,000** Number of those 600,000 who have heartburn **60 MILLION** Number of people who have monthly heartburn **15 MILLION** Number of people who experience daily heartburn, with an individual's chances of developing the condition increasing with age

Drug Development

Better Defense Against Deadly Hepatitis C

A staggering 170 million people worldwide have hepatitis C, a virus that can lead to cirrhosis (scarring and reduced function of the liver), liver cancer, and even death. It's treated with a manufactured form of interferon, which is a protein made naturally by the body that boosts the immune system to help it fight viral infections and also inhibits the ability of viruses to divide and reproduce.

> **The new form of interferon fights hepatitis C better because it stays active longer.**

The goal of interferon treatment is to rid the body of all detectable levels of the virus, so that when treatment stops there is a smaller chance of a relapse. A new experimental form of interferon fights hepatitis C better because it stays active in the body longer.

In a recent trial, when the new interferon, called pegylated interferon alfa-2a (brand name Pegasys), was compared with its predecessor (interferon alfa-2b), Pegasys produced a 56 percent response rate

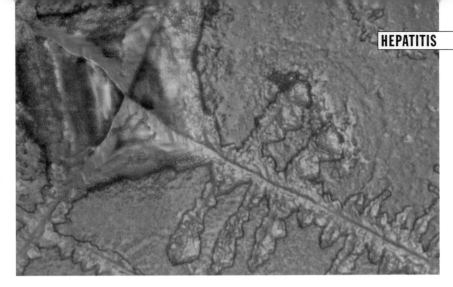

▶ **Interferon, shown here in a micrograph, is a natural protein that helps strengthen the body's immune system and has been used to treat hepatitis C for many years. Now a new form of interferon offers even greater hope to people with this potentially deadly disease.**

(percentage of patients who responded to treatment) at the end of treatment that was sustained over time versus a 45 percent response rate for the older drug. Both drugs were taken in combination with the antiviral drug ribavirin (brand name Rebetol).

How it works. While the old interferon drug has a half-life (the time that elapses before a substance loses one half of its initial effectiveness) of only 7 to 10 hours, Pegasys has a half-life of about 100 hours. It lasts longer because of a process called pegylation. This process attaches polyethylene glycol (PEG) to the surface of the interferon, which slows the rate at which it is absorbed by the body. Just as wearing a mask delays someone's ability to recognize you, the PEG version of interferon has a chemical mask that postpones the

THE ABC'S OF HEPATITIS

TYPE	HOW YOU GET IT	WHO GETS IT	WHAT HAPPENS
A (HAV)	Most commonly spread through food and water contaminated with infected feces; in rare instances, it's spread through contact with contaminated blood	International travelers, daycare children and employees, IV drug users, sexually active gay men, people who live with or have sex with an infected person	Jaundice, fatigue, abdominal pain, appetite loss, nausea, dark urine, diarrhea, and vomiting; usually, it clears up in several weeks
B (HBV)	Spread through contact with infected blood or sex with an infected person; an infected mother can pass it on to her infant during childbirth	IV drug users, hemodialysis patients, health-care workers, people who live with or have sex with an infected person, infants born to infected mothers	Jaundice, fatigue, abdominal pain, appetite loss, nausea, diarrhea, and vomiting; usually, it clears up in three to four months; 5 to 10 percent of adults with acute hepatitis B become chronically infected
C (HCV)	Spread through contact with infected blood; in rare instances it's passed on through childbirth or sex	IV drug users, hemodialysis patients, health-care workers, people who receive transfusions of contaminated blood products, people who have sex with an infected person, infants born to infected mothers	Acute HCV can result in jaundice, fatigue, abdominal pain, appetite loss, nausea, diarrhea, and vomiting; chronic HCV may cause fatigue, but it is usually asymptomatic until it has caused extensive liver damage, including liver scarring (fibrosis) and cirrhosis; in severe cases death may result
D (HDV)	Spread through contact with infected blood	Only those people already infected with HBV, particularly IV drug users	Severe HBV symptoms; 70 to 80 percent of patients with HBV and HDV develop chronic liver diseases, such as cirrhosis
E (HEV)	Spread through food and water contaminated with infected feces	International travelers; people having sex with an infected person	Jaundice, fatigue, abdominal pain, appetite loss, nausea, diarrhea, and vomiting; symptoms usually clear up in several weeks to months

time when it will be recognized by the body chemicals that break it down. Because the drug stays active in the body longer, the hepatitis virus has less opportunity to multiply, preventing liver damage and possibly even reversing prior damage. Another bonus: The drug is injected only once a week versus three times for the traditional treatment.

Availability. Pegasys could receive approval from the U.S. Food and Drug Administration (FDA) by 2002. It was submitted for European approval in February 2001.

RESEARCH ROUNDUP

■ **TATTOOS LINKED TO DANGEROUS DISEASE.** Getting a tattoo can hurt in more ways than one—it can give you the potentially fatal disease hepatitis C. That's the finding of Dr. Robert Haley at the University of Texas Southwestern Medical Center at Dallas, published in the March 2001 issue of the journal *Medicine*. While only 3 percent of the more than 600 American study subjects without tattoos had the disease, a whopping 22 percent of those with tattoos had hepatitis C. Risk increased with the number, size, and design complexity of the tattoos. People with tattoos from commercial parlors were twice as likely as intravenous drug users to have the disease.

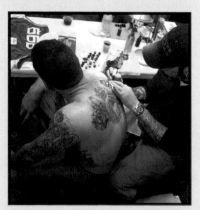

Risky business: Getting a tattoo significantly increases the chances of getting hepatitis C.

Diagnostic Advance
Painless Camera-in-a-Pill Spots Intestine Troubles

▼ **CANDID CAMERA** Now doctors can view your intestinal tract by giving you a very special pill to swallow—one that transmits images as it works its way through your system.

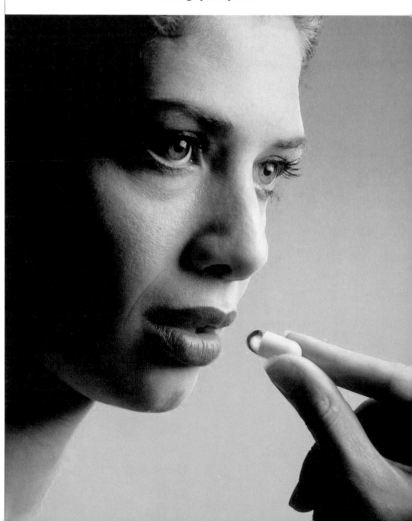

Although the cause of inflammatory bowel disease (IBD) remains a mystery, the symptoms—including bloody diarrhea, pain, fever, and fatigue—are very real for the millions of people who suffer from it. (The term IBD is a general one that encompasses conditions such as colitis and Crohn's disease.) Not only are the symptoms bothersome, but so was the diagnostic test—until a remarkable new camera-in-a-pill arrived on the scene in 2001.

Until now, doctors trying to diagnose IBD had to thread a 4-foot-long tube called an endoscope, outfitted with a tiny video camera, down the throat and into the small intestine to check for abnormalities. The procedure is uncomfortable—often requiring sedation—and its effectiveness is limited by the length and rigidity of the endoscope, which can't always bend into all the nooks and crannies of the intestines or reach far enough down to spot the problem. That's why some people end up needing exploratory surgery.

Enter the Jonah-like M2A capsule. One inch (2.5 cm) long and a third of an inch (8.5 mm) in diameter, it travels the entire 20-foot (6 meter) length of the small intestine as you continue with your daily routine; moving is actually encouraged because it helps the capsule wend its way through the digestive system. A study of 20 patients showed the capsule to be 60 percent effective in uncovering intestinal abnormalities, compared with a 35 percent success rate for the traditional method.

How it works. Your doctor will prescribe the M2A pill to be taken on an empty stomach after a night of fasting. You will be fitted with a data recorder resembling a portable tape player, which you'll wear on a belt around your waist.

The M2A incorporates a light source, miniature color video camera, battery, antenna, and radio transmitter, all in a specially sealed capsule that is resistant to digestive fluids. As the capsule is propelled through the intestinal tract by the normal contractions of the intestine, images of the intestine are captured by the video camera and transmitted by radio frequency to the data recorder.

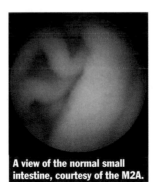

A view of the normal small intestine, courtesy of the M2A.

After approximately eight hours, you return the belt and recorder to the clinic, and the images are downloaded from the recorder so that the doctor can examine them. The images are synchronized to a time code on the screen so that the location of the capsule can be estimated. (Don't worry about returning the capsule to your doctor—it's disposable.)

Availability. The M2A Swallowable Imaging Capsule was approved in the United States, Europe, and Australia in 2001.

RESEARCH ROUNDUP

■ **CROHN'S OR COLITIS? HIGH-TECH DIAGNOSTICS.** Doctors often have a hard time distinguishing between two types of inflammatory bowel disease: ulcerative colitis and Crohn's disease. Colitis causes inflammation of the inner layer of the lining of the intestine, while Crohn's disease can affect any part of the digestive tract. Because treatment for these two conditions is often different, nailing down the diagnosis is important. In the future, magnetic resonance spectroscopy (MRS), an imaging procedure a lot like today's MRIs, may help, according to a study published in February 2001 in the *American Journal of Gastroenterology*.

Proponents of MRS are impressed with the technology but believe that more research—and more funding for research—is needed for the technique to gain wider acceptance. In the study, the imaging tool was almost 99 percent accurate in classifying the diseases as either Crohn's or ulcerative colitis—far better than what doctors can achieve on their own. It may also be able to detect these diseases before they become obvious, and it may even provide clues to their cause.

FAST FACTS
40 PERCENT Likelihood that a second family member will have IBD if a child is diagnosed with the disease **25** Percentage of people who manifest symptoms of IBD before age 20 **15–20 AND 50–80** Ages when patients experience a peak incidence of IBD

STAY TUNED FOR...

Antibiotics Again
One of our oldest drugs may be coming back into vogue for treating Crohn's disease and colitis. For many years, it's been theorized that inflammatory bowel disease is caused by an infection that can be treated with antibiotics. This premise has gone in and out of favor. Now Australian researchers are putting it to the test. Gastroenterologists at 20 centers in Australia have recruited 150 patients for a three-year study. All of the participants will receive the standard treatment (steroids) for flare-ups, but half will also receive a "cocktail" of three antibiotics; the other half will get a placebo. Patients will be monitored for another year to see whether they remain healthy. Doctors hope the results will finally end the debate.

Drug Development

Intestinal Rescue on the Way

Imagine staying home all day for fear that you won't be able to control your bowel movements. Imagine being afraid that a wrenching stomachache and diarrhea could come at any time and having to map bathrooms along your route just in case the moment strikes. This is what life with irritable bowel syndrome (IBS) can be like. The medication options that have been around for years—antispasmodics to prevent diarrhea and fiber to prevent constipation—are not very effective. Recently, though, drugs known as serotonin antagonists have been shown to be effective in treating some cases of the condition, especially diarrhea-predominant IBS.

▼ In irritable bowel syndrome, the intestines spasm rather than contract slowly.

Research from the Mayo Clinic reported in the medical journal *The Lancet* showed that 41 percent of patients treated with one such drug, alosetron (brand name Lotronex), experienced relief from symptoms during the three-month study period compared with 29 percent of the patients taking a placebo (dummy pill). Patients and physicians are hoping that serotonin antagonists may offer a much-needed solution to this hard-to-treat problem.

Unfortunately, alosetron is currently unavailable. The drug was withdrawn from the market in 2001 after it was linked to incidents of ischemic colitis, or restricted blood flow to the colon, and severe constipation. But it may become available again, to be used under more stringent guidelines. New formulations believed to be safer are already making their way through clinical trials. And unlike the original drug, which was effective only in women with diarrhea-predominant IBS, they may be suitable for constipation-predominant IBS too.

For many people who used it successfully, Lotronex was a major advance in treatment, often alleviating many of the debilitating symptoms after just a few doses. Its withdrawal has been a major blow to these people, but the newer formulations seem to have similar beneficial effects.

How it works. Under normal circumstances the intestines slowly contract to move solid substances through the digestive system. But in people with irritable bowels, they move in an inconsistent way—either too fast, resulting in unpredictable bouts of diarrhea, or

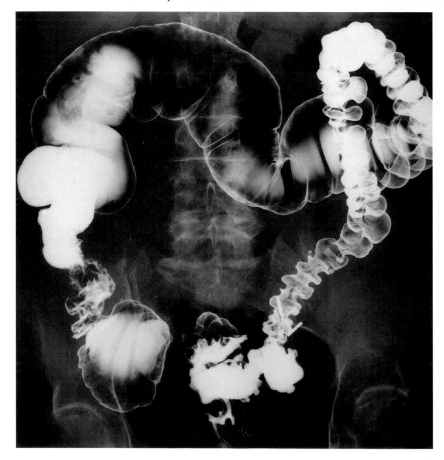

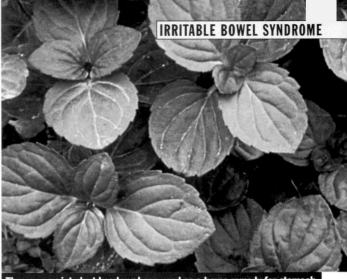

too slow, leading to constipation. The motion of the gut is partially regulated by a neurotransmitter (messenger chemical) called serotonin. Too much serotonin causes the muscles of the intestines to move too quickly, triggering spasms. Serotonin antagonists such as Lotronex work by blocking the uptake (collection) of serotonin by certain chemical receptors in the intestines. Without the chemical signal that instructs the gut to contract, the number of intestinal spasms decreases, leading to less abdominal pain and fewer abnormal bowel movements.

Availability. If Lotronex becomes available again, its use would almost certainly require close monitoring by physicians and it would probably be restricted to patients with the worst symptoms. Similar drugs designed to block the action of serotonin in the intestine are already in advanced clinical trials. One of these drugs, tegaserod (brand names Zelnorm and Zelmac), has cleared phase III clinical trials and is predicted to win marketing approval in Europe and the United States by 2002.

The peppermint plant has long been used as a home remedy for stomach problems; now a study has shown that taking peppermint oil can help children with IBS.

RESEARCH ROUNDUP

■ **ANTIBIOTICS CAN HELP.** New findings suggest that people with irritable bowel syndrome (IBS) may have too much bacteria in their intestines. While bacteria are perfectly normal in the gut, more than three-quarters of patients with IBS had evidence of excessive amounts of bacteria in their small intestines, according to a report in the December 2000 issue of the *American Journal of Gastroenterology*. In the study, after treatment with antibiotics, fewer people complained of bloating, diarrhea, and abdominal pain, and about half no longer had enough symptoms to warrant a diagnosis of IBS.

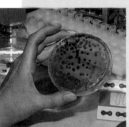

Researchers have found that people with IBS may have too much bacteria in their intestines.

■ **EMOTIONS AND IBS.** A person's emotions and mental state may have an effect on IBS symptoms, according to two new studies published in 2001. As a result of these findings, there is increasing interest in the role of antidepressants in the treatment of this condition. In one of two studies published in the journal *Digestive Diseases and Sciences*, investigators tested the effects of emotionally powerful words on the digestive tracts of women with irritable bowels, including some with psychiatric disorders. In about 75 percent of cases, patients' symptoms seemed to get worse when they heard words associated with anger, sadness, or anxiety.

Alternative Answers
Candy Cane Cure for Kids with IBS

For children suffering from irritable bowel syndrome (IBS), relief may come in the form of a common herb—peppermint. In a study of children aged 8 to 17, published in the February 2001 issue of the *Journal of Pediatrics,* peppermint oil capsules helped relieve symptoms of IBS, including bloating, severe abdominal pain, and cycles of constipation and diarrhea.

In the two-week study, 42 children with IBS were treated with peppermint oil or a placebo (dummy pill). On the first day of the study, all of the children complained of abdominal pain and many also complained of diarrhea, constipation, and gas. Following the two-week treatment period, however, 71 percent of the youths given peppermint oil said they felt "better" or "much better," compared with 43 percent taking the placebo.

Peppermint has long been used as an herbal remedy for indigestion and intestinal problems. Its use as folk remedy has been documented since the eighteenth century, and its use as a remedy for IBS has been studied in adults since the mid-1980s.

> **FAST FACTS**
> **"NORMAL" NUMBER OF BOWEL MOVEMENTS** Anywhere from three times a day to three times a week **UP TO 85** Percentage of IBS patients who report that their symptoms started after a stressful life event, such as a divorce or the death of a loved one **4 FOODS TO AVOID** Beans, broccoli, milk, and alcohol **50** Percentage of people who remain symptomatic five years after their diagnosis

Surgical Solution
"Keyhole" Surgery Better Alternative to Stomach Stapling

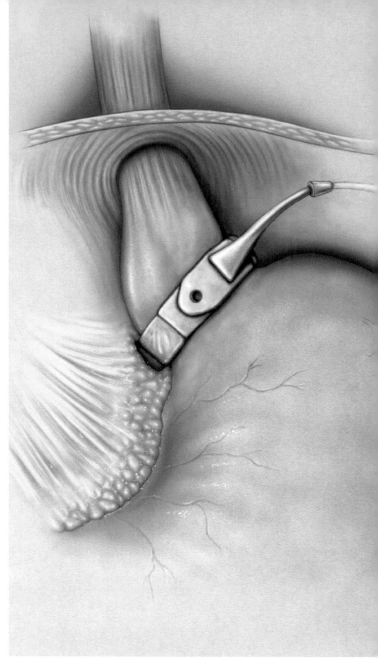

▲ THE BIG SQUEEZE The Lap-Band is placed around the top of the stomach to create a small gastric pouch. A narrow opening allows food to move slowly from the pouch to the lower stomach.

For obese people who have tried dieting, exercise, and drugs, the last resort is usually surgery such as stomach stapling or gastric bypass. These surgeries permanently alter the gastrointestinal tract and usually involve scarring and the risk of infection. Now there's a better alternative to these older, invasive approaches.

On June 5, 2001, the U.S. Food and Drug Administration (FDA) approved a laparoscopic ("keyhole") surgery to close off part of the stomach using the Lap-Band Adjustable Gastric Banding System. The fully reversible procedure has been tested since 1993 in more than 60,000 patients worldwide and leads to an average weight loss of 35 to 68 percent of excess weight over the span of two years.

How it works. An adjustable silicone band is placed around the upper part of the stomach using laparoscopic surgery, in which tiny instruments and a flexible fiber-optic tube are placed through several small incisions. Once the band is in place, its inner lining is filled wtih saline. This inflates the band, closing off the lower part of the stomach and creating a small gastric pouch above it. The small pouch limits the amount of food that can be consumed at any one time and leads to a quicker feeling of fullness. It empties slowly,

> **FAST FACTS**
> **7** Percentage of the total annual healthcare costs in the United States that are connected to obesity-related disability **280,000** Number of preventable deaths in the United States each year that result from obesity-related conditions **100 BILLION** Total annual costs attributable to obesity-related disease in the United States

The smaller gastric pouch limits food consumption and leads to a quicker feeling of fullness.

so the feeling of fullness lasts for several hours. A physician can adjust the band as needed through an access port close to the skin.

Availability. Though it has been tested worldwide, the Lap-Band is available only from surgeons who have been trained to perform the procedure, and most of them are in Europe. Surgeons elsewhere are quickly catching up—meaning that the surgery will be available in most Western countries, including the United States, by 2002.

It is suitable only for people who are at least 100 pounds overweight or twice their ideal body weight and who have failed to lose weight through diet, exercise, or other programs. You will need to go on a special diet for about two weeks following the surgery. Although side effects are much fewer compared with earlier surgical procedures, they may include nausea, vomiting, heartburn, abdominal pain, and band slippage. In tests, side effects caused about a quarter of patients to have the band removed.

STAY TUNED FOR...

Prickly Way to Quash Hunger Pangs

A United Kingdom–based company called Phytopharm has caused some worldwide excitement with the announcement that a South African cactus holds promise for the treatment of obesity. Kalahari natives have long used the rare Hoodia cactus to stave off hunger on hunting trips, and now Western medicine has isolated the active ingredient, code-named P57. The

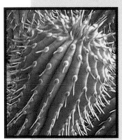

Hoodia extract still has far to go before becoming available, but it cleared its first two preliminary human trials in mid 2001. Pfizer Inc. licensed the worldwide development and marketing rights to P57 in August 1998.

The active ingredient in a South African cactus may prove to be an effective appetite suppressant.

PATIENT PROFILE

Winning the Weight Battle

"I was at the end of my rope. I had tried everything, but nothing worked," recalls Brandi Barber White. "You name it—doctors, weight-loss programs, camps, spas, diet pills, hypnosis, and even fasting—but any time and every time I lost weight I gained it all back, plus some."

Barber had battled with her weight since a life trauma in her early thirties. Five years ago, she caught a glimpse of the surgery that would soon change her life. While watching a television report on an experimental procedure for obesity, Barber was immediately hooked and contacted the manufacturer, Bioenterics, to find out more about Lap-Band. "They sent me some information and I knew that I wanted to do it. There was no cutting of vital organs, no permanent damage, just a 45-minute procedure with little risk. I didn't think I had anything to lose except weight."

At an out-of-control 305 pounds, Barber had a lot of weight to lose. About a year after her surgery she had dropped 175 pounds. "I'm normal now. I love life and I am not living a horrible existence anymore," comments Barber on overcoming the stigma often felt by

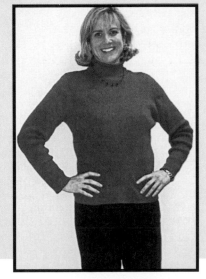

severely overweight people. "I have never been so happy." Of the positive effect that Lap-Band had on her lifestyle, Barber notes, "I must admit I didn't have a diet and exercise plan, but as I started losing weight I felt better and wanted to eat healthier and exercise." Barber now enjoys swimming, water aerobics, kickboxing, yoga, and walks in the park with her husband and twin toddler girls.

When she found out that she was pregnant, Barber had her Lap-Band adjusted in a 15-minute outpatient visit that would allow her to eat more so that her babies could gain enough weight. "The pregnancy was not planned, but we were very excited to find out that we were going to have not one but two little babies" said Barber. "I was worried that I wouldn't be able to gain enough, but it was a little scary to see how quickly the weight could come back on."

Barber attributes the birth of her children to this life-changing procedure. She says, "Without Lap-Band I wouldn't have a husband or my little babies today," and adds, "The best thing about it is that it is totally adjustable to fit your lifestyle in any stage of life."

magine not seeing your grandchild's first smile, or being unable to talk on the telephone or understand more than a few words of conversation. Our eyes and ears connect us to the world around us. When those connections fail, what wouldn't we give to get them back? That's the goal of some of this year's medical miracles, like the implantable hearing aid that is surgically placed under the skin behind the ear canal. This advancement offers people with hearing loss who have difficulty using traditional hearing aids a more comfortable alternative. Other highlights include self-adjusting eyeglasses that could provide corrected vision to millions of people in developing nations who lack access to vision care, as well as an alternative technique to remove cataracts that may be safer than standard procedures. And providing a far-off ray of hope to blind people: The first artificial retinas were implanted in three blind patients—a small step in finding out whether or not the chips can someday help to restore vision.

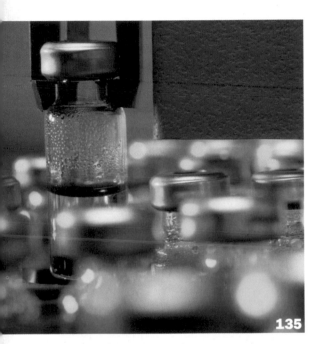

135

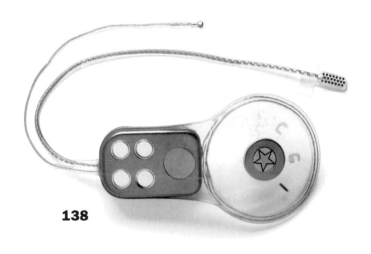

138

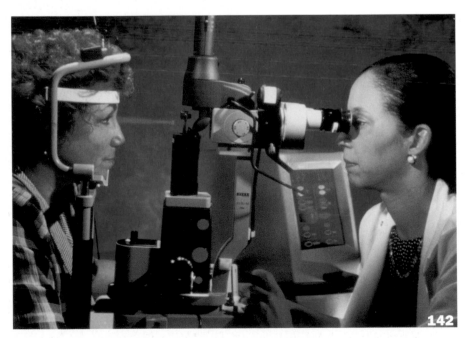

142

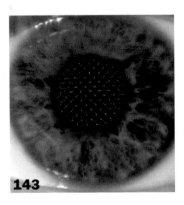

143

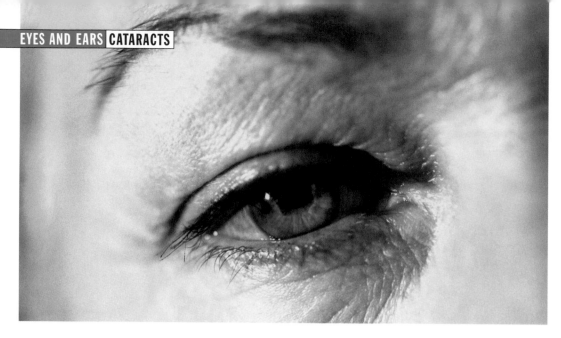

◄ A new surgical procedure may make cataract removal quicker and safer.

Surgical Solution

Laser Device Clears Up Cataracts in Record Time

Cataracts—a progressive clouding of the eye's normally clear lens—can be corrected only by surgery. The most widespread treatment is phacoemulsification, or phaco, which uses ultrasound vibrations to break up the cataract. This technique has been remarkably safe and effective, but now there's a new procedure that offers an alternative.

The probe uses pulsing light to create a shock wave that breaks down the eye's lens.

According to the developers of the Dodick PhotoLysis System, named after Jack M. Dodick, M.D., the surgeon who invented it, it involves a shorter operating time and a smaller incision, and thus may cause fewer complications. The results on 1,000 eyes, published in the journal *Ophthalmology* in April 2001, show the technique to be fast, safe, and efficient. However, more studies are needed to find out if it's actually better than phaco.

How it works. A probe is inserted through a tiny incision. The probe uses pulsing light, rather than the ultrasonic waves of phaco, to create a shock wave that breaks down the eye's lens in just a few minutes, so it can be removed through a suction tube. An artificial lens is then implanted through a separate incision.

Availability. Although similar laser systems have been used in Europe for several years, the Dodick PhotoLysis System is the first of its kind to have U.S. Food and Drug Administration approval for use in the United States. It gained approval in July 2000, but it will take a while before it is fully tested or becomes widely available. The traditional phaco technique is the standard method used in most ophthalmologic offices and has the advantage of a long-term track record.

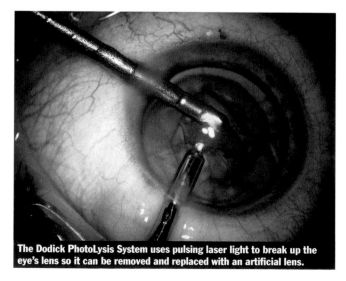

The Dodick PhotoLysis System uses pulsing laser light to break up the eye's lens so it can be removed and replaced with an artificial lens.

RESEARCH ROUNDUP

■ **SMOKING AND CATARACTS.** Kicking the habit—even after many years of smoking—reduces the risk of developing cataracts. A study published in the *Journal of the American Medical Association* on August 9, 2000, showed clear evidence of this. It looked at the effect of smoking on cataract development in a group of more than 20,000 physicians in the United States. The results? Men who quit smoking were 23 percent less likely

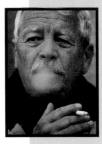

to develop cataracts than were those who continued to smoke. What's more, quitting still had an impact on risk, no matter how heavily the person smoked in the past. The study points out that past vices do leave their mark; some smoking-related damage in the lens of the eye may be irreversible.

■ **EYEING INHALER DANGERS.** If you are a long-time user of steroid inhalers to control asthma, you may be at increased risk of developing cataracts according to a study of more than 200,000 people. In the past, this relationship has been controversial, in part because findings were based on research involving only small groups of people. This recent study found that steroid inhaler users were 30 percent more likely to develop cataracts.

■ **SPARE TIRE TROUBLE.** Researchers have known for some time that there is a connection between excess body weight and cataracts. Now experts at Harvard University have determined that the way excess body weight is distributed is itself a risk factor—with men who carry that extra weight around their middle at a 31 percent greater risk of developing cataracts. Yet one more reason to trim your tummy.

FAST FACTS
400,000 Number of new cases of cataract that develop each year in the United States
50 Percentage of worldwide blindness caused by cataracts

Drug Development
Two New Drugs Offer Options for Glaucoma Patients

The U.S. Food and Drug Administration has approved two new drugs for the treatment of glaucoma, a disease that steals vision bit by bit. In people with glaucoma, fluid builds up inside the eye and causes pressure in the aqueous humor, the clear fluid that fills the space between the lens and the cornea. If this intraocular pressure is not controlled, it can damage the optic nerve (which

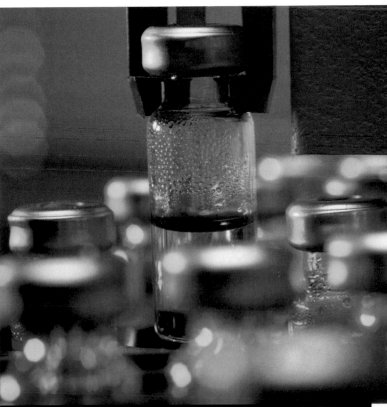

New drugs are now being manufactured for people who do not respond well to standard glaucoma medications.

135

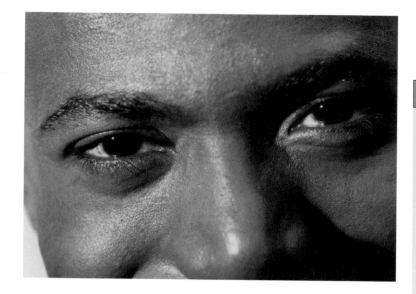

▲ One of the newest glaucoma drugs has been initially shown to be particularly effective in black patients.

RESEARCH ROUNDUP

■ **EARLY WARNING TOOL.** The vexing challenge of diagnosing glaucoma in its early stages, before any significant eye damage occurs, may be much easier in the future, thanks to researchers at Tufts University School of Medicine in Boston.

The team identified a substance in the eye, called ELAM-1, that is present only in eyes affected by glaucoma. This discovery could lead the way for a screening test to detect the disease before any symptoms occur. The team's results were reported in the March 2001 issue of *Nature Medicine*.

■ **CAN YOU TAKE THE PRESSURE?** Most glaucoma drugs reduce the pressure in the eye. But several experimental drugs, called neuroprotective agents, work a different way—by shielding the vulnerable optic nerve from glaucoma-related damage, even as eye pressure builds. One of the drugs, memantine, is already used in Europe for treating certain diseases, including Parkinson's disease and dementia.

How does it work? Injured nerve cells release toxic substances that enter and harm nearby healthy cells. Memantine disrupts this process, limiting the damage that diseased and dying nerve cells can cause. Memantine was also shown to have a protective effect on the eyes of rats and monkeys with glaucoma. Now a four-year worldwide study is under way to test whether the drug can work as a glaucoma treatment in people. Results are expected in 2003.

transmits visual stimuli to the brain) and other parts of the eye, possibly leading to vision loss or blindness.

It's too early to tell whether the two new drugs—bimatoprost (brand name Lumigan) and travaprost (brand name Travatan)—will work better than timolol, the standard glaucoma treatment. But their approval is good news for people who can't tolerate, or don't respond to, timolol. Of particular note, the first studies have suggested that Travatan works better in black patients than in white patients. This is important because, as a group, blacks are four times more likely to have glaucoma. They are also more likely to develop it at a younger age and to go blind from the disease.

These drugs are good news for people who can't tolerate, or don't respond to, timolol.

How it works. Both drugs work by increasing the outflow of fluid in the eye. Possible side effects include a gradual darkening of eye color and eyelid skin and increased thickness and darkness of the eyelashes.

Availability. Bimatoprost and travaprost were approved in March 2001.

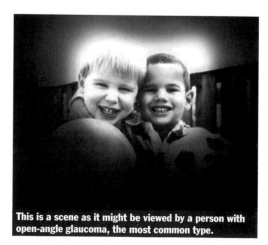

This is a scene as it might be viewed by a person with open-angle glaucoma, the most common type.

FAST FACTS
70 MILLION Number of people worldwide who have glaucoma **5,500** Number of Americans who become blind each year from glaucoma **50** Percentage of Americans who have glaucoma and don't know it **3** Ranking of glaucoma as a cause of blindness worldwide

High-Tech Help

Now Hear This: Implantable Hearing Aid Approved

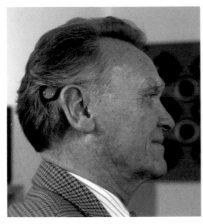
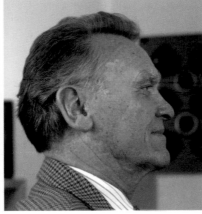

◀ **The processor that picks up sound waves is worn behind the ear and can be concealed under the hair.**

Hearing aids are a real boon to people with hearing loss, but some folks are turned off by traditional devices worn in the ear canal or behind the ear, either because of the way they work or because of the way they look or feel. Some people who own traditional hearing aids don't even wear them. Now there's another option. In August 2000 the U.S. Food and Drug Administration approved an implantable device called the Vibrant Soundbridge for people with sensorincural hearing loss, the most common form of hearing loss. The receiver is surgically placed under the skin behind the ear canal, so the device is more comfortable and less noticeable than a standard hearing aid. Users of the Soundbridge also say it produces a clearer sound, with less electronic feedback and interference from background noise.

How it works. The device has two main parts: a sound processor worn behind the ear and a surgically implanted receiver. The processor picks up sound waves from the environment and transmits them to the receiver, which converts them to vibrations passed via wire to a small electromagnet (the transducer) attached to one of the middle ear bones. The transducer directly vibrates the bones very much the way normal sound does. The operation, which is performed by an ear surgeon, takes about two hours and can be done without an overnight hospital stay. In clinical trials, patients received only one Soundbridge, but now that the device is approved, some patients are opting for implants in both ears.

Availability. As of summer 2001, the Soundbridge was available from over 100 doctors throughout the United States and 1 in Ontario, Canada. The device has been available in parts of Europe since 1998.

The Vibrant Soundbridge

A processor transmits sound waves to the receiver, which converts them to vibrations that travel through the transducer to vibrate the bones of the middle ear.

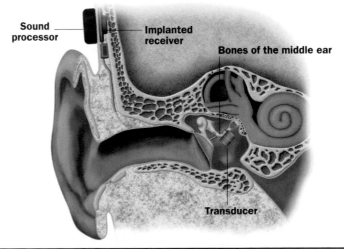

Sound processor

Implanted receiver

Bones of the middle ear

Transducer

BEHIND THE BREAKTHROUGH

A Personal Mission to Help the Hard of Hearing

In 1986, when he started medical school at Stanford University in Palo Alto, California, Geoffrey Ball thought his hearing impairment—the result of a reaction to a drug he was given in early childhood—wouldn't stand in the way of his studies. His first day in the operating room, he learned otherwise.

"With everyone in a surgical mask, I couldn't read lips, so I didn't know what was going on," says Ball. Being a son of the Silicon Valley, Ball decided he'd have to solve the little problem of hearing before he could become a doctor. He figured it would take about two years of experimenting and testing to develop a reliable, comfortable hearing aid that delivered better sound quality than the traditional microphone-plus-amplifier devices he'd worn since the age of seven.

Fifteen years and hundreds of false starts later, the Vibrant Soundbridge won approval from the U.S. Food and Drug Administration. Throughout this long period of trial and error, Ball's chief collaborator was his father, an engineer at National Semiconductor in California, whose many patented inventions include one of the first electronic sound chips.

Much of the work that resulted in the Soundbridge was done with funds granted by the Veteran's Administration, a fact that Ball is quick to emphasize. "People complain about government research money being wasted on things that will never help anyone, but in this case the process actually worked the way it was supposed to." In 1992, he hit on the right formula to make the tiny transducer that functions like the middle ear. Seven years later, Ball had his invention placed in one of his own ears. More recently, he got an implant in his other ear.

Returning to medical school doesn't seem to be in the cards for Ball, who's concluded that his destiny is to design and build devices that will bring sound to the hearing-impaired. The long road he traveled to develop the Soundbridge was, as he puts it, "God's way of saying 'This is what's been planned for you.'"

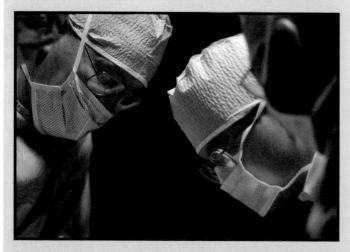

Surgical masks prevented Geoffrey Ball from reading lips in the operating room while he was attending medical school. The predicament inspired him to develop a new, partially implantable hearing aid with the help of his father, an engineer.

High-Tech Help
New Device Lets the Brain Do the Hearing

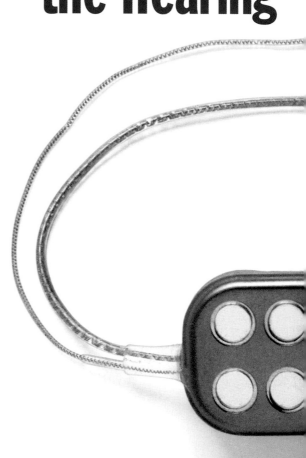

▲ **The Nucleus 24 ABI includes a receiver/stimulator which is implanted under the skin behind the ear and sends electrical impulses through a wire to 21 electrodes implanted in the brain.**

People with a genetic disease called neurofibromatosis type 2 often develop tumors that affect both auditory nerves (the large nerves that transmit sound from the inner ear to the brain). Surgery to remove the tumors usually involves removing parts of the auditory nerve—which results in complete hearing loss. Now a new device, the Nucleus 24 Multichannel Auditory Brainstem Implant (ABI), is allowing people with this form of deafness to hear through their brains instead of their ears.

How it works. An ear surgeon (otologist) places the small receiver/stimulator part of the device under the skin behind the ear and implants the electrode end in the part of the brain known as the cochlear nucleus. A microphone attached to the scalp and a sound processor small enough to carry in a pocket pick up sound waves and change them into electrical impulses that are similar to those the auditory nerve normally conveys. The impulses are sent to the receiver/stimulator, which sends them through a wire to the implanted electrodes. The 21 electrodes use the impulses to stimulate the cochlear nucleus.

Availability. The Nucleus 24 ABI received U.S. Food and Drug Administration approval in October 2000. Currently otologists in at least 10 hospitals and clinics in different regions of the United States are equipped to do the surgery.

[
FAST FACTS
28 MILLION People with impaired hearing in the United States **20** Percentage of hearing-impaired people who could benefit from hearing aids who actually have them **40–50** Percentage of people aged 75 and older with hearing loss **89** Number of seconds an ear can be exposed to noise levels of 110 decibels —the volume of an operating power saw or leaf blower—without risk of damage
]

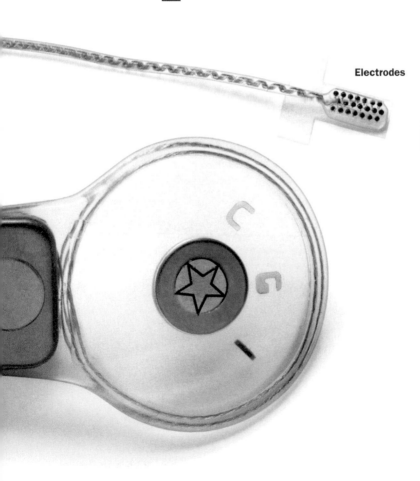

Electrodes

Receiver/Stimulator

STAY TUNED FOR...

Invisible Hearing Aids

Miraculous as they are, implantable hearing devices (such as the Vibrant Soundbridge) all have at least one component that is worn outside the body. But the next-generation devices are a different story. One, the Implex TICA, recently became available in parts of Europe and is now being tested in the United States. It consists of three totally implanted components, modeled on the physiology of the normal-functioning middle ear. Normally, sound waves enter the ear canal, where they vibrate the eardrum, which in turn vibrates three tiny "hearing bones" in the middle ear. These vibrations are transferred to the fluids of the inner ear, which stimulate sensory hair cells, which produce electrical signals perceived by the brain as sound. The sensor of the Implex TICA is inserted beneath the skin of the ear canal, close to the eardrum, where it picks up sound signals and amplifies them electronically. This allows it to mimic the chain reaction of mechanical vibrations and send them directly to the middle ear bones—avoiding the need for the "loudspeaker" that conventional hearing aids use.

High-Tech Help

First Artificial Retinas Implanted in Blind Patients

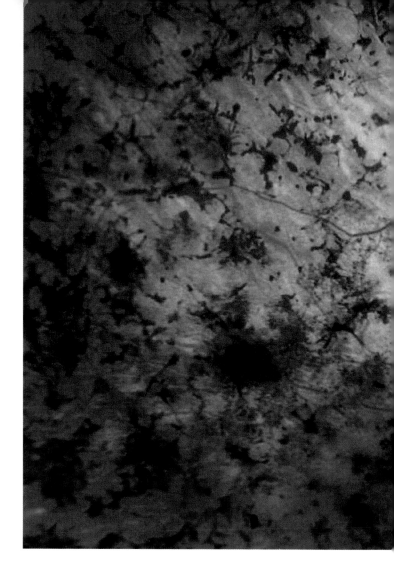

A rtificial vision took a step toward reality in June 2000, when three blind patients were implanted with the first artificial retinas. The Artificial Silicon Retina (ASR), invented by brothers Vincent Chow and Alan Chow, M.D., of Optobionics, is a microchip designed to replace damaged photoreceptor cells—the eye's light-sensing cells, also known as rods and cones. These cells are found in the retina, a delicate membrane located in the back of the eye. In a normal-functioning retina, the rods and cones convert light into electrical signals, which the retina sends back to the brain so that we can see.

The patients who received the ASR are participants in an FDA-approved feasibility and safety study (a study to determine whether the chips can be safely implanted and not create side effects). They had volunteered to receive the ASR because they had lost nearly all their vision to retinitis pigmentosa, a disease that causes the loss of photoreceptor cells in the retina.

Implanting the ASR

The new retinal implant is a microchip implanted under the retina that responds to light stimulation and electrically activates overlying retinal cells.

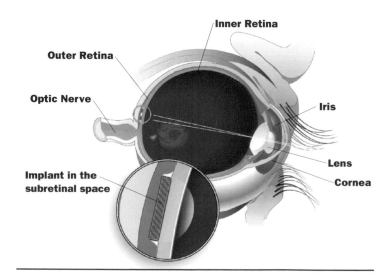

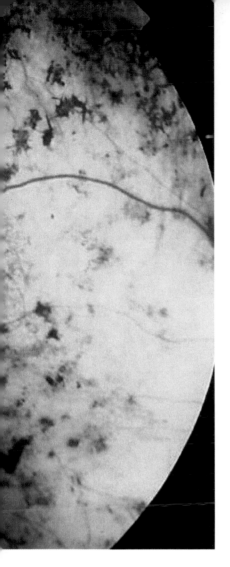

BEHIND THE BREAKTHROUGH

With New Company, New Hope in Sight

Alan Chow, M.D., a pediatric ophthalmologist, was particularly concerned about a young patient whose eyesight was rapidly deteriorating because of retinitis pigmentosa. Chow had read hundreds of papers on how the cells of the retina convert the analog signals of light into the electrochemical signals of the nervous system. He believed that a prosthesis could be developed that could stimulate the patient's remaining still-functioning photoreceptors. Over Thanksgiving dinner, he presented his idea to his brother Vincent Chow, an electrical engineer.

Thus began the development of the Artificial Silicon Retina (ASR). The Chow brothers created their own company, Optobionics, of Wheaton, Illinois, to develop the ASR, with Alan Chow as president and CEO and Vincent Chow as vice president of engineering. The U.S. Food and Drug Administration has given Optobionics permission to implant the ASR in 10 patients for preliminary safety and feasibility studies. So far, six patients have received the device.

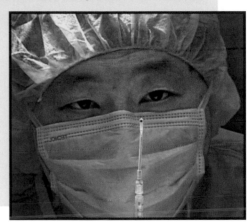

Dr. Alan Chow in the operating room preparing the ASR for implantation.

▲ In this magnified image of an eye with retinitis pigmentosa, the dark clumps of pigment indicate the disease.

One year after the implantation, all three patients reported that they were not experiencing any ill effects from the device. According to David McComb, Chief Information Officer of Optobionics, "The chips are tolerating the eyes, and the eyes are tolerating the chips." After getting the good news, doctors at Optobionics implanted the ASR in three more patients in July 2001. If all goes well, the next phase of research will determine whether the chips can restore some degree of visual function.

Optobionics is not alone in the quest to develop a functional artificial retina. Several other groups in the United States, Germany, and Japan are also looking into this type of device. Some groups are developing fully implanted chips similar to the ASR. Others are investigating chips that work in conjunction with computers, cameras, and other devices outside the body.

How it works. The ASR is surgically implanted under the retina in a location known as the subretinal space, so that the chip underlies the eye's healthy nerve cell network. The chip is only 2 mm in diameter and is thinner than a single strand of human hair yet it contains some 3,500 microscopic solar cells. These cells respond to light stimulation by generating electrical impulses. The electric current then stimulates overlying still-functioning retinal cells, essentially activating the patient's own visual system.

Availability. The ASR is in the earliest phase of testing. After the next phase, in which researchers will see how well the device works, the ASR could become available in as little as five years. People who think they may be candidates for the ASR and would like to participate in the FDA-approved study can fill out a questionnaire online and submit it to Optobionics at www.optobionics.com.

The chips are designed to treat the group of conditions known as outer retinal disease. They cannot treat retinal conditions, such as glaucoma, in which the nerve fibers leading to the optic nerve are damaged. They are presently intended only for people who have lost most or all of their vision, and the current design of the chip is unlikely to give more than the most basic level of sight.

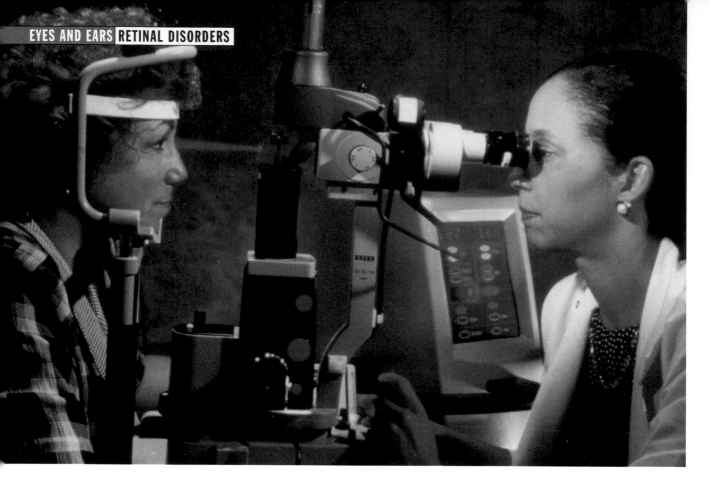

▲ A new treatment for retinal damage uses laser light to activate medication targeted to the eye.

Drug Development
Drug Slows Vision Loss in CNV Patients

The drug verteporfin (brand name Visudyne) slows the deterioration of vision in people who have suffered damage to the eye from choroidal neovascularization (CNV), the growth of abnormal blood vessels behind the center of the retina. It has been in use in the United States, parts of Europe, and elsewhere since 2000 for patients with CNV caused by some forms of age-related macular degeneration (AMD, the leading cause of blindness in people over 50). And now it has been approved, in parts of Europe, for patients with CNV caused by severe myopia (near-sightedness), a rare condition, but one which can affect people as young as 30.

How it works. The treatment is a two-step process that can be performed in a doctor's office. First, verteporfin is injected into a vein in the patient's arm. The drug is activated by shining a weak laser light into the patient's eye for about 90 seconds. The activated drug affects the abnormal blood vessels in the retina but does not appear to damage normal vessels. Although the drug does not actually restore vision, it does slow down—and in some cases even stop—the process of deterioration. On average, people in clinical trials received five treatments each over a two-year period.

Availability. Verteporfin has been approved for CNV caused by severe myopia in parts of Europe and is still awaiting approval in the United States for this condition.

[
FAST FACTS
13 MILLION Number of people in the United States who have signs of age-related macular degeneration
50,000 Number of new cases of choroidal neovascularization (CNV) caused by severe myopia that occur each year in the world
]

High-Tech Help
Adjustable Glasses for the Masses

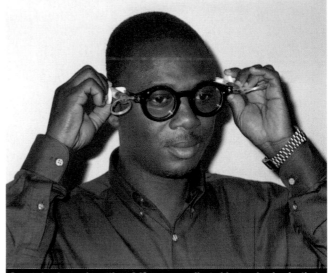

A completely new invention, AdSpecs are adjusted by turning knobs that control the flow of silicone oil into the lenses.

Dial into better vision in less than a minute. That's the promise of revolutionary new adjustable spectacles called AdSpecs—glasses that could bring clearer vision to millions of people in developing nations who don't have access to trained ophthalmologists or prescription lenses. The wearers adjust the curvature of the lenses themselves simply by turning knobs on the glasses' temple pieces, or "stems," until they can see clearly.

The spectacles are the brainchild of Dr. Joshua Silver, a physicist at Oxford University who developed them over the course of 15 years. According to his company, Adaptive Eyecare, the glasses can correct the vision of 90 percent of the typical population (people requiring correction of up to +6 or –6 diopters). The design is so innovative that it won *Popular Science*'s Medical Technology Grand Award in its *Best of What's New 2000*.

How it works. The spectacles use a completely new lens technology that, in a sense, mimics the way the eye works to get clear vision—by changing the curve of the lens. The wearer does this by turning the temporary knobs attached to the stems of the glasses. The knobs control the flow of silicone oil, contained in a set of syringes attached to the lenses, into the lenses. This changes the lenses' curve, increasing or decreasing the correction power for a wide range of near or distance needs.

The knobs and syringes are temporary—they are meant to be snapped off and discarded after the glasses are adjusted. The design allows the adjustment to be performed only once, but a model under development will allow for repeated adjustments.

Availability. The spectacles were field-tested in Ghana, Nepal, Malawi, and South Africa by the British Government's Department for International Development. Adaptive Eyecare is now taking orders for the spectacles from international aid organizations and nations interested in providing inexpensive eye care for their citizens.

STAY TUNED FOR...

20/10 Vision

Most people who undergo LASIK are happy to come away with 20/20 vision. Now, a process called adaptive optics is being investigated to offer LASIK that can correct vision to better than 20/20—even as sharp as 20/10. While there are people who are naturally endowed with vision better than 20/20, this is the standard benchmark for visual acuity in everyday life.

The new process, called wavefront-guided LASIK, promises to improve on nature by more precisely matching vision correction to each person's eye irregularities. During the process, a light is shone into the eye. As this light

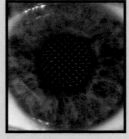

A new laser-correction technique measures tiny aberrations in the eye and may lead to LASIK that corrects to better than 20/20 vision.

reflects off the various surfaces of the eye, including the cornea, lens, and retina, tiny aberrations are identified. Measurements of these aberrations can then be used to guide a LASIK procedure that sculpts the cornea to correct for the focusing imperfections of the eye's surfaces—giving the eye an extremely high degree of visual efficiency. Another possible application for this technology is to create customized contact lenses that compensate for the thinning of the cornea as a result of an eye disease called keratoconus. Currently several companies are testing wavefront-guided systems, but the procedure is not yet commercially available.

We are more likely to die from heart disease than from any other condition. Fortunately, advances in this area are some of the most exciting in medicine. A major milestone: In July 2001, the first fully implantable artificial heart was placed in a middle-aged man. There's also good news for heart attack survivors: For the first time in history, stem cells transplanted into a person's heart actually brought damaged heart muscle back from the dead.

Other highlights include a "super-aspirin" for angina that may help people avoid surgery. And for those who require a stent, a new procedure helps prevent restenosis, the crisis U.S. Vice President Dick Cheney experienced in March 2001. Plus new hope for the recovery of motor skills in stroke survivors, a clever computer designed to help you lower your blood pressure by changing your breathing, and a laser surgery for varicose veins that's less expensive than traditional surgery—and more effective.

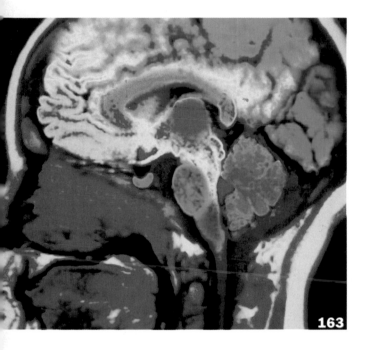

163

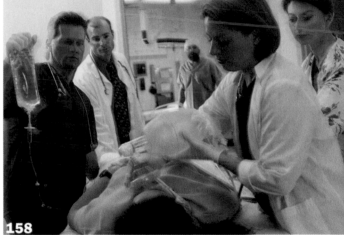

158

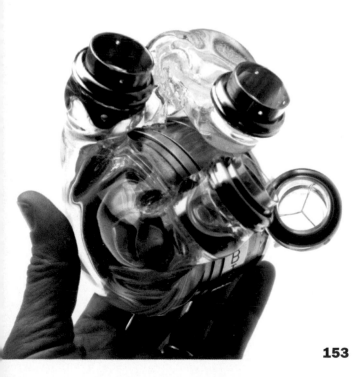

153

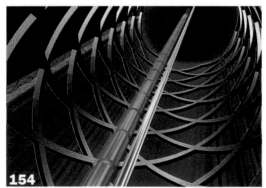

154

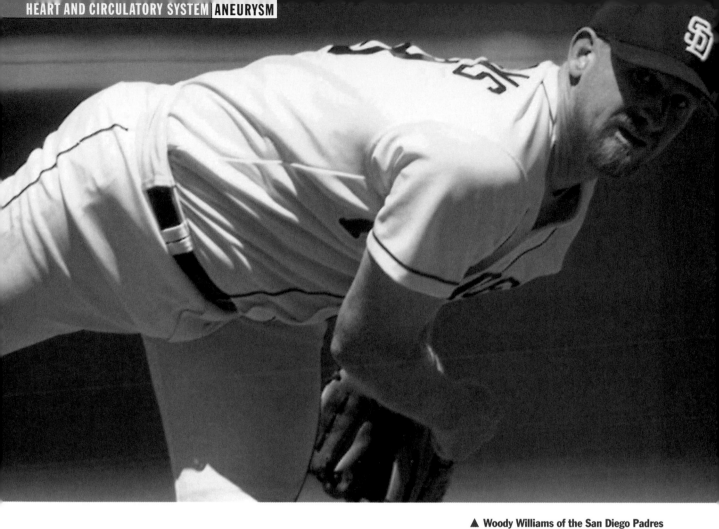

▲ Woody Williams of the San Diego Padres returns to pitch after recovering from surgery for an aneurysm in his armpit. One day antibiotics may make aneurysm surgery unnecessary.

Drug Development
Antibiotics for Aneurysms

An aneurysm is a swelling and expansion of a blood vessel, which, like a balloon, can eventually burst if left untreated. The culprit is usually an enzyme called MMP, which dissolves the proteins in the artery wall that give it strength and stability. After several years, as the artery walls thin and the bulge of the aneurysm grows, surgery is often needed to replace the damaged section—and that can be a tricky, dangerous procedure. Fortunately, now there may be a better solution. The first phase of clinical trials using the antibiotic doxycycline has proved highly successful in preventing, or at least delaying, surgery.

How it works. The antibiotic seems to attack MMP and prevent it from destroying the artery walls. In a six-month study involving 36 patients, at Washington University School of Medicine in St. Louis, Missouri, researchers found that doxycycline lowered levels of MMP by a whopping 80 percent. This is potentially lifesaving news for people who suffer from aortic aneurysms. A burst aorta, the biggest artery in the body, can be fatal.

Availability. The second phase of clinical trials using doxycycline began in July 2001 at nine medical centers across the United States. Widespread use of this drug will depend on the outcomes of what will be a four-year study.

[
FAST FACTS
15,000 Number of people who die each year from a ruptured aortic aneurysm **50 to 70** Percentage of people receiving emergency surgery for a burst aneurysm who die as a result of the rupture
]

Surgical Solution
Laser Surgery Improves Life for Chest Pain Patients

I f you suffer from severe angina and have failed to find relief from medications, coronary artery bypass surgery, or angioplasty (the use of a balloon placed inside the coronary artery to widen it), your doctor may suggest a recently developed surgery. It involves drilling tiny holes directly into your heart to help the oxygen-starved muscle receive oxygen-rich blood. But the idea of additional chest surgery—an incision in the chest through which a laser is placed to drill the holes—is not a pleasant prospect. The good news is the advent of a newer technique for placing holes in the heart from *inside* the body, using a laser threaded through a small catheter inserted in the groin.

"My doctor gave me a choice: They could either open me up again or try something new."

The technique is PMR (percutaneous myocardial revascularization, previously called PTMR). Unlike its older cousin, called TMR (transmyocardial revascularization, the through-the-chest technique), PMR does not require a chest incision, which means a lower risk of infection and complications, a shorter hospital stay, and the use of a local anesthetic instead of general anesthesia.

Now, the results of a recent clinical trial on PMR show that it really works to relieve angina. The study, led by a team at Massachusetts General Hospital in Boston and reported in *The Lancet* on November 18, 2000, found that the procedure (in conjunction with anti-angina medication) reduced angina in 34 percent of patients and was associated with better scores on exercise tests and an improved quality of life compared with those who received only medication.

How it works. In PMR, a surgeon makes a small incision in the groin and threads a thin catheter through a blood vessel in the leg up into the left ventricle of the heart. Using precise cuts with a handheld laser beam, the doctor drills tiny holes in the heart muscle. The holes appear to restore blood flow to starved parts of the heart and may also boost angiogenesis, the growth of new blood vessels, within the heart muscle.

Not all studies agree, however, on whether PMR improves blood flow, and how PMR works to relieve angina is still under debate. A recent study comparing patients who had received the laser treatment with a group who had a sham procedure (the same catheterization, but without the actual use of the laser) revealed that both groups improved. This effect has led some researchers to feel that the benefits of the procedure could be due to a "placebo" effect (a response to the procedure that is not attributable to the actual treatment).

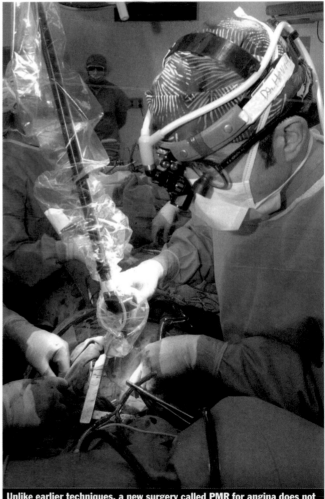

Unlike earlier techniques, a new surgery called PMR for angina does not involve a chest incision.

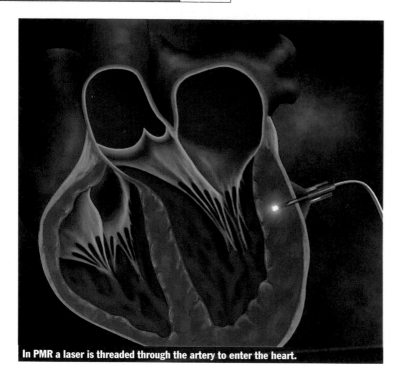

In PMR a laser is threaded through the artery to enter the heart.

Availability. PMR was approved for use in Europe during the late 1990s. In July 2001, citing safety concerns, the Circulatory Devices Panel of the U.S. Food and Drug Administration (FDA) did not recommend approval of PMR. The panel acknowledged, however, that the technique relieved angina. The manufacturer is now working with the FDA to correct these concerns.

PATIENT PROFILE

Surgical Success Story

"My heart pain was constant," recalls Robert Reed. "It felt like a stack of bricks was lying on my chest." Though Reed had never actually had a heart attack, he began having serious problems with his heart when he was in his late 30s. When doctors discovered that three of Reed's arteries were completely clogged, he underwent three-way bypass surgery. But the pains came back, and only a few years after the bypass, doctors discovered that his arteries had become 100 percent clogged again.

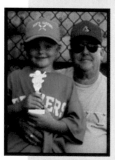

Reed with grandson

Reed had an angioplasty, but that helped only for a short time. He says, "I had to do something, and my doctor gave me a choice: They could either open me up again or try something new...I went for the new procedure."

Reed chose to undergo the minimally invasive laser procedure known as PMR (percutaneous myocardial revascularization). "No pain," he reports. "You are awake the whole time. The whole procedure lasted less than an hour." Reed says that he felt much better "right away" after undergoing PMR, and that he felt better and better as the weeks went by. He can even ride a bicycle again, and he enjoys taking long walks with his wife, Judy. He says he wouldn't hesitate to recommend PMR to anyone else. Says Reed, "It probably saved my life."

Drug Development
Super-Aspirin May Prevent Cardiac Death

A new anti-clotting drug called clopidegrel (brand name Plavix) may soon be added to the treatment regimen for patients with a serious form of chest pain known as unstable angina, reported researchers at the March 19, 2001, meeting of the American College of Cardiology. Nicknamed the super-aspirin, clopidegrel is prescribed along with old-fashioned aspirin and seems to boost its heart-protective effect.

The CURE (Clopidegrel in Unstable Angina to Prevent Recurrent Ischemic Events) trial found that taking clopidegrel along with aspirin reduced the risk of death from cardiac problems (including heart attack and stroke) by 20 percent in the more than 12,000 patients in 28 countries who took it compared with taking aspirin alone. Most of the patients in the study also received standard heart medications for their cardiac condition. The benefits from taking clopidegrel started within two hours and were maintained throughout the 12-month study. Salim Yusuf, M.D., Ph.D., from McMaster University in Ontario, Canada, led the research.

How it works. In serious heart problems like angina and mild heart attacks, pain often arises from blood clotting and thickening, which blocks blood flow to the heart. Like aspirin, anti-clotting medications help reduce the number and size of clots in the blood vessels, "thinning" the blood so it flows more readily.

Availability. Because clopidegrel has already been used as a treatment for other heart problems, it is currently available by prescription.

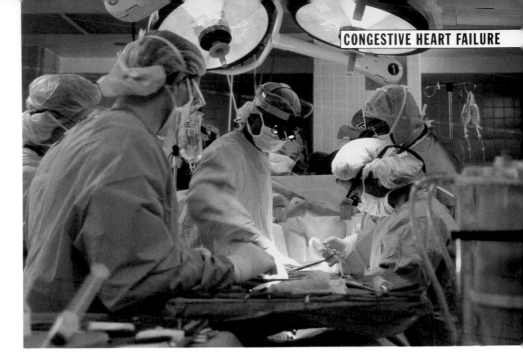

▶ **HELP FOR THE HEART**
Surgeons at the University of Chicago successfully implanted the CardioVad System in a patient with congestive heart failure.

High-Tech Help
Wearable Aid for Failing Hearts

Imagine a battery-powered device that helps your heart so it doesn't have to work so hard. Now imagine being able to strap the device in yourself — and take it off when you want. Thanks to the ingenuity of Adrian Kantrowitz, M.D., it's a reality. Kantrowitz, the first U.S. surgeon to transplant a heart and the developer of many noted heart devices and techniques, has been working on this new technology for 30 years, and he reported the promising results of the first five implants of his device, called the CardioVad System, at a conference of the American Society for Artificial Internal Organs on June 7, 2001.

Held as the next generation of heart-assist devices, the CardioVad doesn't entirely take over the work of the heart. Instead, it picks up only half the work, so a weak and failing heart can rest but not waste away. The system was designed for permanent use by patients who have chronic congestive heart failure with frequent hospitalizations and poor quality of life but who, because of age or a poor medical condition, are not considered candidates for a heart transplant. It is one of the current pack of "destination" devices being developed for heart failure patients in contrast to the "bridge" devices designed to assist patients only until a heart becomes available.

What is particularly special about the CardioVad is that a patient can take off the vestlike device for fairly lengthy periods of time. One patient, who has been using the device since October 2000, removes it for about three hours twice a day without any ill effects. For quality of life, mobility, and self-esteem, the vest is a vast improvement over other assist devices.

How it works. The CardioVad starts with a balloon sewn into the heart's aorta. One tube connects this balloon to an external battery. This battery and an air pump are contained in a vest that weighs about 10 pounds (45 kilograms). When the heart relaxes between beats, the balloon in the aorta inflates, pushing blood out to the rest of the body. A second tube connects to an external computer that monitors the heart's rhythm and electrical activity; the computer can speed up or slow down the heart's pumping action as needed to meet the body's changing demands.

Availability. The CardioVad System is now being tested at two centers in the United States and is set to enter the next stage of testing—100 patients in 10 institutions—toward the end of 2001. In the future, look for heart-assist devices like the vest devised by Kantrowitz that can be worn for even shorter periods of time—say, for 10 hours, rather than all day. Patients could wear such devices overnight while they sleep and be free of them during the day.

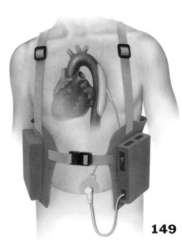

▶ **LIFE VEST**
This removeable device eases the burden of diseased hearts.

High-Tech Help
Heart "Jackets" May Keep Risk in Check

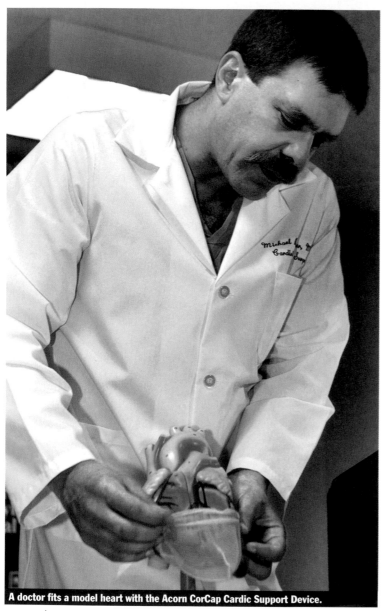

A doctor fits a model heart with the Acorn CorCap Cardic Support Device.

Polyester jackets aren't exactly au courant—unless you're one of the first patients who gets to wear one on your heart. In the summer of 2000, surgeons at the University of Pennsylvania in Philadelphia began wrapping hearts enlarged by heart failure in a polyester jacket, called a cardiac support device. The hope is to save lives while reducing the need for heart transplants. The jacket is being used in clinical trials on patients with both congestive heart failure and valve disease in the United States, Germany, and Australia.

How it works. Big hearts aren't healthy hearts: They represent a vicious circle of inefficiency, as cardiac muscle grows to try to keep up with demand. The cardiac support device works like support hose, physically restraining heart tissue and, hopefully, preventing the heart from getting bigger as heart disease progresses. Only time will tell how well the cardiac jackets wear over the years.

Availability. This experimental device was approved for sale in parts of Europe in September 2000. Clinical trials in the United States began in summer 2000, and the U.S. Food and Drug Administration may approve the device as early as 2003. Worldwide, more than 75 implants have been performed so far.

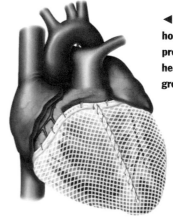

◄ Like support hose, the jacket prevents diseased hearts from growing larger.

[
FAST FACTS
46,980 Number of deaths from congestive heart failure in the United States in 1998 **2,197** Number of heart transplants performed in the United States in 2000
]

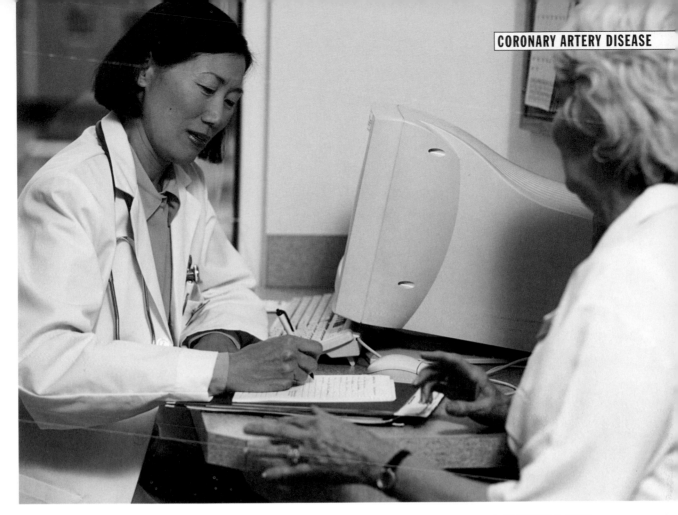

▲ **CUSTOMIZED CARE**
**Thanks to new guidelines,
more people at risk for
a heart attack will be
identified and treated.**

Progress in Prevention
New Cholesterol Guidelines Should Mean Fewer Deaths from Heart Disease

New guidelines issued by the National Cholesterol Education Program of the U.S. National Heart, Lung, and Blood Institute, in May 2001, lower the threshold of who is considered at risk of coronary artery disease (CAD). As a result, millions more people will receive treatment that could save their lives.

In the past, many Americans who had a high risk of a heart attack were not identified, so they failed to receive aggressive treatment. The new guidelines should make a big difference: The number of Americans on dietary treatment for high cholesterol could increase from about 52 million to about 65 million, and the number who have been prescribed a drug to lower cholesterol could rise from about 13 million to about 36 million. With appropriate treatment, fewer deaths as a result of heart disease should occur. As in the past, emphasis is placed on lowering LDL cholesterol, the "bad" cholesterol (the fatlike substance in the blood that can clog up and stiffen the arteries). But the new guidelines go even further. Here are some key points worth noting.

- **Better identification of who is at risk of CAD and heart attack.** A new "risk assessment tool," a risk calculator, is used to examine a variety of medical and lifestyle factors (such as your cholesterol levels, whether you smoke or have diabetes or high blood pressure, and your family history of heart disease) to determine your risk of having heart problems. Of particular interest, the new guidelines state that type 2 diabetes poses as serious a risk for heart attack as heart disease itself. By looking at all your risk factors, your doctor can customize a treatment plan for your risk level.

- **A Therapeutic Lifestyle Changes (TLC) plan that combines more intense use of nutrition, exercise, and weight control to treat elevated blood cholesterol.** The new TLC diet calls for daily intake of less than 7 percent of calories from saturated fat and less than 200 mg of dietary cholesterol; up to 35 percent of daily calories can come from total fat, as long as most of it is unsaturated fat, which does not play a part in raising cholesterol levels. Foods that are high in fiber, such as cereal grains, legumes (for example, beans and peas), and many vegetables and fruits, are encouraged, as well as certain margarines and salad dressings that contain plant compounds called stanols and sterols (substances found to lower cholesterol levels).

- **More stringent guidelines for HDL, the "good" cholesterol that helps prevent cholesterol from building up in your arteries.** In the past, HDL was considered dangerously low at 35 mg/dl or less. Now, having a level of even 40 mg/dl or less is considered a major risk factor. A level of 60 mg/dl or higher is protective against CAD.

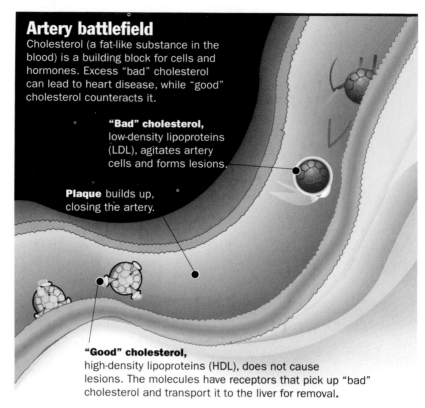

Artery battlefield

Cholesterol (a fat-like substance in the blood) is a building block for cells and hormones. Excess "bad" cholesterol can lead to heart disease, while "good" cholesterol counteracts it.

"Bad" cholesterol, low-density lipoproteins (LDL), agitates artery cells and forms lesions.

Plaque builds up, closing the artery.

"Good" cholesterol, high-density lipoproteins (HDL), does not cause lesions. The molecules have receptors that pick up "bad" cholesterol and transport it to the liver for removal.

- **Better recognition and treatment of high triglyceride levels.** Triglycerides are fats in the blood that play an important part in heart disease. The new guidelines recommend treating even levels that are considered "borderline-high" (a level of 150 mg/dl or higher).

- **Recommendation against using hormone replacement therapy (HRT) as an alternative to cholesterol-lowering drugs.** Unlike cholesterol-lowering drugs, HRT has not been shown to reduce the risk of major coronary events (such as heart attacks) or deaths in postmenopausal women with heart disease. In fact, HRT is known to increase the risk of thromboembolism (the blocking of a blood vessel by part of a blood clot) and gallbladder disease.

So speak to your doctor at your next checkup about getting a full cholesterol workup. In addition, as always, pay careful attention to the nutrition labels on packaged food—a good place to see how much saturated fat, cholesterol, and calories are contained in what you eat.

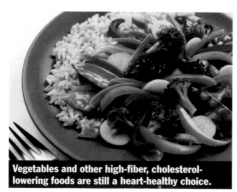

Vegetables and other high-fiber, cholesterol-lowering foods are still a heart-healthy choice.

High-Tech Help
Man Receives the First Totally Implantable Artificial Heart

A major milestone has been reached in the quest for a completely implantable artificial heart. The AbioCor Implantable Replacement Heart, approved in January 2001 for experimental use in humans, is the first artificial heart that can be fully enclosed in the body—no wires or pumps are visible, and there is no loud motor to be heard by confused passersby. And in July 2001, the first recipient of the heart made headline news after his successful surgery.

In July 2001, the first recipient of the heart made headline news.

The heart will be used only in people with extremely diseased hearts who have end-stage coronary artery disease (CAD) or congestive heart failure where death is imminent. How long the heart will work in humans is still unknown. The initial goal of the surgery is to keep the patients alive for at least 60 days. Without surgery, the first recipient had an estimated 80 percent chance of dying within 30 days.

How it works. Implanted in the chest along with its rechargeable battery coil, the AbioCor has two pumps, like the body's own left and right ventricles. A battery pack worn outside the body runs the heart for several hours at a stretch, although the artificial heart can also pump itself for 30 minutes without recharging (so, for instance, a patient can take a shower).

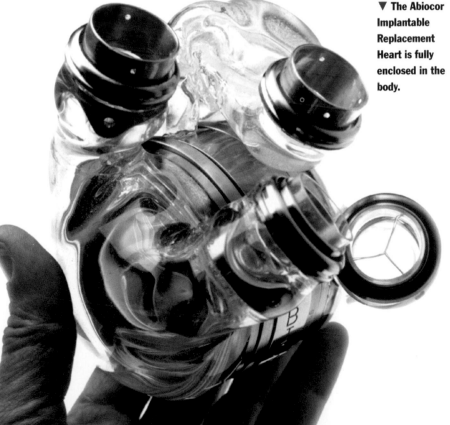

▼ The Abiocor Implantable Replacement Heart is fully enclosed in the body.

Once the heart is implanted, no wires or tubes extend from the skin, virtually eliminating the risk of infection, a prime reason earlier artificial hearts failed. Instead, external batteries charge the heart directly through the skin. Computerized feedback mechanisms respond to the body's need for a faster or slower heartbeat.

Unlike the body's natural heart, which circulates blood in a pump/rest cycle, the AbioCor moves blood constantly through the body, bringing the added benefit of a lower risk of clotting disorders and stroke.

Availability. So far, U.S. Food and Drug Administration approval extends only to the experimental use of the heart in five patients. The results will determine the fate of future trials.

High-Tech Help
Clearer Future for Stents

S tents are the tiny wire-mesh tubes placed inside blocked coronary arteries to prop them open after bypass surgery or angioplasty. The problem is that an estimated 1 in 4 of these devices becomes inflamed and blocked with scar tissue in a process called restenosis. Several new advances were made in 2000 to help prevent, or at least delay, restenosis. (This was U.S. Vice President Dick Cheney's medical crisis in March 2001, as his coronary artery disease continued to advance even after several bypass surgeries.)

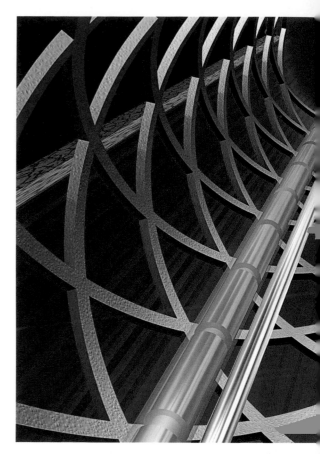

► A new technique to keep stents clear begins with the insertion of a catheter into the stent.

Zapping stents with radiation. In 2000, positive clinical studies led to U.S. Food and Drug Administration (FDA) approval of two new radiation devices—one delivering gamma radiation, the other beta radiation—designed to help keep stents clear by curbing the regrowth of the artery wall. In the radiation treatment, gamma or beta radiation in the form of a bead-like "string of pearls" is precisely measured by a team of specialists, which includes a radiation oncologist and a medical physicist as well as a cardiologist. The beads are then inserted through an arterial catheter into the stent. After 5 to 10 minutes of beta radiation treatment or 10 to 20 minutes of gamma radiation treatment, the radiation beads are removed.

The two manufacturers of the radiation devices, Cordis Corporation and Novoste Corporation, are working to make their devices available to cardiologists, but the procedure is not yet widely available in every hospital setting. Future reports will evaluate longer-term safety and efficacy and seek to confirm whether radiation keeps a stent clear longer than other methods.

Several new advances were made in 2000 to help prevent, or at least delay, restenosis.

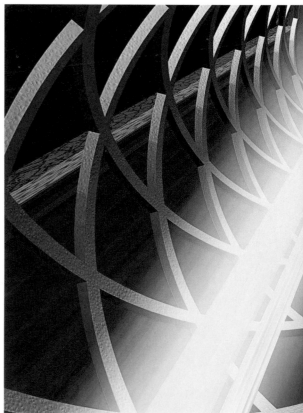

► Next, radiation is delivered through the catheter, which keeps the artery walls from closing up around the stent.

Teflon coatings. Another new stent development was the use of rapamycin (a drug that suppresses the immune system and also acts against fungus) or the anticancer drug paclitaxel as a special coating for the tube to inhibit scar tissue growth within the stent. Drug-coated stents are currently undergoing clinical trials in the United States, and preliminary results show that they are more effective than noncoated stents in preventing restenosis.

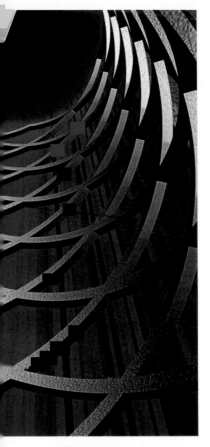

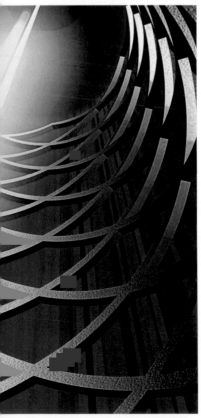

Diagnostic Advance
New MRIs for Early Heart Disease Detection

A new imaging technique may soon replace angiography as a way to map the coronary arteries, as reported in *Circulation: Journal of the American Heart Association* on August 1, 2000. Angiograms are X rays of the blood vessels using the help of an injected dye, but the constant waves of blood flowing through the arteries hide the actual vessel walls themselves—so it's like trying to see the details of coastline rocks beneath crashing waves. The new technique is a special form of MRI (magnetic resonance imaging) that lets the doctor see right through the blood (in other words, it "blacks out" the blood), so the subtleties of the blood vessel walls—and any dangerous buildup of plaque inside—are visible.

Studies show that up to 70 percent of heart attacks happen in people whose blood vessels look normal or only mildly narrowed on an angiogram. The new technique, nicknamed a "black blood MRI," is an exciting step forward in the early detection of coronary artery disease (CAD) and the prevention of heart attacks, especially because of its non-invasive nature.

How it works. As CAD progresses, plaque and fatty deposits build up inside the artery walls and can thicken them from less than 1 mm in a healthy person to 4 mm in someone with CAD. This new,

RESEARCH ROUNDUP

■ **FISH FOR THE HEART.** Omega-3 fatty acids have made it to the big time: the American Heart Association's (AHA's) recommended diet. Found in fatty fish such as salmon, omega-3s lower the level of triglycerides in the blood, as well as the risk of blood clotting. The AHA suggests eating at least two 3-ounce servings each week of salmon, tuna, sardines, and other fish containing omega-3s.

■ **MAYBE MIRACLES DO WORK.** The results of the MIRACL (Myocardial Ischemia Reduction with Aggressive Cholesterol Lowering) trial, published in the April 4, 2001, issue of the *Journal of the American Medical Association,* showed that the cholesterol-lowering medication atorvastatin (from the class of drugs known as statins) lowered angina by 26 percent, cut stroke by 50 percent, and lowered the risk of cardiac death and heart attack by 16 percent if given in high doses to hospitalized patients right after the coronary event. For the more than 3,000 patients in the trial, follow-up studies will determine just how long their miracles will last.

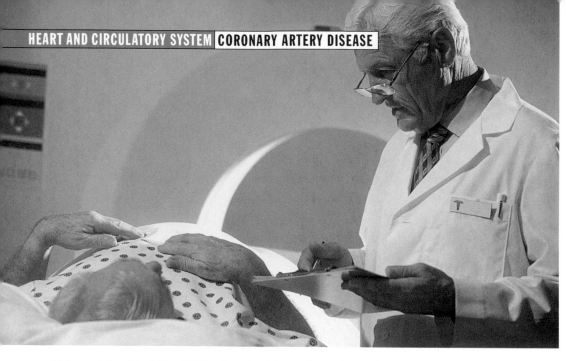

◀ A new MRI technique may soon replace angiography as a way to examine coronary blood vessels.

high-resolution black blood MRI gives physicians a direct view of the structure and thickness of artery walls, without the blood flow in the way. Vulnerable plaque—those bits that are more likely to break off and cause a heart attack—can be identified before they rupture.

Availability. Researchers at the Mount Sinai School of Medicine in New York, who reported the new MRI technique in August 2000, note that further research over the next two to three years is needed to perfect the test and its effectiveness as a screening tool, but that it may appear in U.S. medical centers within the next five years.

Surgical Solution
Adult Stem Cells Used to Grow New Heart Tissue

The promise of genetic medicine is being fulfilled in tiny increments—increments as small as a single cell. The year 2000 saw the first human recipient of a breakthrough stem cell transplant procedure in which stem cells from a man's thigh muscle were transplanted into his heart. Stem cells are immature cells capable of morphing into new kinds of cells (such as heart muscle cells). Doctors hoped that the stem cells would induce damaged heart muscle, considered dead after a heart attack, to begin contracting again. And it may have worked.

Philippe Menasché, M.D., performed the cell transplant at Hôpital Bichat in Paris and reported his five-month follow-up results in *The Lancet* on January 27, 2001. The scarred heart muscle showed signs of contracting on an echocardiogram, but the results are not clear-cut because the same patient also had bypass surgery, which may have contributed to the muscle's ability to contract. Still to come are the results of a similar procedure performed in May 2001, at the University of California Medical Center in Los Angeles.

STAY TUNED FOR...

Gentler Angioplasty
Phase II clinical trials are under way in Little Rock, Arkansas for an experimental angioplasty technique called photoangioplasty. It uses a light-sensitive chemical called Antrin to help clear blocked arteries. Antrin is injected into the patient's artery and is activated by a special type of non-visible light, called far-infrared light, inserted into the artery via fiberoptic wires. Rather than working mechanically as angioplasty does, the light triggers a reaction in the chemical, which helps "melt" away the fatty buildup of plaque in the artery. The new technique was developed, in part, as a response to one of the unfortunate side effects of angioplasty: The balloon-insertion surgery can damage the delicate walls of the arteries—and thus lead, ironically, to a worsening of coronary artery disease.

FAST FACTS
600 Typical number of days the first patients of temporary heart transplants lived **70** Approximate percentage of transplant patients who survive five years after transplant **700,000** Number of angioplasties performed each year in the United States

Progress in Prevention
Trial to Shed Light on Preventing Life-Threatening Blood Clots

Results of the PREVENT trial (Prevention of Recurrent Venous Thromboembolism), under way at 60 clinical sites throughout the United States, may shed more light on preventing idiopathic, or unexplained, deep vein thrombosis (DVT) and pulmonary embolism (blood clots that may inexplicably form in veins and travel up to the lungs, causing a life-threatening condition). The trial, due to run through May 2003, is testing the effectiveness of long-term, low doses of the blood-thinning drug warfarin (Coumadin) to prevent recurrence of clots and pulmonary embolisms in patients who have had these problems in the past.

Currently, patients who have had DVT and pulmonary embolism are given warfarin for only three to six months, but 1 of every 3 people who complete the warfarin therapy develops another DVT or embolism within five years. Long-term therapy with warfarin is not without risks, however, as some patients may experience episodes of bleeding from the blood-thinning medication, ranging from nosebleeds to major bleeding ulcers. The 800 patients included in the study will be people who have experienced idiopathic DVT or pulmonary embolism and have already received standard short-term therapy for their condition.

The PREVENT trial will evaluate long-term use of low-dose warfarin for both effectiveness and safety. Researchers hope that it will safely prevent new clots from forming in patients who have this condition.

1 in 3 people who complete warfarin therapy develops another DVT or embolism within five years.

Deep vein thrombosis

In deep vein thrombosis, blood clots can form in the veins of the legs. These can become life-threatening if they break loose and block blood flow in the lungs (pulmonary embolism).

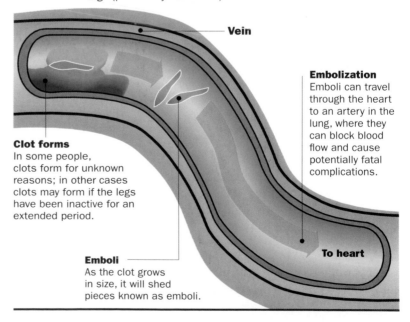

Vein

Embolization
Emboli can travel through the heart to an artery in the lung, where they can block blood flow and cause potentially fatal complications.

Clot forms
In some people, clots form for unknown reasons; in other cases clots may form if the legs have been inactive for an extended period.

To heart

Emboli
As the clot grows in size, it will shed pieces known as emboli.

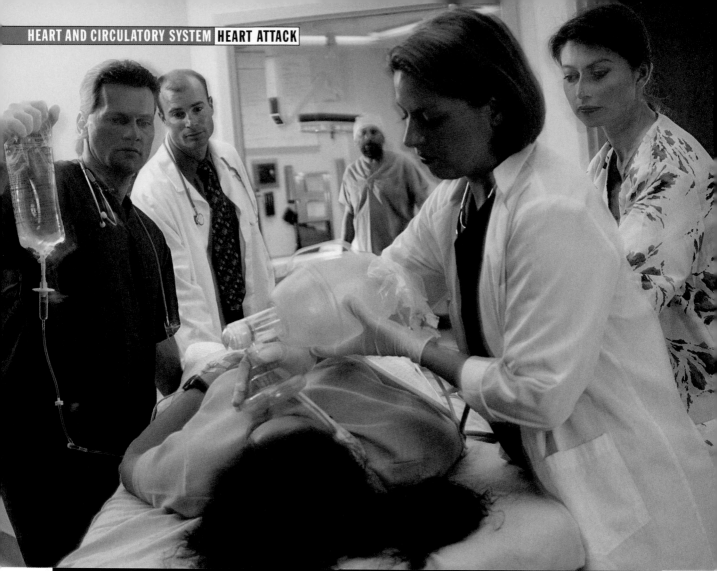

The new clot-busting drug works in just five seconds and has given ER doctors a lifesaving tool against heart attack.

Drug Development
New One-Shot Clot Buster

Clot-busting drugs, also known as thrombolytics, were introduced in the late 1980s and saved countless heart attack victims' lives. Advances since then have brought even better drugs to the ER. But until now, it took an hour-and-a-half transfusion of t-PA (tissue plasminogen activator), the most widely used thrombolytic agent of the past decade, to stop a heart attack. Enter tenecteplase (TNKase). This clot-buster can be administered over five seconds in one dose—with the same lifesaving results. Further, it comes packaged in a new, needleless injection system to protect health care workers from HIV and other blood-borne diseases.

How it works. Tenecteplase dissolves the clot that caused the heart attack. It works by activating the body's own anti-clotting mechanisms. More specifically, it triggers the body to produce plasmin, which dissolves the structure of the clot. Once the clot is broken down, blood can again flow freely to the heart. An added advantage: The new drug targets just the clot, rather than globally thinning the blood, which can cause excessive bleeding.

Availability. The U.S. Food and Drug Administration approved the use of tenecteplase in people in summer 2000. Marketed by the genetic research firm Genentech, the drug is currently under scrutiny in four major clinical trials in the United States. More than 9,000 patients are being evaluated to further define with what other drugs it is best used. Tenecteplase is currently awaiting approval for use in European countries.

High-Tech Help
Safer Angioplasty on the Way

H eart attacks are often the result of coronary artery disease (CAD). But occasionally, they are a nasty, little-talked-about side effect of cardiac care. Angioplasty, performed roughly 750,000 times every year, carries a nearly 5 percent risk of causing a heart attack. During the procedure, plaque is shifted away from artery walls—but it may run amok to block a smaller blood vessel down the line. When performed on patients who have bypass grafts and stents in place, angioplasty carries an even higher risk (15 percent) of heart attack. Now new gadgets called embolization protection devices may reduce

Angioplasty carries a nearly 5 percent risk of causing a heart attack.

▼ SAFETY NETS
These devices are part of a new generation of tools to trap rogue pieces of plaque before they can cause a heart attack.

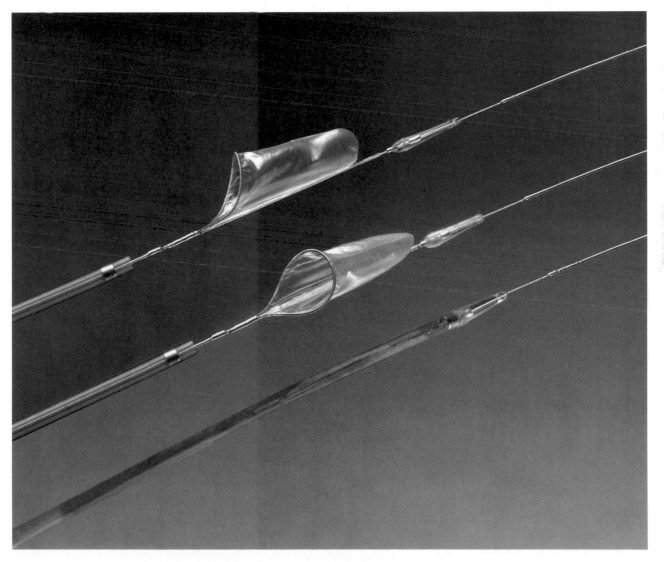

the danger. One such device, the FilterWireEX, features a filter to trap broken pieces of plaque before they can cause trouble.

How it works. The filter is threaded into the blood vessel before the angioplasty. About the size of a pencil tip, it catches pieces of debris loosened by the surgery, some big enough to see without a microscope. Doctors testing the new device report being amazed at the pieces of broken clots they can now see stirred up after angioplasty. They estimate that the new filter catches 93 percent of plaque debris.

Availability. The FilterWireEX has been approved for use in parts of Europe; it is still awaiting approval in the United States but is expected to be available for general use in 2002. Another debris catcher, the PercuSurge, which works with a balloon to catch the debris and a suction device to retrieve it, was approved for use in the United States in mid-2001.

How the FilterWireEX Works

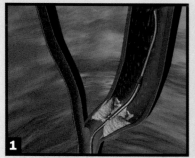

The FilterWireEx is inserted into a blood vessel prior to angioplasty.

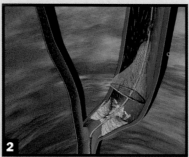

Once in place, the filter is opened.

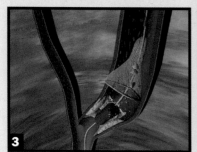

Floating debris is caught in the filter during angioplasty.

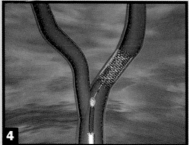

The FilterWireEx is easily retrieved after angioplasty.

RESEARCH ROUNDUP

■ **MENSTRUATION–HEART ATTACK LINK.** A woman's menstrual period may cause more than just a bad mood. Researchers at Laval University in Quebec studying sudden, unexpected heart attacks in women found that their subjects were significantly more likely to have heart attacks either during their menstrual periods or just afterward, when their estrogen levels were low. The study, reported at the American Heart Association's Scientific Sessions 2000, is still preliminary. Future research will try to filter out the effects of other risk factors, such as diabetes and smoking.

■ **WEEKEND WARRIOR WARNING.** What's the most likely day of the week to have a heart attack? For men between ages 25 and 54, it's Saturday or Sunday according to a new study from France, published in the September 2001 issue of *Heart*. Why the weekend trend? According to the researchers, it could be due to so-called weekend warrior syndrome—engaging in strenuous physical activity on the weekends after sitting at a desk all week. Good advice is to exercise throughout the week, and always warm up before launching into vigorous exercise.

FAST FACTS
1.1 MILLION Number of Americans who suffer a heart attack each year **40** Percentage of people who have a heart attack who die from it **90** Percentage of heart disease deaths in women that occur after menopause **$214 BILLION** Estimated amount that heart disease and heart attacks cost the United States in the year 2000 alone

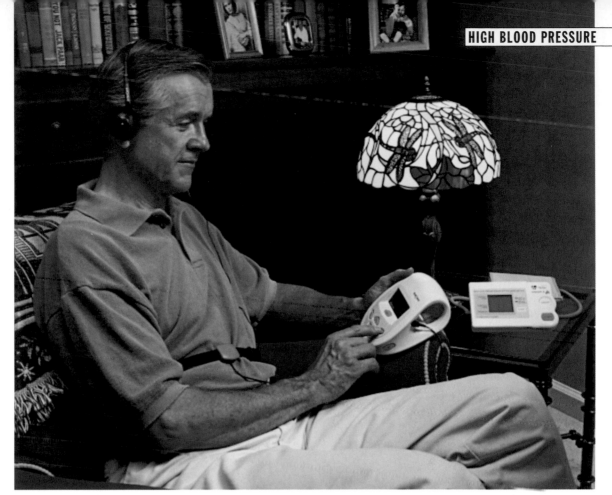

▲ BREATHE EASY
Now people can lower
high blood pressure
by listening to
the RespeRate's
musical tones.

High-Tech Help
Deep Breathing Lowers High Blood Pressure

Sometimes the simplest things are the most effective. RespeRate—the first device to be approved by the U.S. Food and Drug Administration (FDA) to treat high blood pressure, or hypertension—teaches patients how to lower their blood pressure by breathing deeply. It analyzes their breathing patterns and plays musical tones to help them achieve the slow, deep breathing shown to reduce blood pressure when practiced daily.

How it works. Heart rate, breathing, and blood pressure are so entwined that a change in one automatically affects the others. RespeRate, used once a day for 10 to 15 minutes, monitors breathing with a monitor worn around the midsection of the body. At the same time, the patient listens to musical tones. Both the monitor and

> **"I was flabbergasted, because I approached it with the idea that it was some sort of voodoo. And of course it isn't—it really does work."**

161

headphones are connected to a device (about the size of a compact disc player) that analyzes the breathing pattern and emits sounds to guide the patient to breathe at a slower rate. The device also stores readings that can be transferred securely to the patient's own RespeRate website so that patients can review their progress and print reports to bring to their doctor. There are no risks or side effects other than an enjoyable sense of calm.

Availability. The RespeRate is available throughout the United States, by prescription only. Its designers advise that the device should be used in conjunction with an overall high blood pressure treatment plan, which may also include antihypertensive drugs, a low-sodium diet, and an exercise program. The RespeRate costs $399.

PATIENT PROFILE

Resperate Really Works!

"When it was first suggested to me, I thought, 'Well, this really sounds hokey,'" says Paula Carney, a retired airline agent in her early 70s. She was talking about the RespeRate, a device that looks like a compact disc player attached to an elastic belt worn around the midsection of the body. When Carney was only in her 50s, her doctor had warned her that her high blood pressure was leading her toward a stroke. She quit her "pressure-cooker" of a job, and "the blood pressure came down some." She began taking medication ("that brought it down some more") and embarked on an exercise program ("that brought it down some more—but it was still in the high range").

Carney heard about the RespeRate while listening to a fine arts radio station in her hometown, Chicago. "They [Rush-Presbyterian Hospital] were looking for people for this study and I thought, 'Oh, that sounds like me... Maybe this will help.'" She arranged to participate in the eight-week-long study, and the researchers gave her a RespeRate to use at home every day, as a supplement to the medications she takes.

"During the first week I used it, my systolic pressure came down 10 points and the diastolic pressure came down 5 points—and I decided that that was just phenomenal," said Carney. "I spend 15 minutes of my day just sitting there all relaxed, listening to these tones and breathing with them... I do it usually in the afternoon. I come home from the gym, have my shower, my lunch, and do the RespeRate."

Carney finds that the effects continue long after her daily 15 minutes are up. She explains: "The blood pressure readings I've been getting are right in the normal range. I got one reading as low as 119/70. I thought, 'Oh my God, my blood pressure hasn't been that low since I was a child...' I was flabbergasted, because I approached it with the idea that it was some sort of voodoo. And of course it isn't—it really does work."

Alternative Answers
Therapy Helps the Brain Recover after a Stroke

The conventional wisdom used to be that after a stroke, affected areas of the brain were completely dead, unresponsive to later treatment. Not so, say researchers in a joint American-German study on the treatment technique called constraint-induced movement therapy (CI therapy) that was published in the journal *Stroke* in June 2000.

In CI therapy, pioneered by Edward Taub, Ph.D., a stroke patient's healthy limb is held fast so the "bad" arm has to re-learn simple tasks like picking up pennies or sorting beans. In the study, all patients made significant gains in the use of their affected arm. Earlier studies showed similar results. What's new about this study is that the damaged section of their brain involved in the movement showed physical changes—an increase in size and brain activity—that were still apparent in a six-month follow-up.

Now Taub and his group are extending the reach of CI therapy to a wider range of patients. Some of the trials being carried out involve the use of this therapy to increase arm function caused by brain injury, as well as to increase leg function after incomplete spinal cord injury and fractures of the hip.

How it works. CI therapy involves restraining the less affected arm in a sling or mitt for 90 percent of waking hours for two to three weeks while simultaneously spending many hours every weekday on continuous physical therapy for the "bad" arm.

It's not yet known exactly how the process works, but researchers believe it's likely that the brain's nerve cells rewire themselves so that

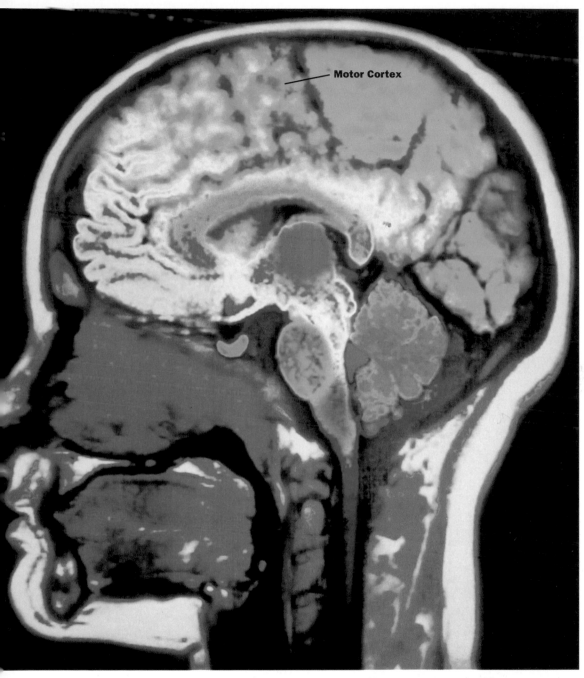

Motor Cortex

◄ **BRAIN CHANGES**
Damaged sections of the brain's motor cortex—a small area on the outer covering of the brain that controls movement — showed repair following constraint-induced movement therapy, a type of physical therapy for stroke patients.

damaged areas can function again and different areas can be recruited to help in producing movement of the affected arm. Mapping the brain of post-stroke patients by a technique called transcranial magnetic stimulation showed anatomical proof of the improvement.

Availability. CI therapy is currently available at several centers around the United States. The University of Alabama at Birmingham, where the research was conducted, has recently opened a clinic for administering CI therapy.

"When we showed it produced a large effect on the brain, then a lot of investigators and clinicians, many of whom are involved in work on the nervous system, felt that they could no longer ignore it."

BEHIND THE BREAKTHROUGH

Fresh Thinking Turned Therapy on Its Ear

Edward Taub, Ph.D., the psychologist-neuroscientist behind constraint-induced movement therapy (CI therapy), came to the field indirectly—from work in monkeys. The leap from teaching monkeys to reuse limbs that had lost all sensation to physical therapy rehabilitation for stroke patients came after 20 years of primate research, so Taub was able to approach the field of physical rehabilitation with a fresh, never-before-used point of view.

"When you look back at it now, it's really obvious, it's totally simple," he said. "We restrain the non-affected arm and train the affected arm, thereby inducing the person to use the arm over and over again."

This was the opposite of what had always been done in rehabilitation, wherein the patient was trained to use the less-affected arm "to get the job of life accomplished" but with the result that non-use was stamped into the affected limb. In other words, not using the limb contributed to its inability to function, and dependence on the unaffected limb increased.

Taub said that it was in the mid-1970s that he realized that his behavioral techniques could be applied to human physical therapy. He didn't realize that his approach was "not the way you do rehabilitation." Rather, "it was the opposite of how you do rehabilitation."

Even though his therapy had been shown to be clinically effective in previous articles, said Taub, it was the publication of the June 2000 *Stroke* article that resulted in thousands of requests for information. "When we showed it produced a large effect on the brain, then a lot of investigators and clinicians, many of whom are involved in work on the nervous system, felt that they could no longer ignore it," Taub stated.

Work is continuing at the University of Alabama at Birmingham and other sites around the United States using CI therapy for a variety of conditions, including traumatic brain, spine, and hip injuries; cerebral palsy in children; and hand movement problems in musicians (focal hand dystonia).

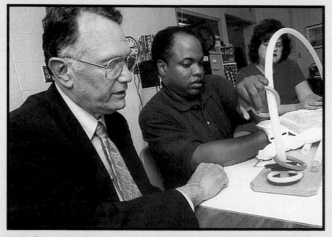

Help for stroke victims: Dr. Edward Taub, who pioneered constraint-induced movement therapy (CI therapy), works with a patient to rehabilitate his affected arm.

High-Tech Help

Helping Hands for Stroke Survivors

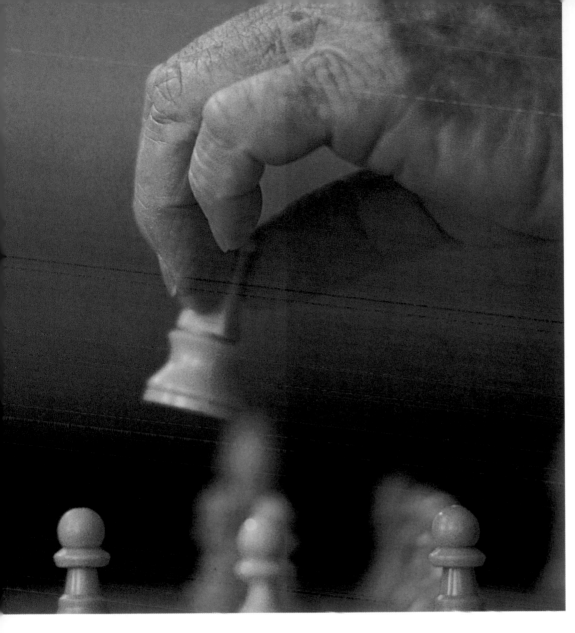

◄ SMOOTH MOVE
A new therapy
uses electrical
stimulation to
restore hand
control after
a stroke.

Recovering lost use of the hands is a prime focus of stroke rehabilitation so patients can gain independence and hold a fork, a newspaper—even a grandchild. Now doctors have a more precise rehabilitation therapy at their disposal, developed by researchers at the University of Florida in Gainesville led by James H. Cauraugh, Ph.D. The technique is simple but bears a tongue-twisting name: electromyography-triggered neuromuscular electrical stimulation. Simply put, it helps revive the hand/brain connection as the brain builds new nerve pathways.

A study reported in June 2001 in the journal *Stroke* showed a dramatic gain in strength, speed, and control of the hand and arm—especially with extension movements of the hand and wrist— critical in regaining independent living after experiencing a stroke.

Spontaneous recovery for many people is seen in the first six months to a year after a stroke. But, after a year, patients are typically dropped from therapy in the belief that no further gains can be made. Cauraugh notes that "these people are typically dismissed by their insurance companies because motor recovery

FAST FACTS
600,000 Number of people who have a stroke annually in the United States **4.5 MILLION** Number of Americans who live with the crippling after-effects of stroke **Stroke** The third leading cause of death in the United States, behind heart disease (number 1) and cancer (number 2)

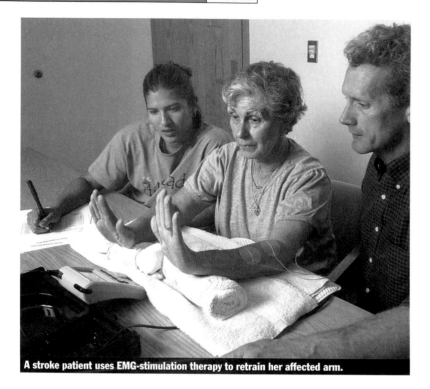

A stroke patient uses EMG-stimulation therapy to retrain her affected arm.

appeared to plateau." This therapy works with stroke patients a year or more after their stroke, targeting the delicate hand and wrist movements needed to perform basic daily tasks.

How it works. Small electrodes on a person's forearm monitor muscle activity as he or she tries to extend the wrist or fingers. After the patient moves as far as possible, the machine fires a small, painless electric impulse to help complete the movement. The device measures the movement and the electrical activity and makes precise adjustments as patients gradually become able to do more of the work themselves. Researchers believe it's the effort from the patient combined with the electrical trigger from the device that makes the therapy work.

Availability. While the latest study tested the technique in only 11 patients, stroke experts are thrilled at the ray of hope the device provides. Further, because EMG stimulation causes no side effects, risks, or complications, it's likely to become an increasingly widespread rehab technique as more stroke centers fine-tune the use of the equipment. Recently, Cauraugh received funding from a branch of the American Heart Association to sponsor the continuation of his research in this area.

> **Stroke experts are thrilled at the ray of hope the device provides.**

STAY TUNED FOR...

A Drug to Reduce Brain Damage

Preliminary animal testing of a new drug dubbed NXY-059 shows dramatic results in reducing brain damage after stroke. After inducing a stroke in lab rats in order to block blood flow to the brain, the new drug was administered in varying doses and at different time intervals after the stroke. The highest dose reduced brain damage by more than 80 percent. Doses administered after five minutes reduced damage by 50 percent. After 240 minutes, damage was still reduced by 35 percent. NXY-059 is thought to act by interrupting a sequence of brain-damaging chemical events that occur in the brain after a stroke. British studies have shown similar results in monkeys.

Trials reported in March 2001 that tested the safety of NXY-059 in people have revealed that the drug is well tolerated when given to patients with acute stroke (the early stage of a stroke). Future clinical trials will test how effective the drug is in people.

Stem Cell Miracles

Researchers at Albert Einstein College of Medicine in New York, working with rats, recently transplanted stem cells into their damaged brains after inducing stroke to see whether the stem cells— those magicians found in embryos and bone marrow that can transform into any kind of cell the body needs—would mature into new nerve cells and other healthy brain tissue. And they did.

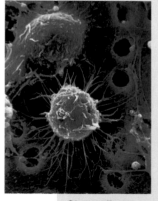

Now, researchers are investigating what factors, such as scar tissue in the brain after stroke, or the particular location of the damage, help or hinder stem cell growth. A better understanding of these factors might someday enable human stem cells to be used to grow new brain tissue in people after they have experienced a stroke.

Stem cells are primitive cells that can develop into many types of tissue.

Surgical Solution

New Laser Surgery for Varicose Veins

Femoral artery

Femoral vein

Laser

Greater saphenous vein

An intense red light is used to aim the laser before the heat is turned on.

▶ EVLT uses heat to seal off the greater saphenous vein, which eliminates the cause of varicose veins.

L aser therapy has been widely available for what are called spider veins, those tiny varicose veins on the surface of the skin, often on the face, that look like creepy crawlers. But for the bigger, gnarly varicose veins caused by broken valves in the deep veins of the leg, only surgery or sclerotherapy (injecting a chemical into the vein to close it up) had been tried—until now. In March 2001, researchers led by Robert J. Min, M.D., at Cornell University in New York, reported excellent results with a new laser surgery technique called EndoVenous Laser Treatment (EVLT). While surgery to "strip" the bad vein fails 10 percent of the time, and sclerotherapy needs to be repeated in 50 percent of patients, EVLT showed a remarkable 99 percent success rate that held up almost completely one year later.

How it works. Laser is a form of light that, unlike sunlight or light bulbs, can be narrowly focused into a scalpel-sharp beam. A surgeon can direct this laser beam at the deep leg vein that's causing the backup of blood, and use its heat to seal off the vein. Smaller, surrounding veins then pick up the work of the sealed vein. Min notes that although there is some bruising and soreness after the procedure, there are no complications, and EVLT has "lower risks, no scars, and a shorter recovery period" when compared with surgery.

Availability. Finding a surgeon trained in the new procedure and a medical center with the expensive, high-tech laser equipment to do it are half the battle. The other is coming up with the $2,000 to pay for it, since medical plans often consider varicose veins a cosmetic problem. Traditional surgery, though, would cost closer to $6,000, so it may be money well spent. Min expects the laser surgery to quickly gain popularity, with thousands of patients undergoing the procedure over the next year.

FAST FACTS
50 Percentage of people over age 50 who suffer from varicose veins **Leg crossing** One probable cause of tiny spider veins **50** Percentage increase in risk of leg ulcers or blood clots in the legs in people who have varicose veins **Pregnancy** Common trigger of varicose veins

MENTAL HEALTH

Patients at more than a dozen medical centers are wearing tiny, implantable generators as part of a study to see if brain stimulation can jolt a person out of the depths of depression. And because this ailment is being recast as a chronic condition, like asthma, people who suffer its periodic lows can now take a once-a-week formulation of the antidepressant Prozac to keep them on an even keel. Other exciting breakthroughs in the field of mental health: Alcoholics may be able to stem the craving for that next drink by taking a drug currently given to chemotherapy patients to stop nausea. And people suffering from obsessive-compulsive disorder could one day soon gain control of their symptoms by taking a certain painkiller. Finally, if you're trying to quit smoking, don't go it alone. According to the latest report from the U.S. Surgeon General, your chances of succeeding are much greater if you get help from your doctor, a counselor, or a support group—and use one of the medications available to help you kick the habit.

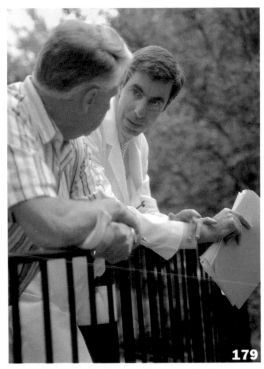

179

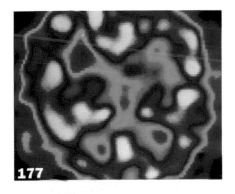

177

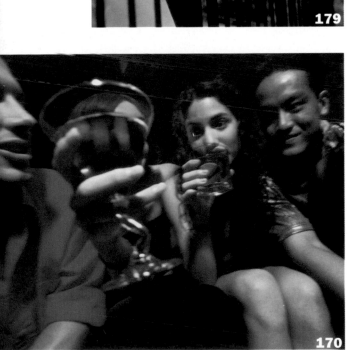

170

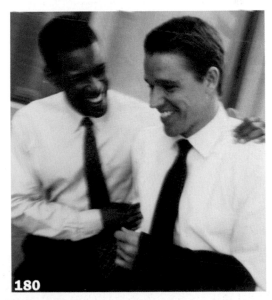

180

Drug Development
Drug Curbs Craving for Alcohol

What if an alcoholic could turn off the craving for that next drink simply by popping a pill? Soon certain alcoholics may be able to. The drug, called ondansetron (brand name Zofran), is currently used to treat nausea in chemotherapy patients. Now a study conducted at the University of Texas Health Science Center at San Antonio, published in the *Journal of the American Medical Association* on August 23, 2000, suggests that it can stem the cravings experienced by people with early-onset alcohol dependence—the hardest type of alcoholism to treat.

Early-onset alcoholism occurs before age 25 and tends to be particularly tenacious and severe. Compared with people who develop alcoholism at a later age, people with early-onset alcoholism are more likely to have a family history of alcoholism and to engage in antisocial behavior. Early-onset alcoholism tends to be quite resistant to behavioral therapy alone, making a drug alternative even more crucial to successful treatment.

The Texas study followed 271 alcoholics and compared ondansetron at three different dosages with a placebo. All participants received weekly group cognitive-behavioral therapy—which aims at changing thought patterns that trigger or increase anxiety—as well as the drug. People taking the middle dose experienced the best results; they went

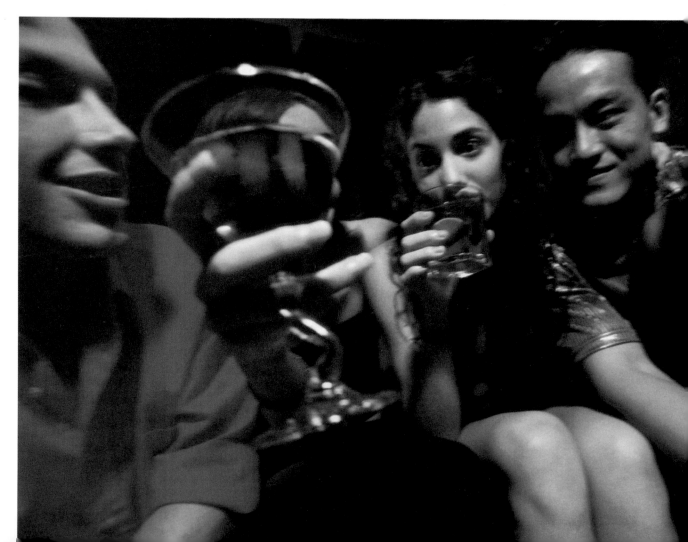

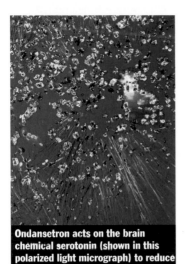

Ondansetron acts on the brain chemical serotonin (shown in this polarized light micrograph) to reduce the craving for alcohol.

longer without drinking and had fewer drinks overall. Participants with late-onset alcoholism did not gain any significant benefits from ondansetron.

How it works. Chemicals within the brain, called neurotransmitters, transmit messages concerning mood, thoughts, memories, sleep patterns, pain, pleasure, and emotional well-being. Two neurotransmitters—serotonin and dopamine—are believed to be particularly important in regulating emotion and behavior in all people. Those who develop early-onset alcoholism seem to have a biologic predisposition to alcoholism, and their craving for alcohol is thought to be caused by an imbalance between dopamine and serotonin. The drug ondansetron works on the transmission of serotonin in the brain, thereby restoring the chemical balance between the two neurotransmitters.

Availability. Ondansetron has been approved by the U.S. Food and Drug Administration for chemotherapy-induced nausea. More studies must be carried out before it can be prescribed for alcoholism.

◀ Alcoholism that starts before age 25 is especially hard to overcome. An existing nausea drug may help.

FAST FACTS

50 Percentage of people who relapse at least once after receiving treatment for alcoholism
25 Percentage of Americans who need treatment for alcohol and substance abuse who will receive it **25** Percentage of deaths in 15- to 29-year-old males in Europe attributable to alcohol
14 MILLION Number of Americans who have been diagnosed as alcohol dependent or alcohol abusers

STAY TUNED FOR...

Relapse Insurance

The drug acamprosate (brand name Campral) is widely used in Europe to help recovering alcoholics avoid relapse. Now it is undergoing clinical trials in the United States. Like other medications that work to head off relapse in recovering alcoholics, acamprosate reduces the intensity of craving and curbs the pleasurable effects of drinking, allowing people to remain abstinent until they can muster sufficient self-motivation.

Unlike disulfiram (brand name Antabuse) and other drug treatments, acamprosate will not cause unpleasant reactions—specifically, vomiting—when any type of alcohol is ingested. Nor will it produce many of the other serious or intolerable side effects associated with other drugs.

Acamprosate offers an option for recovering alcoholics for whom other medications don't work. Because it is not substantially metabolized in the liver, it can be used even when a patient has liver disease. And it doesn't appear to interact with other medications frequently used to treat alcoholism or with antidepressant, antianxiety, or hypnotic (sleep) medications.

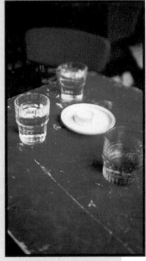

A new drug may help recovering alcoholics stay sober.

Final Answers

The U.S. National Institute on Alcohol Abuse and Alcoholism (NIAAA) has launched a nationwide study to compare the effectiveness of behavioral treatments alone with the effectiveness of these treatments in combination with drugs to treat alcohol dependence. Based in 11 universities and named COMBINE (Combining Medications and Behavioral Interventions), this extensive research effort reflects the NIAAA's belief that the first priority of research needs to be identifying and developing effective treatments for alcoholism. The NIAAA is recruiting over 1,300 people to participate in this study; recruitment began in early 2001 and will continue for two years. People interested in participating can call 866-80-STUDY to find out if they are eligible.

Key Finding
Do Cigarettes Make You Nervous?

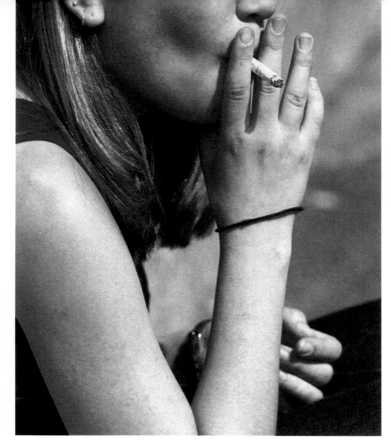

The common conception is that cigarettes settle the nerves. But a recent study looked at the links between smoking and anxiety disorders in adolescence and young adulthood and found that heavy cigarette smoking during adolescence increases the risk of developing generalized anxiety disorder (feelings of excessive anxiety accompanied by physical symptoms), agoraphobia (irrational fear of going out in public), and panic disorder.

Published in the November 8, 2000, issue of the *Journal of the American Medical Association,* the study found that for people who smoked 20 or more cigarettes per day, there was a 20.5 percent risk for developing generalized anxiety disorder versus 3.7 percent in nonsmokers; a 10.3 percent risk of agoraphobia versus 1.8 percent in nonsmokers; and approximately 8 percent risk for panic disorder versus less than 1 percent in nonsmokers. On the other hand, youngsters who smoked fewer than 20 cigarettes per day were not at increased risk for early-adulthood anxiety disorders. Nor was there a noticeable correlation between smoking and social anxiety and obsessive-compulsive disorder, a chronic condition in which a person is plagued by intrusive, recurrent thoughts and displays uncontrollable repetitive behavior.

Both cigarette smoking and anxiety disorders become increasingly common during the teenage years. That fact makes it difficult to discern whether having an anxiety disorder leads to increased smoking or whether smoking leads to anxiety disorders. Nevertheless, there is a growing body of literature suggesting that smoking is one of the factors that lead to the development of these disorders.

▲ A new study shows that people who smoke heavily as teens are at higher risk for anxiety disorders.

RESEARCH ROUNDUP

■ **TREATING PANIC DISORDERS.** The importance of psychotherapy in treating panic disorders was reaffirmed in a study reported in the December 2000 *Medical Journal of Malaysia.* This study found that people whose treatment combined therapy with medication did best, both immediately and over time. People who were on medication alone—in this case fluvoxamine (brand name Luvox)—showed significant improvement over time but did not show as much improvement as people who received only cognitive-behavioral therapy. In addition, whenever therapy was added to the mix, less medication was needed than when medication was used alone.

FAST FACTS
2 : 1 Ratio of women to men who are likely to have a panic disorder, generalized anxiety disorder, agoraphobia, or specific phobia **DEPRESSION, EATING DISORDERS, SUBSTANCE ABUSE** Other disorders that are likely to occur along with anxiety disorders **13** Percentage of people between the ages of 18 and 54 who suffer from anxiety disorders **2** Percentage of people between 18 and 54 who experience a panic disorder in any given year

Drug Development

Like Asthma, Depression May Be Chronic Illness

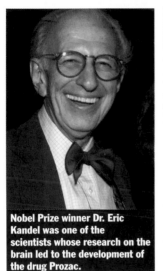

Nobel Prize winner Dr. Eric Kandel was one of the scientists whose research on the brain led to the development of the drug Prozac.

For years, the medical and psychiatric communities have approached depression as if it were an episodic condition: Treat the lows when they hit, then when things even out again, suspend treatment. However, a study published in the March 2001 issue of the *Archives of General Psychiatry* suggests that even people who have "recovered" from depression after successful treatment are likely to relapse. People who have experienced one bout of depression stand a 50 percent chance of relapse. After two bouts, the chance of relapse goes up to 80 percent, and after three episodes, the chance of becoming depressed again is 90 percent.

As a result, scientists and clinicians are rethinking depression, recasting it as a chronic illness, much like asthma, diabetes, or high blood pressure. This, in turn, would affect treatment, meaning that the goal would be to manage the condition rather than necessarily cure it. And now the company that manufactures the antidepressant fluoxetine (brand name Prozac) has developed a new, once-a-week formulation of the drug, making long-term use less cumbersome and making it more likely that patients will stick with their drug regimen.

How it works. The new formulation of fluoxetine (brand name Prozac Weekly) has a special coating that dissolves only once the pill works its way down to a segment of the intestines where the pH exceeds 5.5 (the pill does not dissolve in the more acidic—lower pH—environment of the stomach). The release of the drug is therefore delayed by up to two hours compared with the daily formula, and the effects last for the entire week.

Availability. Approved by the U.S. Food and Drug Administration in March 2001, Prozac Weekly is suitable for preventing relapse in people who have already successfully treated their depression.

STAY TUNED FOR...

Better Treatments for Bipolar Disorder

The U.S. National Institute of Mental Health is sponsoring the largest research study for bipolar disorder ever conducted. The Systematic Treatment Enhancement Program for Bipolar Disorder (STEP-BD) is a $22 million, five-year outpatient study aimed at assessing and improving current treatments for bipolar disorder. Coordinated through Massachusetts General Hospital in Boston, trials are being conducted in 17 U.S. cities. For more information, visit the website www.nimh.nih.gov/studies/STEP-BD.cfm, or e-mail stepbdinfo@mail.nih.gov.

Pacemaker for the Brain

Cyberonics of Houston, Texas, has named 2002 as the year we'll see the results of a major study on vagus nerve stimulation (VNS) for the treatment of depression. The vagus nerve, located in the neck, carries important information to and from the brain—information that regulates sleep, heartbeat, and mood, among other things. The 94 participants in the study are patients with chronic depression who have been implanted with the VNS generator. The tiny device, which is inserted under the skin of the upper chest, acts like a pacemaker for the brain; it sends mild electrical impulses along tiny wires to stimulate the vagus nerve for 30 seconds every five minutes throughout the day and night. These nerve impulses in turn stimulate areas of the brain thought to be connected to mood.

Depression therapy

Originally designed to treat severe epilepsy, a pacemaker-like device has been found to relieve some symptoms of severe depression.

❶ A small generator that emits electrical signals is placed in the patient's chest.

❷ Signals stimulate the vagus nerve, which relays messages between the brain and the organs.

❸ The vagus nerve extends deep into the area of the brain that is thought to regulate mood and emotion.

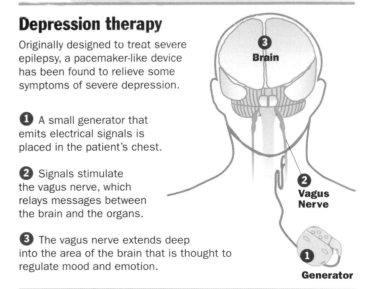

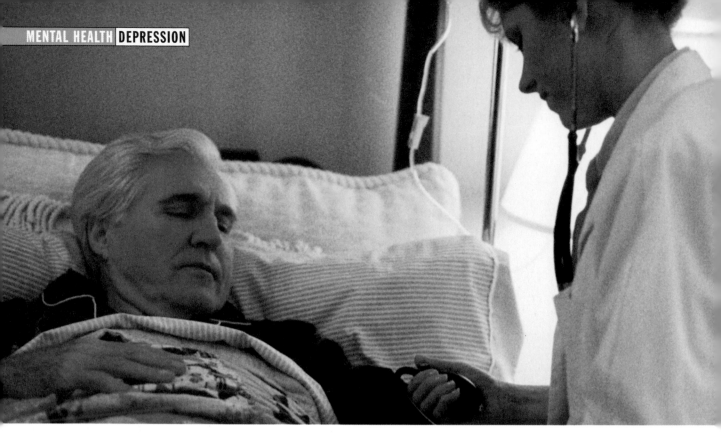

Key Finding
Depression Is Bad for Your Health

▲ If you have heart disease, diabetes, or another ailment, depression can make your condition worse.

There's new evidence that your mood affects your physical health. During a March 2001 forum held by the National Institute of Mental Health, clinicians and researchers presented new evidence that depression strongly influences the course of other major illnesses, including cancer, diabetes, heart disease, stroke, HIV/AIDS, and Parkinson's disease. People who live in the shadow of depression are less likely to lead healthy lifestyles—they tend not to eat as well, get enough sleep, or exercise. They also lack the motivation or energy to comply with complicated treatment plans.

Researchers also found that on the cellular level, depression disrupts various neurotransmitters (brain messenger chemicals) such as serotonin and dopamine. This disruption affects, among other things, the progression of Parkinson's and other neurological (nervous system) diseases. Depression also triggers the release of stress hormones that can act on the cardiovascular system and affect blood clotting, contributing to heart disease. And depression can suppress the immune system, making it harder for the body to fight back against cancer and HIV/AIDS.

With this new research, it is becoming ever clearer that, for the millions of people suffering from depression, seeking timely and effective treatment isn't just about improving their mood—it's about protecting their health.

> **FAST FACTS**
> **MAJOR DEPRESSIVE DISORDER** Leading cause of disability in the United States and in many parts of the world
> **9.5** Percentage of adults affected by clinical depression each year **70** Percentage of those suffering from major depression who can fully recover if properly treated

RESEARCH ROUNDUP

■ **SHINING THE SPOTLIGHT ON SAD.** When it comes to using light therapy for seasonal affective disorder (SAD), it's not just the wattage but the timing that counts. Researchers at Columbia University's College of Physicians and Surgeons and the New York State Psychiatric Institute found that when treatments are timed to correspond to the body's internal clock, the antidepressant effects are dramatically heightened. Doing it early in the morning is best—specifically, 30 minutes of intense, bright light (with no ultraviolet radiation).

■ **DETECTING BIPOLAR DISORDER IN CHILDREN.** Bipolar disorder, also called manic-depressive disorder, isn't usually identified until late adolescence or early adulthood. But a study published in October 2000 indicates that recognizing the signs early on—perhaps even in infancy— could bring about early intervention. When medical records of adults with bipolar disorder were reviewed, researchers found telling "clusters" of symptoms that often dated back to the earliest years of life, including episodes of depression, irritability, and sleep problems. Identifying these symptoms in children may lead to early treatment for bipolar disorder. It may also help avoid unnecessary detours in addressing the problem, such as mistaking the condition for attention deficit-hyperactivity disorder.

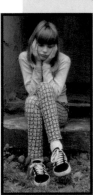

A recent study has shown that symptoms of bipolar disorder often appear in childhood.

■ **PREVENTING RELAPSE AFTER SHOCK TREATMENT.** Depression that is severe, recurrent, and unresponsive to other treatments often yields to electroconvulsive therapy (ECT). Unfortunately, the occurrence of relapse is common within six months following ECT. A new study out of New York State Psychiatric Institute has found that the use of the antidepressant nortriptyline in conjunction with lithium greatly counters the risk of early relapse.

Drug Development
Painkiller is New Weapon against Obsessive-Compulsive Disorder

The painkilling drug tramadol (brand name Ultram) is an unexpected new weapon in the fight against obsessive-compulsive disorder (OCD), a chronic and often disabling condition characterized by recurrent and intrusive obsessions, impulses, and often by uncontrollable repetitive behavior. While not a cure, tramadol may relieve between 30 and 60 percent of OCD symptoms according to a small study conducted at the University of Florida in Gainesville.

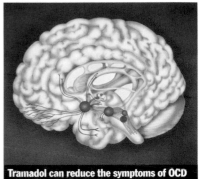

Tramadol can reduce the symptoms of OCD by binding to the brain's opiate receptors.

How it works. Tramadol is an analgesic (pain reliever) with a mode of action that is not completely understood. It is as effective as opiates (narcotics) in relieving pain, but it is not nearly as addictive as these drugs. It has been discovered that many people with OCD have a particularly sensitive opiate system—a part of the analgesic center of the brain. By binding to the opiate receptors, tramadol can reduce the symptoms of OCD.

The potential benefits of tramadol must be carefully weighed against possible, though rare, side effects, including light-headedness, nausea, headache, increased anxiety, and rapid heart rate. In addition, tramadol should not be taken with alcohol or used with other central nervous system depressants or antidepressant drugs.

Availability. Tramadol has been approved by the U.S. Food and Drug Administration for pain relief and is now being tested in OCD.

RESEARCH ROUNDUP

■ **EQUATION FOR SOLVING OCD.** When it comes to treating OCD, medication plus therapy most often equals success. Researchers in Great Neck, New York, report that children and teenagers with OCD who participated in cognitive-behavioral therapy (which aims at changing thought patterns that trigger increased anxiety) and who took fluvoxamine (brand name Luvox) improved significantly in comparison to children who received only medication. A two-year follow-up study found that all patients, including those who received only medication, continued to improve, but those who used both medication and therapy noticeably improved more.

Drug Development
Schizophrenia Drug Gets a Second Look

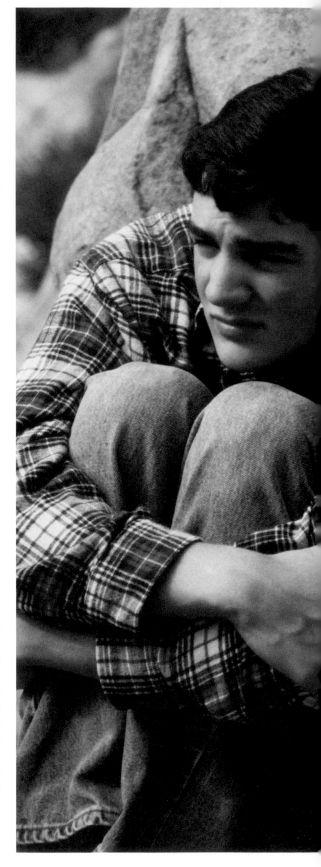

Many of the most popular medications used to treat schizophrenia have been around since the 1950s. However, in recent years, "atypical" anti-psychotic medications have been gaining currency in treating schizophrenia, especially in its early stages. Indeed, a new study shows that these drugs may actually work better than the "typical" ones.

A recent collaborative effort between Chinese and American researchers suggests that clozapine (brand name Clozaril) works faster and more effectively than the conventional treatment chlorpromazine (brand name Thorazine). Patients are also more likely to stick with clozapine because it causes fewer and less problematic side effects. In fact, it appears that people who are treated immediately with clozapine are more likely to recover from the illness and less likely to experience a second episode, as long as they stay on the medication.

> **Patients are more likely to stick with clozapine because it causes fewer and less problematic side effects.**

How it works. The atypical anti-psychotic medications target specific brain chemicals differently than the older typical anti-psychotic drugs do. For example, clozapine binds to different receptors for the brain chemical dopamine, and it affects serotonin, another brain chemical, as well. A higher-than-normal level of dopamine in particular seems to affect reality perception. Clozapine helps correct the chemical imbalances that cause the type of disordered thought associated with schizophrenia.

Availability. Clozapine has been available for over 10 years, but in some countries, including the United States, its use has been restricted due to a rare but dangerous side effect called agranulocytosis. This condition causes a dramatic drop in white blood cell production that interferes with the body's ability to ward off disease. When the drug is prescribed, it is necessary to monitor for this effect weekly. If agranulocytosis develops, treatment is promptly stopped; in most cases, this reverses the problem. The American-Chinese study argues for the use of clozapine as a first-line choice of treatment, specifically for people who can follow the rigorous monitoring required.

▶ **A recent study casts new light on what drugs work best in treating schizophrenia.**

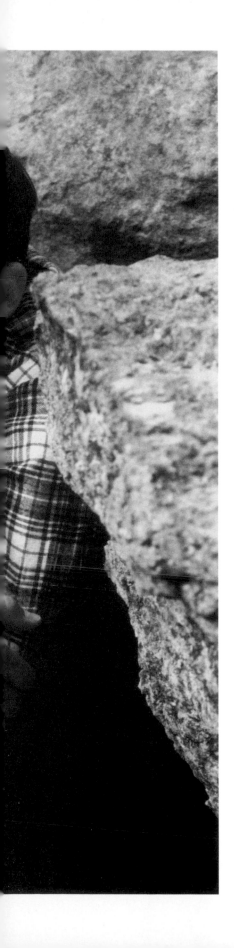

Drug Development
Anti-Psychotic Medication Finally Wins Approval

Ziprasidone (brand name Geodon) has joined the ranks of "atypical" anti-psychotic drugs in the arsenal against schizophrenia. Despite the fact that the U.S. Food and Drug Administration (FDA) refused to approve the drug in 1998, the agency has now okayed it, asserting that the possible benefits outweigh the risks. The agency's reservation is due to a possible link between the drug and QT prolongation—a heart rhythm irregularity that can cause a potentially fatal heart condition called torsade de pointes. Aside from this potential problem, ziprasidone's side effect profile is better than other similar medications. It does not

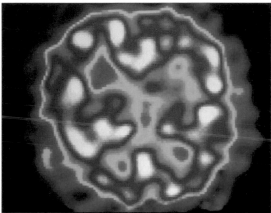

An imbalance in the brain chemical serotonin (highlighted in this MRI brain scan) seems to play a part in schizophrenia.

RESEARCH ROUNDUP

■ **ESTROGEN FOR SCHIZOPHRENIA.** Scientists have long noted that women with schizophrenia tend to have their first psychotic episode at a later age than men. Women are also prone to relapse following childbirth and during menopause. All this suggests a link between low estrogen levels and susceptibility to schizophrenia. Now an Australian study has confirmed that wearing an estrogen patch may reduce schizophrenia symptoms in women. In the study, women began improving after wearing the patch for only four or five days. At the end of 28 days, the results were dramatic. Women who wore a patch and took anti-psychotic drugs improved even more. If the study's findings hold, doctors will likely recommend that women with a history of schizophrenia receive hormone replacement therapy as they approach menopause to prevent psychotic relapse or to increase the therapeutic effects of anti-psychotic drugs.

increase the risk of developing type 2 diabetes, and neither does it cause weight gain—a side effect that prompts many people to decide to stop taking their medication.

How it works. Scientists are not certain how ziprasidone works. It is thought to reduce schizophrenia's "positive" symptoms (such as

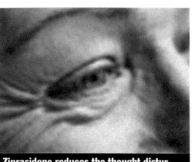

Ziprasidone reduces the thought disturbances of people with schizophrenia and helps them experience pleasure again.

visual and auditory hallucinations, delusions, and thought disturbances) by blocking the action of the brain chemicals serotonin and dopamine at specific chemical receptors in the brain. The drug also improves the "negative" symptoms of schizophrenia such as social withdrawal, apathy, lack of motivation, and an inability to experience pleasure. However, because ziprasidone takes two to four weeks to achieve an effect, scientists feel that the drug's affect on the serotonin system may be complex and indirect.

Availability. Approved by the FDA in February 2001, ziprasidone is available in the United States as well as in other countries. It is marketed as Zeldox in Sweden and in other parts of Europe.

STAY TUNED FOR...

A Blood Test for Schizophrenia

Scientists at the Weizmann Institute in Israel are on the verge of developing a blood test that may yield early and precise diagnosis of schizophrenia. According to a report published in the January 16, 2001, issue of *Proceedings of the National Academy of Sciences,* it may now be possible to measure the number of dopamine receptors in the blood of schizophrenics. Postmortem (autopsy) and PET brain scan analysis of patients have indi-

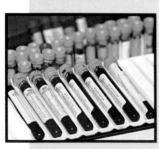

cated a high count of dopamine receptors in the brains of people with schizophrenia—a sign of excessive activity of the brain chemical dopamine. But a simple method to measure dopamine receptors in the brain is not available. Now a blood test that measures the molecules involved in generating dopamine receptors could provide an easy and reliable marker for schizophrenia. Whenever diagnosis is made early, treatment can be immediate and therefore more effective. Further studies will be conducted to determine whether the levels of these receptors relate to how the disease progresses. If this is the case, a blood test could monitor changes in the patient's condition as well as diagnose it at the onset.

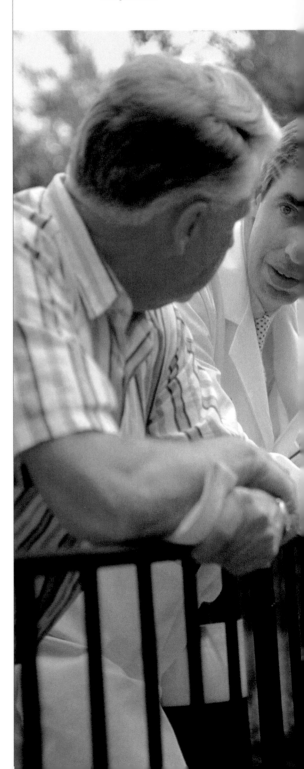

▼ People have greater success in quitting smoking when their doctors are involved in the process.

Progress in Prevention

Trying to Quit? Your Doctor Could Be Your Best Friend

W hen it comes to quitting smoking, your doctor can help. That's one of the messages in the U.S. Surgeon General's latest report on curbing tobacco use. According to the report, whenever a doctor recommends and monitors a multiple-approach smoking cessation plan, the likelihood that the patient will be successful increases.

The report is the first of its kind to provide an in-depth analysis of the effectiveness of various methods to reduce tobacco use. It is unequivocal in its assertion of the importance of the human factor in promoting smoking cessation. Tobacco dependence counseling that involves person-to-person contact, either through individual, group, or telephone counseling, was found to be uniformly effective. In fact, the greater the human contact, the more likely it is that efforts to quit will be successful.

What works. The government panel found three types of counseling and behavioral therapies to be particularly effective:

- **Practical counseling,** such as problem solving, skills training, or cognitive-behavioral therapy
- **Support groups**
- **Social support** outside of treatment, such as regular phone contact or a buddy system.

A number of medications exist to help people quit. The panel recommends that, unless there is some contraindication, all patients attempting to kick the habit should be offered one of these drugs.

Five first-tier medications have been shown to increase long-term success rates:

- **Bupropion SR**
- **Nicotine gum**
- **Nicotine inhaler**
- **Nicotine nasal spray**
- **Nicotine patch.**

Two second-tier medications have been shown to be effective when first-tier medications do not work:

- **Clonidine**
- **Nortriptyline.**

Overall, the Surgeon General's guidelines are based on the firm belief that anyone who wants to quit can—especially when health care professionals get involved. That belief is backed up by the panel's search of electronic databases, which yielded the conclusions of 6,000 published scientific articles on the subject of tobacco-use intervention.

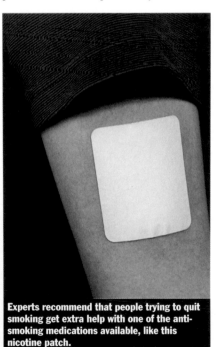

Experts recommend that people trying to quit smoking get extra help with one of the anti-smoking medications available, like this nicotine patch.

Alternative Answers

Friends—Nature's Stress Busters

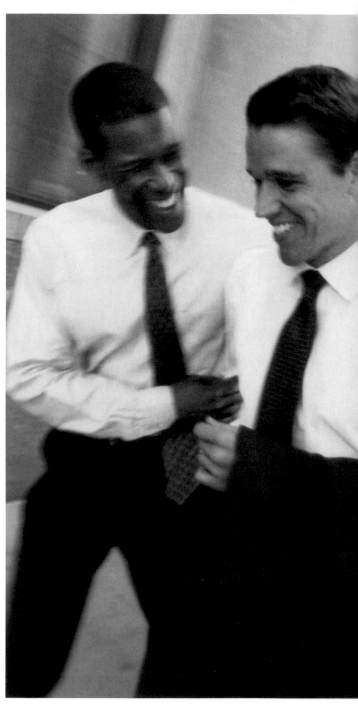

▼ A new study indicates that in men the anti-stress hormone oxytocin is enhanced by friendship.

There's no question that having a good friend around during times of stress can help relieve the pressure. Now researchers at the University of Zurich, Switzerland, are beginning to understand just how friendship acts to trigger and enhance chemicals in the brain that, in turn, help people cope with stress better.

The results of this study, presented at the March 2001 meeting of the American Psychosomatic Society, suggest that a single hormone, called oxytocin, plays a key role in protecting us from the physical costs wrought by stressful situations. And friendship seems to enhance the stress-busting benefits of the hormone.

> **Oxytocin plays a key role in protecting us from the physical costs wrought by stressful situations. And friendship seems to enhance the stress-busting benefits of the hormone.**

Boosting nature's defenses. Oxytocin is the body's own anti-stress hormone. Like adrenaline, it is generated in response to a real or perceived threat. The hormone not only guards against stress and anxiety, it also fosters maternal and social attachment. Scientists have long noted that animals with high blood levels of the hormone tend to be calmer, more relaxed, and more social.

In women, oxytocin is enhanced by the female hormone estrogen. Oxytocin is the reason a woman may feel calm and relaxed when breast-feeding, since the baby's sucking stimulates the release of the hormone in the brain and bloodstream in both mother and child. This encourages milk production and lowers levels of the stress hormone cortisol in the breast milk.

In contrast, oxytocin is inhibited by male hormones. Therefore, it may not induce calm as effectively in men — unless, according to the study, they have the support of a good friend during stressful times.

Helping men cope. The study followed 40 healthy men who received either the hormone oxytocin or a placebo as a nasal spray, with or without social support from their best friend, prior to being asked to perform a stressful task (giving an unrehearsed speech or doing mental arithmetic before an audience). The friends were instructed to offer moral support during a 10-minute period before the event. Stress levels were then gauged with a questionnaire and by measuring cortisol levels in the saliva.

The researchers found that when men were given oxytocin and had the support of a friend, they experienced a reduction in stress similar to that experienced by nursing women. Even more interesting, the nasal spray by itself—without the friend's support—provided no benefit, but having the best friend present (without the oxytocin) was the second-best technique.

Investigators are currently researching the uses of oxytocin-related drug interventions—that is, medications that would help counteract the effects of our highly stressful and, at times, anxiety-provoking lives. In the meantime, finding solace in the company of others is still the best cure for what stresses us.

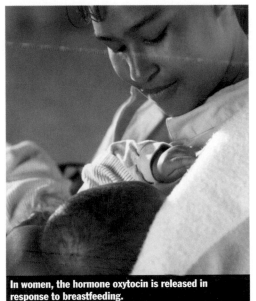

In women, the hormone oxytocin is released in response to breastfeeding.

RESEARCH ROUNDUP

■ **STRESS THERAPY.** Does stress have a hold on you? Try a stress management technique such as autogenic training (a self-relaxation practice), biofeedback, anxiety management, and type A hostile behavior reduction. According to a report published in the April 23, 2001, issue of the *Archives of Internal Medicine*, the benefits of all of these techniques show up almost immediately in the form of lower blood pressure. Specifically, researchers found that adults with high blood pressure had significantly lower pressure after only 10 weeks of therapy. At a six-month follow up, blood pressure levels were still lower. In addition, several people who showed no immediate benefits had lower blood pressure readings later on.

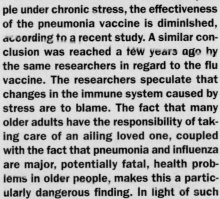

A recent study confirms that stress management techniques, like self-relaxation, really work.

■ **STRESS AND VACCINES.** In older people under chronic stress, the effectiveness of the pneumonia vaccine is diminished, according to a recent study. A similar conclusion was reached a few years ago by the same researchers in regard to the flu vaccine. The researchers speculate that changes in the immune system caused by stress are to blame. The fact that many older adults have the responsibility of taking care of an ailing loved one, coupled with the fact that pneumonia and influenza are major, potentially fatal, health problems in older people, makes this a particularly dangerous finding. In light of such health implications, the investigators recommend that doctors direct their vaccine candidates toward stress reduction programs and that patients try to get the vaccine during a low-stress period.

FAST FACTS
75 TO 90 Percentage of all doctor's visits that are for stress-related ailments and complaints
PROBLEMS AT WORK The life stressor that outranks financial and family problems as the culprit in health complaints **75** Percentage of employees who believe that work is more stressful than it was a generation ago **STRESS** Risk factor to which the six leading causes of death——heart disease, cancer, lung ailments, accidents, cirrhosis of the liver, suicide——are all linked

MUSCLES, BONES, AND JOINTS

I t's hard to walk tall when your bones are brittle or your joints are crippled with arthritis pain, but new developments in the past year should help. On the arthritis front, there's finally proof that people who take the natural supplement glucosamine to ease pain and slow the deterioration of joints are doing themselves a favor. New research provides a better understanding of the mysterious diseases chronic fatigue syndrome and fibromyalgia, which may some day lead to effective treatments. And a better test for Lyme disease can tell you once and for all whether or not you have the condition—even if you've had the Lyme disease vaccine. If you have persistent or recurrent Lyme disease, there's new reason to think twice about taking more antibiotics. For people with severe osteoporosis, a new surgical technique promises to make life a little easier. Finally, thanks to a recent discovery about lupus, one company is testing a drug that could nip the disease in the bud.

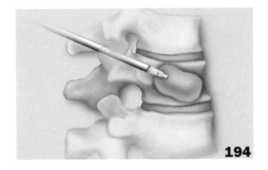

194

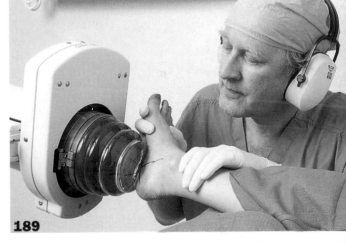

189

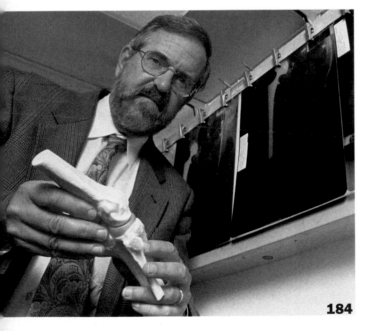

184

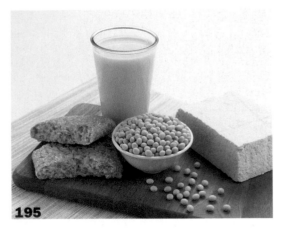

195

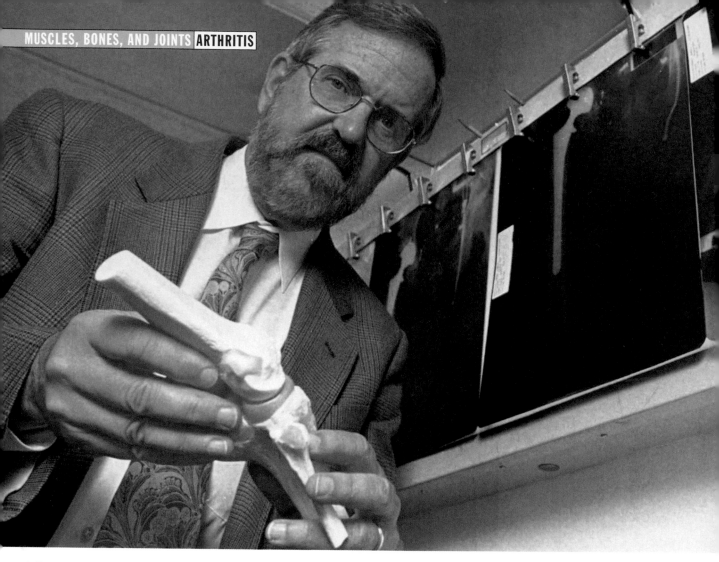

Alternative Answers

Study Backs Use of Glucosamine for Arthritis

C hances are you know someone who takes glucosamine for arthritis. The dietary supplement became an overnight sensation when it was hyped in *The Arthritis Cure* in 1997. Since then, its popularity has continued to grow. But does it work?

New evidence says yes. In January 27, 2001, the journal *The Lancet* published results from a three-year study that examined the benefits of taking glucosamine for osteoarthritis (the most common type of arthritis, characterized by the breakdown of the cartilage of a joint). The study, conducted by a team of researchers in Belgium, Italy, and the United Kingdom, followed 212 patients with osteoarthritis. Half of them took 1,500 mg of glucosamine sulfate every day for three years, and the other half took a placebo (a sugar pill). The result? Glucosamine slows the progression of arthritis. The people who took the supplement maintained better joint function and experienced less pain than those in the placebo group, who experienced further loss of cartilage.

What is glucosamine? Glucosamine is a naturally occurring amino sugar found in relatively large amounts in the joints and connective tissues, where the body uses it to

◀ **David S. Hungerford, M.D., is among the orthopedists who have championed the use of glucosamine and chondroitin for people with arthritis. Now studies are confirming that these supplements really do work.**

form the larger molecules needed for cartilage development and repair. The supplement form is derived from tissue found in crab, lobster, and shrimp shells; therefore, people who are allergic to shellfish should talk to their doctor before taking glucosamine. Another caveat: Not all glucosamine products necessarily work as well as the one used in the study. Because dietary supplements are unregulated, the quality and content of products vary widely.

Adding chondroitin to the mix. Should you take glucosamine alone, or combined with the other popular joint-maintenance supplement, chondroitin? Researchers may soon know the answer. A large study, the first of its kind, is under way to determine whether these substances are more effective taken alone or in combination. A total of 1,588 people will be enrolled at 13 different clinical centers around the United States. The study is being conducted by two branches of the National Institutes of Health (NIH)—the National Center for Complementary and Alternative Medicine (NCCAM) and the National Institute of Arthritis and Musculoskeletal and Skin Disease (NIAMS)—and is being funded largely by money earmarked by Congress. The final report is due March 2005.

New hope for stiff joints

New research suggests that the progression of osteoarthritis, a form of arthritis characterized by cartilage deterioration, can be slowed by taking the nutritional supplement glucosamine sulfate.

HEALTHY JOINT

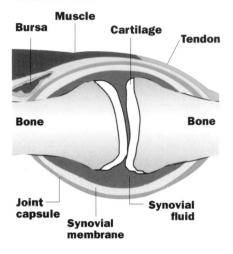

OSTEOARTHRITIC JOINT

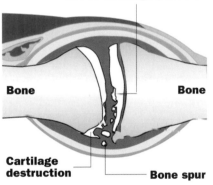

Glucosamine is a simple naturally occurring molecule that plays a significant role in the structure of cartilage and other connective tissues.

Alternative Answers
Have a Little Faith— Studies Show It Helps

There's one alternative to painkillers for arthritis pain that you won't find at your local drugstore, although you might find it at your local house of worship. Researchers from seven leading medical universities and institutes around the United States recently reported that people who used positive religious and spiritual strategies such as meditation and prayer in order to feel closer to God and to help them cope with their disease were able to decrease the amount of pain they experienced on a daily basis.

In the study, published in the *Journal of Pain* in April 2001, 35 people who were diagnosed with rheumatoid arthritis were asked to maintain a record of their daily routines. In this diary they noted their spiritual and/or religious experiences, their moods, and their levels of arthritis pain, as well as how they coped with that pain. The results suggested that people who practiced daily positive spiritual experiences were more likely to be in better moods and have a stronger social support network. These two factors seemed to help them deal with the pain of their condition.

Wrote the researchers in the report, "One might expect that people coping with chronic illness or chronic pain might find it difficult to maintain a positive outlook or feel connected to God or the beauty of life. The results of this study suggest otherwise."

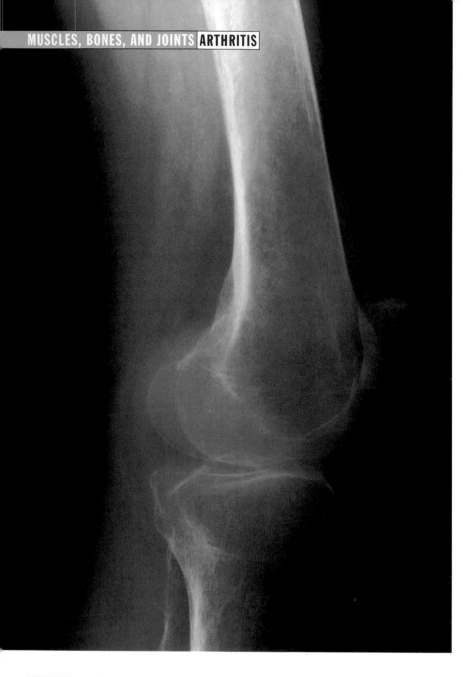

◄ **Arthritis mainly affects cartilage, which has no pain sensors. So why does it hurt? The answer may lie in the bone marrow.**

Key Finding
Feeling It in Your Bones— But Why?

The source of arthritis pain has puzzled researchers for years because arthritis primarily affects bone-cushioning cartilage, which is devoid of any pain-sensing fibers. But a study published in the *Annals of Internal Medicine* on April 3, 2001, has pinpointed a possible culprit.

In the study, researchers from Boston University School of Medicine found that the MRIs of participants who had painful osteoarthritis more often showed lesions (abnormalities or bruising) on their bone marrow, the spongy tissue found in the large bones of the body, than those with nonpainful osteoarthritis. Of the 351 patients with knee pain, 78 percent had lesions, but only 30 percent of the 50 patients without knee pain had lesions; in addition, large lesions were found almost exclusively in those with knee pain. No correlation was found between the severity of pain and the presence of lesions.

As is often the case, the study provides more questions—such as what causes the lesions in the first place—than it does answers. But the finding may help explain why people with arthritis feel more pain at night than during the day: Bone marrow lesions incurred during daytime activity may have a delayed reaction, causing more discomfort hours later.

Scientists are hoping that further investigation of bone marrow lesions will lead to improved treatment of osteoarthritis.

RESEARCH ROUNDUP

■ **BAD NEWS ABOUT CHUNKY HEELS.** New research published in *The Lancet* on April 7, 2001, revealed that high-heeled shoes with wide ("chunky") heels are just as hard on your knees as stilettos. The study's authors found that both types of shoes applied equal amounts of pressure to the knees. Compared with walking barefoot, the wide heels increased pressure on the inside of the knee by 26 percent—and this increased pressure on the knee may lead to injury in a joint prone to osteoarthritis.

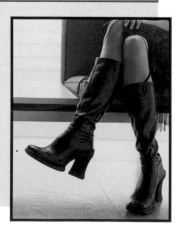

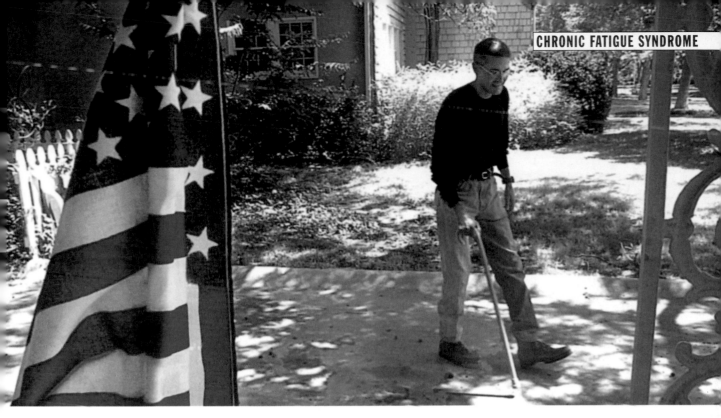

▲ A new study is looking at CFS in Gulf War veterans.

Diagnostic Advance
Gulf War Veterans Provide Clues to Chronic Fatigue Syndrome

Patients whose symptoms are not easily explained are sometimes told, "It's all in your head." All too often, this has been the fate of those who complain of unrelenting fatigue, joint and muscle pain, and memory or concentration problems, among the other symptoms of chronic fatigue syndrome (CFS). Now, a new study shows that the condition may have measurable signs as well as subjective symptoms—ones that may eventually lead to a better understanding of CFS.

It's not all in your head. The study looked at a group of people with an alarmingly high rate of CFS: Gulf War veterans. Up to 45 percent of the vets display symptoms of CFS. This study compared 51 vets with chronic fatigue and 42 without. All were given math tests and asked to present a speech, which was video-taped. These tests were expected to raise the vets' blood pressure. (Blood pressure should rise as a normal response to stress.) But in the group with chronic fatigue, the increase in blood pressure was much lower—even though they perceived the test to be just as stressful and challenging as did the other group. The vets with CFS symptoms—particularly those who had complained of the most severe symptoms—also had more difficulty with the cognitive tests.

These findings support earlier research, which has shown that at least one subset of chronic fatigue sufferers has associated cardiovascular problems, while another appears to have problems related to the immune system. Identifying the causes of these problems is an important step toward targeting treatment for each group. As for the Gulf War veterans, researchers agree that further study is needed to identify the cause of symptoms, with chemical exposure at the top of the list of likely suspects.

> **FAST FACTS**
> **800,000** Estimated number of people in the United States who have CFS **90** Percentage of people who have CFS but have not been diagnosed or treated **3 : 1** Ratio of women to men with CFS **6** Number of months that symptoms must be present before a diagnosis of CFS is made

Key Finding

Fibromyalgia Patients "Remember" Pain All Too Well

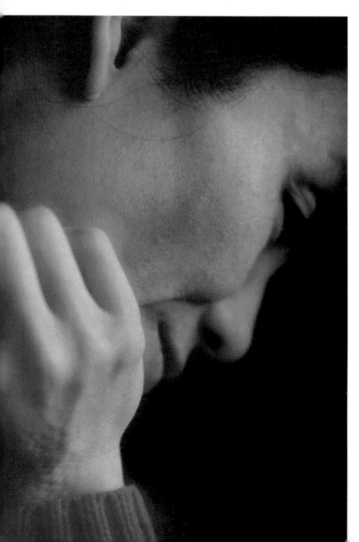

Fibromyalgia, a chronic condition characterized by fatigue and widespread pain in the muscles, ligaments, and tendons, has for some time been associated with problems within the central nervous system (the brain and spinal cord). Now a recent study from the University of Florida suggests that the symptoms of fibromyalgia may be caused by faulty pain processing in the spinal cord, resulting in a central nervous system that "remembers" pain sensations for an abnormally long time.

The study compared pain responses in healthy volunteers and people with fibromyalgia. When the researchers applied heat stimuli to the hands of both groups, the people with fibromyalgia experienced both residual pain, or pain that "hung on" much longer than normal, and a greater amount of overall pain. Normally, pain sensations quickly subside between stimuli, but "pain memory" appeared to be longer in people with fibromyalgia. Because of this, each subsequent stimulus was like adding insult to injury, resulting in greater and greater pain sensations.

If these results can be duplicated elsewhere, scientists may be able to develop better tests to diagnose this debilitating ailment. In the future, patients may be given drugs that target this faulty system of processing pain rather than the all-purpose painkillers and antidepressants that are often prescribed today.

▶ Researchers are discovering that people who suffer from fibromyalgia feel painful sensations for longer than normal.

STAY TUNED FOR...

Qigong for Pain Relief

Mind/body medicine may be the next step toward relieving the pain of fibromyalgia. Researchers from the University of Maryland Complementary Medicine Program are currently studying the effects of the Chinese art of qigong, which combines meditation, movement, and breathing exercises to improve the body's energy and powers of self-healing. One hundred fibromyalgia sufferers will be randomly split into two groups, with one practicing qigong once a week and the other attending a self-help group that educates them about their condition.

This study is a follow-up to an earlier, much smaller pilot study on 20 women, which indicated that weekly qigong sessions helped to relieve fibromyalgia symptoms. The results of the new study are expected at the end of 2001.

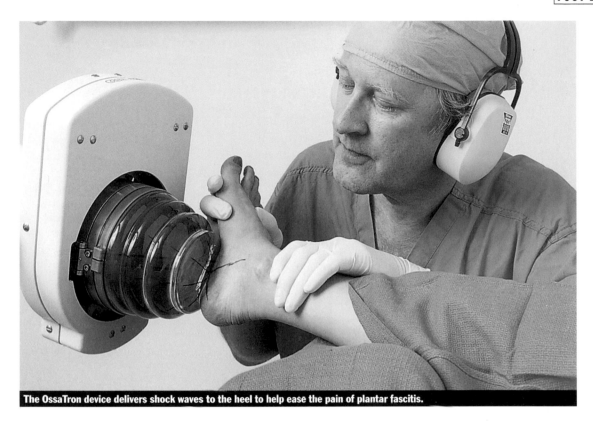

The OssaTron device delivers shock waves to the heel to help ease the pain of plantar fascitis.

High-Tech Help
Shocking Treatment Relieves Foot Pain

A Swiss device originally used to treat kidney stones provides a less extreme alternative to the surgery usually recommended for stubborn cases of plantar fascitis, a painful, chronic heel condition. One of the primary symptoms of this foot disorder is a sharp, shooting pain in the heel after you stand up. It generally occurs when there's too much stress on the heel bone as a result of ill-fitting shoes or walking incorrectly. The U.S. Food and Drug Administration (FDA) approved the device, called OssaTron, in October 2000.

How it works. OssaTron uses shock waves directed into the heel area to break up damaged tissue. "It is successful in up to 80 percent of cases, giving sufferers the chance to return to a happy and pain-free life," says John Ogden, M.D., who pioneered the use of this device in the United States. "The treatment itself is painful— I've tried it," says Ogden. It therefore requires local anesthetic or conscious sedation.

Although the pain of plantar fascitis may initially disappear, it typically returns three days after treatment. Then it usually takes three to four weeks before improvement is seen—the time it takes for new blood vessels and tissues to grow. Occasionally a second treatment may be required, and in these cases the success rate is close to 90 percent.

FAST FACTS
10,000 Average number of steps we take each day **115,000** Average number of miles—about four times around the earth's circumference—walked in a lifetime **80** Percentage of women who wear shoes that are too small for their feet

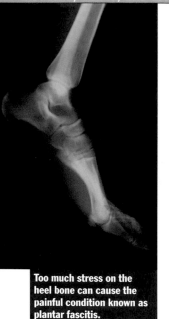

Too much stress on the heel bone can cause the painful condition known as plantar fascitis.

Availability. The FDA has approved OssaTron for patients who have failed to find relief using other kinds of treatments for a period of six months. (It is widely recognized that this kind of heel pain may go away on its own or with other treatments such as orthotic inserts, over-the-counter painkillers, and plain old rest.) There are currently a limited number of the half-million-dollar devices in the United States, but more may be available pending FDA approval for other indications (OssaTron is currently being tested for its effectiveness in tennis elbow and the delayed healing of tibial fractures). It is available in parts of Europe under the name ReflecTron and is increasingly reimbursed by insurance in certain countries.

RESEARCH ROUNDUP

■ **HELP FOR HAMMERTOES.** A study published in the journal *Foot and Ankle International* found that patients who underwent surgery of the PIP joint (the joint between the first and second bones of the toe) to correct hammertoe deformities were pain free for at least five years after the procedure. This is the first study on the long-term results of this common surgery for hammertoe deformity, which involves the curling of the small toes, characterized by the toes flexing downward at the first joint.

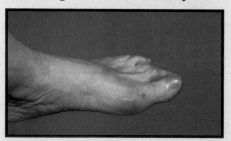

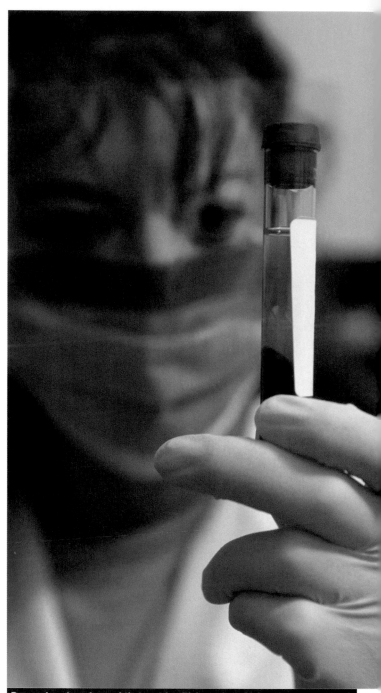

Researchers have learned that people with lupus have higher-than-normal levels of a certain protein, which may cause the immune system to overreact.

FAST FACTS
1 MILLION Estimated number of Americans with lupus **9 : 1** Ratio of women to men with lupus **30** Percentage of lupus patients who are photosensitive (sun exposure causes further symptoms of the disease) **3** Number of times African-American women are more likely to develop lupus than white women **21** Number of different symptoms commonly associated with lupus

Key Finding
Critical Discovery May Lead to Lupus Treatment

Researchers have learned that people with lupus have abnormally high levels of a certain protein (BLyS), and this discovery could lead to new treatments for the disease. Developing a way to limit the production of the protein could help not only lupus patients, but also people with other autoimmune diseases, such as rheumatoid arthritis.

In people with lupus, the immune system goes haywire. It produces antibodies to the body's own healthy tissues, thereby destroying them. (Antibodies are molecules that identify invaders such as viruses and bacteria and mark them for destruction by other immune system cells.) Two years ago, a team of researchers from the University of Alabama and Human Genome Sciences discovered a protein called BLyS (B lymphocyte stimulator) that stimulates the release of these antibodies by white blood cells (lymphocytes) called B cells. Now studies have shown that people with lupus have higher-than-normal levels of BLyS, which may be what triggers the immune system's ill-conceived attacks.

Human Genome Sciences is developing a genetically engineered antibody tailored to block the effect of BLyS. It is now in preclinical (animal or basic research) trials. The company plans to start clinical trials sometime in 2001. In addition to potentially treating lupus, there is one more possible benefit to the discovery: Elevated levels of BLyS might help identify the disease in people who haven't yet shown any symptoms.

How BLyS works in the body

The protein known as BLyS stimulates the release of antibodies by white blood cells called B cells. In lupus, these antibodies attack healthy cells.

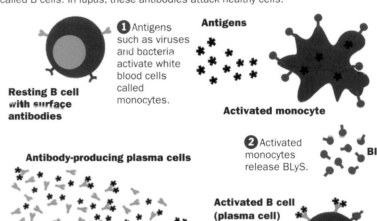

Resting B cell with surface antibodies

1 Antigens such as viruses and bacteria activate white blood cells called monocytes.

Antigens

Activated monocyte

2 Activated monocytes release BLyS.

BLyS

Antibody-producing plasma cells

Activated B cell (plasma cell)

3 BLyS stimulates B cells to become plasma cells, which produce antibodies.

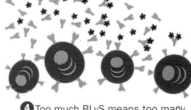

4 Too much BLyS means too many antibody-producing plasma cells.

RESEARCH ROUNDUP

■ **MORE INSIGHTS INTO THE CAUSE OF LUPUS. In** lupus, the immune system turns against the body's own tissues, viewing them as dangerous invaders and damaging the organs in the process of "defending" the body against them. Now researchers at the University of California, San Diego School of Medicine, have identified a gene mutation that causes a remarkably similar autoimmune disease in mice. This discovery may help scientists better understand the disease in humans.

The mutation occurs in an enzyme important to the formation of carbohydrates, called N-glycans, found on the surfaces of cells. These carbohydrates help the immune system distinguish between friends and foes of the body's own tissue. Mice bred to lack the gene for this enzyme had significantly fewer N-glycans than normal, and the ones they did have were oddly shaped. The study suggests that faulty glycan construction may also play a part in the onset of human autoimmune diseases such as lupus. This is the first time that an autoimmune disease has been linked to glycans, providing new insights into these diseases as well as suggesting new diagnostic tests for lupus.

Diagnostic Advance

More Accurate Lyme Disease Test Puts Confusion to Rest

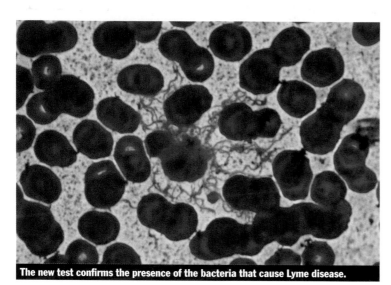

The new test confirms the presence of the bacteria that cause Lyme disease.

In the fall of 2000, a more accurate test became available—one that can be used to confirm cases of suspected Lyme disease. The new test, called C6 Lyme Peptide ELISA, has been shown to dramatically reduce the number of false-positive results compared with earlier tests; this is especially important for those people who have had the Lyme disease vaccine, since they test false positive with other tests. And because the new test is so sensitive, it can be used two to four weeks earlier than older tests.

How it works. Researchers believe that part of the reason the bacteria that causes Lyme disease (*Borrelia burgdorferi*) can evade the immune system is its ability to change its genetic composition. But recently, scientists identified a portion of a surface protein (the C6 peptide), present on every known strain of the bacteria, that remains constant. The new test identifies antibodies produced in response to this part of the protein.

Availability. The test became available in the United States in September 2000.

Lyme disease is notoriously difficult to accurately diagnose. Because its symptoms include fatigue and swelling of the joints, it is often confused with other diseases, such as lupus and chronic fatigue syndrome. It's estimated that Lyme disease often goes undiagnosed 10 times more than it is diagnosed. But that may soon change.

STAY TUNED FOR...

Tick-free Deer

A five-year U.S. federal study is being conducted on the use of an experimental deer feeder. The four-poster feeder coats the heads and necks of wild deer with insecticide as they feed. It includes a bin of corn and four paint rollers treated with insecticide. The deer must brush their head, neck, and ears against the rollers to get at the corn. The device has already triggered steep declines in the population of young ticks in Maryland and Connecticut. In Maryland, samplings at three test sites indicated drops of 50 to 78 percent in numbers of immature ticks since 1998. The Northeast Regional Tick Control Project, which is sponsoring the deer feeders, will continue until 2003 at sites in New Jersey, Maryland, Connecticut, New York, and Rhode Island.

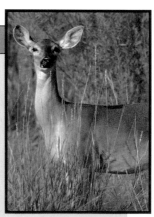

[
FAST FACTS
145,000 Number of Lyme disease cases reported to the U.S. Centers for Disease Control and Prevention between 1980 and 2000 **90** Percentage of Lyme disease cases reported in the United States since 1982 that occurred in the Northeast
]

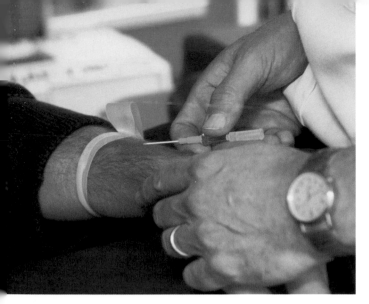

Key Finding
Persistent Lyme Disease: A Horse of a Different Color

The effectiveness of antibiotics for treating Lyme disease is well accepted by the medical community, with a 90 percent cure rate often cited for a course of antibiotics. But treatment for those patients whose Lyme disease persists or recurs after antibiotics is controversial. Should a second course of drugs be used to knock out the disease when the first treatment fails? Or are more antibiotics useless because patients are experiencing a new, secondary disorder, in which the body's immune system is attacking its very own cells?

A study published in the July 12, 2001, issue of the *New England Journal of Medicine* found no difference in improvement between patients given antibiotics and those given a placebo to treat chronic Lyme disease. In fact, the study was cut short because the patients receiving the antibiotics were not improving.

Stay tuned. Not all doctors are in agreement, however, that chronic or recurring Lyme disease indicates a new disorder that should not be treated with antibiotics. Brian Fallon, M.D., of Columbia University, in New York, is studying the effectiveness of 10 weeks of intravenous antibiotics in patients with persistent Lyme disease who have cognitive symptoms, such as memory loss and difficulties in thinking. This study will be combined with one using brain imaging to examine what types of changes Lyme disease causes in nerve cells and blood vessels within the brain, and whether the antibiotic has any effect on them.

▲ **Doctors disagree whether intravenous antibiotics help cases of persistent Lyme disease. A recent study concluded they don't.**

Progress in Prevention
Vaccine for Children Is under Review

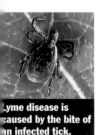

Lyme disease is caused by the bite of an infected tick.

Children make up about 40 percent of the reported cases of Lyme disease, but so far they have not been able to receive the vaccine that has been available to adults since 1998. Now GlaxoSmithKline, the company that developed the vaccine, is testing a pediatric version on children between the ages of 4 and 15.

How it works. The LYMErix vaccine triggers an immune response in the body to the bacteria that ticks carry and transmit by their bites.

Availability. The pediatric form of LYMErix has passed through the clinical trials phase and was submitted for final review and approval by the U.S. Food and Drug Administration (FDA) in 1999. The process may be completed by the end of 2001. However, some experts in the medical and FDA community feel that the LYMErix vaccine was approved prematurely for adults, and they have expressed concern over the vaccine's long- and short-term safety. Over the past year, there have been several reports of people developing a severe form of chronic arthritis after receiving the vaccine. In January 2001, FDA advisors agreed that more data was needed to determine the safety of LYMErix, which may have some bearing on the approval of this vaccine for use in children.

RESEARCH ROUNDUP

■ **HOW GOOD IS THE LYME DISEASE VACCINE?**
The Lyme disease vaccine (LYMErix) may be less effective than we thought. Researchers have discovered that more than one kind of protein spreads the disease via the bloodstream. LYMErix targets only one of them; therefore, researchers are beginning to question how protective the vaccine really is. They cite the need for a new vaccine with a chemical element that can attack all of these kinds of proteins, not just one.

Surgical Solution

Balloons for Osteoporosis Patients

Osteoporosis makes the bones in your body so brittle that they break easily. The hip is a common site of fracture, but the small bones called vertebrae that make up the spine are also very vulnerable. Even normal activities—such as picking up a grandchild or stepping off a curb—can cause a painful break in vertebrae made brittle by osteoporosis. These bones are stacked on top of one another, so when one breaks, the spinal column above it curves forward in response. If the bones heal in the collapsed position, a curvature of the spine (sometimes called a "dowager's hump") can result, which can interfere with daily living and even with breathing.

To fix vertebral fractures, there's a new, minimally invasive surgery called kyphoplasty. First introduced in 1998 and now becoming more widely available, it involves placing a balloon (similar to that used by heart surgeons to open clogged arteries) into the fractured vertebra and lifting the vertebra back into place. Recent studies show that kyphoplasty is over 90 percent successful in relieving the pain caused by these fractures; the studies

> **FAST FACTS**
> **28 MILLION** Number of Americans who are affected by osteoporosis **80** Percentage of those affected by the disease who are women
> **20** Percentage of bone mass women can lose in the first five years following menopause
> **1.5 MILLION** Number of fractures a year caused by osteoporosis in the United States

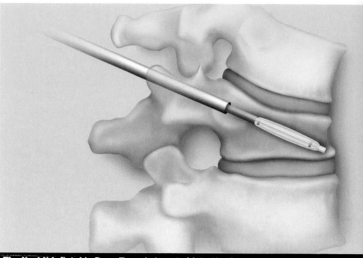
The KyphX Inflatable Bone Tamp is inserted into the damaged vertebra.

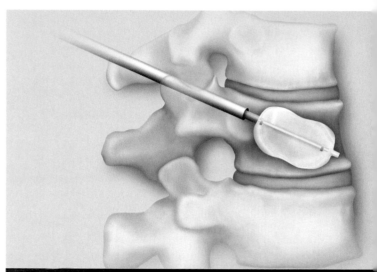
The balloon is inflated to raise the collapsed portion of the bone.

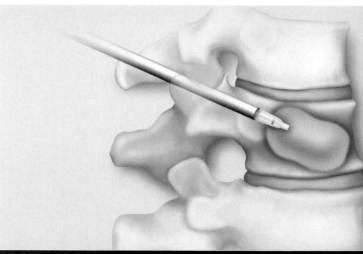
The balloon is deflated and removed, leaving a cavity that can be filled with an approved bone filler of the physician's choice.

Recent studies show that kyphoplasty is over 90 percent successful in relieving the pain caused by vertebral fractures. It may also restore lost height.

also indicate that the technique can restore some of the height lost because of bone compression.

How it works. A tiny drill is used to create a channel in the fractured bone. Then a balloon is placed inside the channel and inflated. This elevates the collapsed bone back into its normal position. The surgeon can then fill the cavity with a special bone cement, which reinforces the bone and prevents future fractures. Kyphoplasty is similar to an older procedure, vertebroplasty, which uses a needle to insert cement into the damaged vertebrae without the use of a balloon to first clear a space.

Availability. The Kyphon Inflatable Bone Tamp, known as the KyphX, was cleared for use in the United States in 1998 and in parts of Europe in 2000. As more doctors are trained in its use, the procedure will become more readily available. It can be performed on an inpatient or outpatient basis and has best results within the first two months of the fracture.

RESEARCH ROUNDUP

■ **HOW LOW CAN YOU GO?** Though estrogen replacement therapy helps with preventing bone loss, it can cause many potentially dangerous side effects, such as gallbladder disease, blood clots, and in some cases breast cancer. Now a new study has shown that a low dose of estrogen may be just as effective in improving bone density, with fewer side effects than the higher doses, when given to women aged 65 and older. The study was published in the *Journal of Clinical Endocrinology and Metabolism* in December 2000.

Nutrition Tip
Soy Keeps Bones Strong

You probably know that drinking milk can help keep your bones strong. But could downing a glass of soy milk do the same? Or eating tofu? Probably so. New research findings published in the January 2001 issue of *Obstetrics and Gynecology* suggest that a diet rich in soy may help women retain strong bones and reduce the risk of painful and debilitating fractures.

In the Japanese study, led by Yoshiaki Somekawa, M.D., researchers found that among women in both early and late postmenopausal stages, those who consumed the most soy foods, such as tofu, boiled soybeans, and soy milk, had significantly denser bones than women who consumed the least soy foods. Women in early postmenopause also had significantly fewer backaches and aching joints.

How It works. Soybeans are a rich source of isoflavones, plant-based estrogenlike compounds found predominantly in legumes and beans. When estrogen levels plummet during menopause, women are at increased risk of the bone-thinning disease osteoporosis. (Estrogen is thought to play a key role in the formation of new bone.) Consuming a lot of soy foods appears to combat the bone-thinning effects of low estrogen levels.

Availability. Soy is widely available as fresh, dried, or frozen soybeans; tofu; soy milk, ice cream, and cheese; and also comes in powdered form.

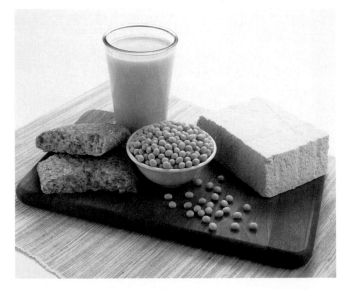
▼ A diet rich in foods made from soy may help prevent bone loss.

Topping the list of breakthroughs this year in sexual and reproductive health is a new family of AIDS drugs that offer an alternative to protease inhibitors, the "miracle" antiviral drugs that fight the deadly disease, but with serious side effects. What's more, researchers are hot on the trail of an AIDS vaccine, and there's reason to believe that one of the vaccines now being tested might actually succeed. In other news, more and better options for contraception are on the horizon, including a convenient birth control patch that works just as well as the Pill. And the stigma surrounding sexual dysfunction is disappearing as new treatments become available, including a Viagra-like drug for both men and women that may hit the European market soon. There is also new evidence that a popular herbal remedy may help ease the symptoms of PMS.

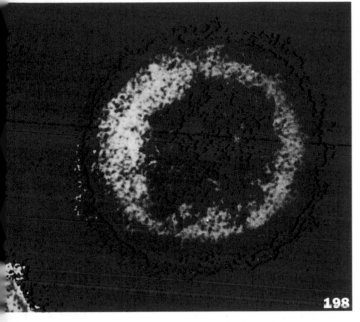

198

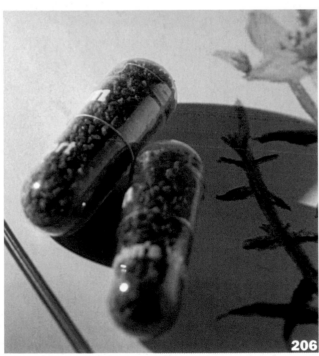

206

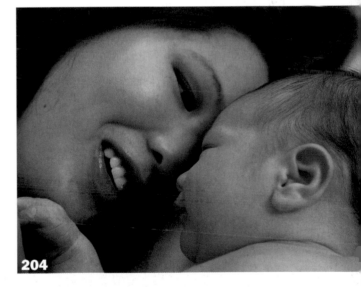

204

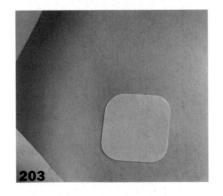

203

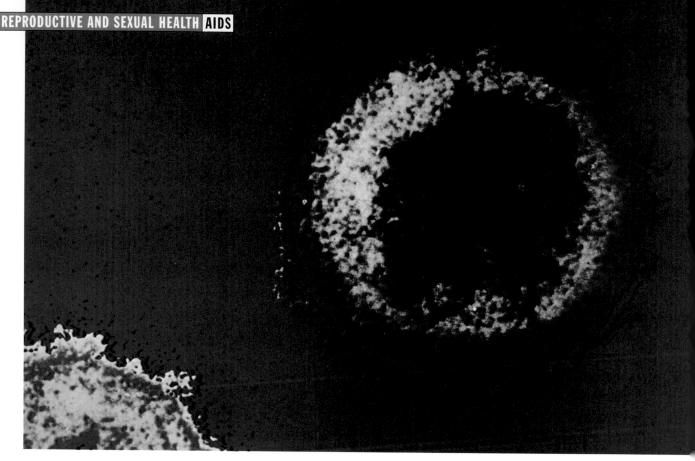

Drug Development
Building a Better AIDS Drug

The final decade of the twentieth century saw the introduction of protease inhibitors, drugs that became part of the famous "AIDS cocktail" that extended the life of thousands of patients infected with human immunodeficiency virus (HIV), the virus that causes AIDS. Unfortunately, it was discovered that long-term use of these drugs takes a toll on the body—causing nausea, vomiting, diarrhea, pancreatitis (inflammation of the pancreas), and, in some cases, kidney failure. The search continues for drugs that will help people infected with HIV stay healthy, without the serious and sometimes life-threatening side effects. A new family of drugs known as entry inhibitors holds promise.

How they work. Entry inhibitors prevent the entry of HIV into healthy immune cells. Of the three types of entry inhibitors, fusion inhibitors are the furthest along in development. Fusion inhibitors act as a decoy to trap the virus and bind to it, preventing it from binding to the body's immune cells.

Availability. Still experimental, entry inhibitors are not yet available by prescription. Research on one of them, a drug called T-20, has progressed to the point that the drug has received fast-track designation by the U.S. Food and Drug Administration. The results of clinical trials released in early 2001 show that T-20 is well tolerated by patients and is effective in preventing HIV from replicating (copying itself) in the body. The drug is now in phase III clinical trials, the last phase before it can be marketed. It could be available within the next few years.

▲ HIV attacks healthy immune cells, but the newest experimental drugs, called entry inhibitors, prevent the virus from getting inside.

Drug Development

Finally, Hot on the Trail of an AIDS Vaccine

It's been almost two decades since the link between HIV and AIDS was discovered by Drs. Luc Montagnier and Robert Gallo, working in France and the United States. Since that time, cases of HIV and AIDS have skyrocketed, with current worldwide estimates running at more than 36 million HIV-infected men, women, and children (in addition to the 23 million who have already died as a result of AIDS since the disease was first recognized). Since the 1980s, scientists have been struggling to develop an effective vaccine to treat the disease, with little success. Now, exciting new discoveries as well as more funding and research collaborations have energized the search.

Currently, more than 20 different AIDS vaccines are being tested around the world. The HIV Vaccine Trials Network, a division of the U.S. National Institutes of Health, oversees a global network of clinical trial sites; their website at www.scharp.org/hvtn/ provides a comprehensive overview of current vaccine research and clinical trial locations.

Vaccine success in monkeys. One study published in the journal *Science* in March 2001 provided new evidence that AIDS can be controlled by vaccine. According to the researchers at Emory University in Atlanta, Georgia, 24 monkeys inoculated with a combination of vaccines stayed healthy after they were infected with human and monkey HIV viruses. In contrast, a control group of four unvaccinated monkeys all developed high levels of the virus in their bodies and then progressed to AIDS. It should be noted that the vaccines did not keep the virus

More than 36 million men, women, and children in the world are infected with HIV.

entirely at bay: Vaccinated monkeys became infected, but the vaccinations triggered enough of an immune response to keep the virus in check. As a result of this study, the vaccine is being fast-tracked, and clinical trials in humans are planned for 2002.

BEHIND THE BREAKTHROUGH

Teaming Up to Fight AIDS

While in the past AIDS research has been done by many dedicated scientists all working in isolated laboratories, Robert Gallo, M.D., head of the Institute of Human Virology (IHV) in Baltimore, Maryland, had a new vision—a collaboration of top scientists working together to develop an AIDS vaccine. The idea led to The Waterford Project, a "virtual lab" that uses the latest Internet technology to link scientists and their research.

This joint effort brings together the most brilliant minds, such as Warner Greene and Tom Coates of the University of California, San Francisco, and Harvard University's Bruce Walker and Max Essex, all with one goal—to focus on AIDS vaccine research. Other researchers include Gallo's team at IHV.

Project leaders believe the greatest benefit of collaboration is speed. The research, which received initial funding from the John D. Evans Foundation (Evans, the co-founder of the cable network C-SPAN, was instrumental in pulling the project together), can move forward without scientists having to convince an outside group that the idea is worth sponsoring.

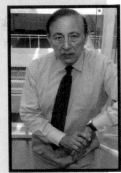

Dr. Robert Gallo has united AIDS researchers in a "virtual lab" where they share their latest work.

Testing of vaccine begins in humans. Another combination vaccine developed by a team of Kenyan and British scientists that has proved successful in monkeys has now begun testing in people in England and Kenya. Part one of the vaccine is a simple DNA vaccine, which contains proteins found in the AIDS virus. This vaccine reminds the immune system to fight back if infection occurs. Part two, given weeks later, is based on a virus used in a smallpox vaccine. This second vaccine mimics a viral infection and triggers an immune reaction. Initial clinical trials to test for safety are being carried out on each part separately. If the vaccines are found to be safe, the next step will be to see whether using both components in the same people will effectively stop the virus.

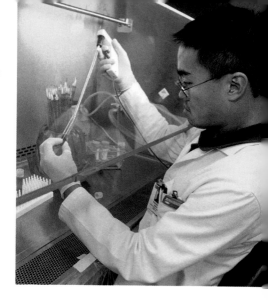

▶ One of the most exciting areas of AIDS research is the work being done to find vaccines against HIV, the virus that causes AIDS.

AIDS VACCINE CLINICAL TRIALS

SPONSORS	LOCATION	STAGE OF CLINICAL TRIAL
VaxGen, U.S. Centers for Disease Control and Prevention	U.S., Canada, Netherlands	Phase III, interim results possible in November 2001
VaxGen, Thai Ministry of Public Health	Thailand	Phase III, injecting drug users
Aventis Pasteur, VaxGen, NIH, Medical Research Foundation of Trinidad, National Laboratory of Research in Haiti, Federal University of Rio de Janeiro, U.S. military	Thailand, Haiti, Trinidad and Tobago, Brazil, U.S.	Three separate phase II trials
IAVI, Oxford University, University of Nairobi	U.K. and Kenya	Phase I
Italian NIH, Germany's Research Center for Biotechnology	Italy	Phase I, fall 2001
AlphaVax, IAVI, NIAID, Johns Hopkins University, University of Natal	U.S. and South Africa	Phase I, 2001
Therion, NIAID	U.S.	Phase I, fall 2001
Chiron, NIAID	U.S.	Phase I, 2002
Wyeth-Lederle, NIAID	U.S.	Phase I, 2002
Merck	U.S.	Phase I, spring 2001
French National Agency for AIDS Research	France	Phase I
NIAID, Protein Sciences	U.S.	Phase I, end of 2001
NIAID, University of New South Wales, Australia	Australia	Phase I, 2002
EuroVax	Switzerland and U.K.	Phase I, 2002
ABL, NIAID	U.S.	Phase I, 2002
Institute of Human Virology, IAVI, NIAID	Maryland and Uganda	Phase I, 2002
Emory University, NIAID	U.S.	Phase I, 2002

What are the phases of a clinical trial?

■ **In phase I,** a new drug or treatment is given to a small group of people (20–80) for the first time to evaluate its safety, determine a safe dosage range, and identify side effects.

■ **In phase II,** a larger group of people (100–300) is given the drug or treatment to see if it is effective and to further evaluate its safety.

■ **In phase III,** the drug or treatment is given to a large group of people (1,000–3,000) to confirm its effectiveness, monitor side effects, compare it with commonly used treatments, and collect information that will allow the drug or treatment to be used safely.

Abbreviations NIH, National Institutes of Health; IAVI, International AIDS Vaccine Initiative; NIAID, National Institute of Allergy and Infectious Diseases; ABL, Advanced BioScience Laboratories, Inc.

Drug Development

Hormone-Releasing IUD Offers Five Years of Contraception

If you're looking for long-term contraception, ask your doctor about Mirena, a hormone-coated intrauterine device (IUD) that provides worry-free contraception for at least 5 years. The small T-shaped piece of soft plastic is inserted in the uterus by a health-care provider during an office visit. Mirena works for 4 years longer than Progestasert, another hormonal IUD that has been available for more than 20 years, although it needs to be replaced sooner than the copper IUD, which provides 10 years of contraception.

Mirena, as well as Progestasert, is less likely to produce the increased menstrual bleeding and cramping associated with the copper IUD. In fact, the hormonal IUDs are associated with lighter menstrual bleeding and less painful periods. Women who have already had a child will have the greatest success with Mirena because pregnancy has stretched the uterus, and this reduces the chance of uterine cramping or expulsion of the IUD.

How it works. After Mirena is inserted, it releases a continuous low level of the hormone levonorgestrel, which is also in birth control pills, directly into the uterus. Although exactly how this hormone prevents conception is unclear, Mirena probably works by thickening the cervical mucus (blocking sperm's passage through the cervix), preventing sperm movement, and thinning the lining of the uterus (reducing the chance of an egg implanting there). The effectiveness of Mirena is comparable to sterilization.

Availability. After more than 10 years of use in Europe, Mirena received U.S. Food and Drug Administration approval in December 2000. Although currently approved for use only as a contraceptive, doctors may also choose to use Mirena as an alternative to hysterectomy in women with a condition called menorrhagia, or excessive menstrual flow.

Use of Mirena (and other IUDs) is not risk-free; some women may develop inflammation of the fallopian tubes, which can lead to complications, including infertility. A woman in a monogamous relationship is much less likely to experience this complication.

> **Women who have already had a child will have the greatest success with Mirena.**

▶ **Mirena, a new hormone-coated intrauterine device, can be left in place for up to five years.**

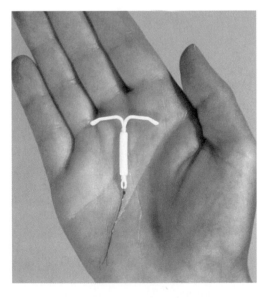
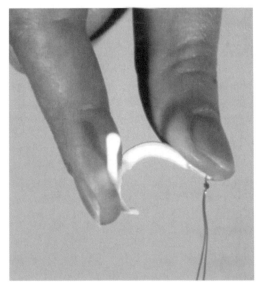

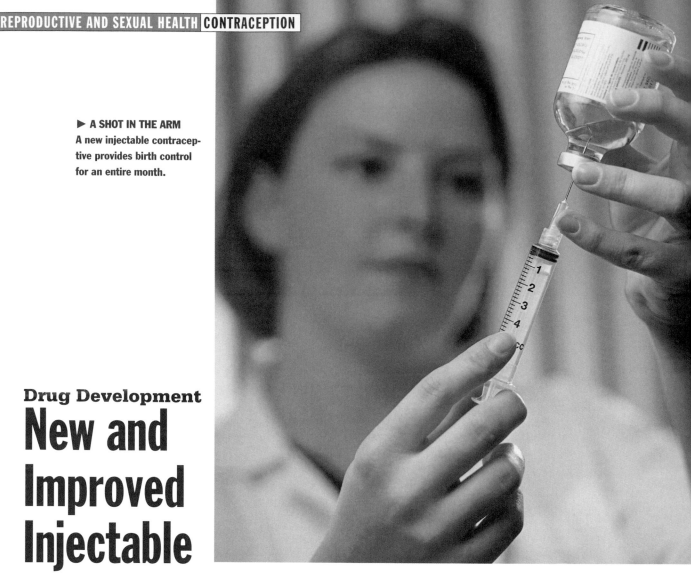

▶ **A SHOT IN THE ARM**
A new injectable contraceptive provides birth control for an entire month.

Drug Development
New and Improved Injectable Contraceptive

For women who want the convenience of a monthly contraceptive injection, Lunelle could be just the ticket. Most women are able to achieve pregnancy within four months after they stop using Lunelle, which makes it attractive for those who are planning to start or add to a family. As an added benefit, Lunelle makes periods much lighter, and it causes fewer side effects (such as irregular bleeding) than Depo-Provera.

How it works. During the first five days of a woman's menstrual cycle, a health-care provider injects a combination of progestin and estrogen into the muscle of the arm, thigh, or buttock. These hormones prevent ovulation, thicken the cervical mucus (making it difficult for sperm to pass) and thin the lining of the uterus (making it less conducive to the implantation of a fertilized egg). Three weeks after the injection, the woman's period begins.

Availability. Lunelle was approved by the U.S. Food and Drug Administration in October 2000. In a few areas of the country, certain pharmacists are certified to administer the shot, making the contraceptive more convenient for busy women, who may not have time to visit their doctor each month. A self-administered injection is also a possibility in the future. While self-administration is already an option in other countries, the U.S. National Women's Health Network believes that convenience should not be placed above health and at this time recommends that women who use Lunelle continue to get periodic checkups from their physicians.

> **Lunelle causes fewer side effects than Depo-Provera.**

Drug Development
The First-Ever Contraceptive Patch

Ortho-Evra, the world's first contraceptive patch, makes birth control easier than ever before—and just as effective. It works on the same principle as the hormone replacement patch, delivering a constant low level of progestin and estrogen through the skin into the bloodstream. Recent studies indicate that Ortho-Evra works as effectively as oral contraceptives to prevent ovulation.

How it works. About the size of a matchbook, each contraceptive patch is worn for one week (usually on the upper arm, abdomen, or buttocks) and then replaced with a fresh patch for the first three weeks of the menstrual cycle. No patch is worn during menstruation.

Availability. Ortho-Evra was submitted to the U.S. Food and Drug Administration for review in December 2000. It could be approved by the end of 2001.

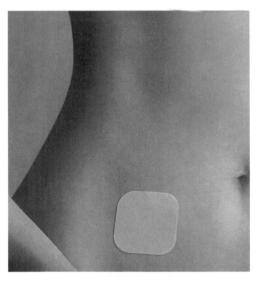

▲ The contraceptive patch works as well as the Pill and is easier to remember to use.

STAY TUNED FOR...

Birth Control Ring

Nuvaring, a flexible plastic contraceptive ring that a woman inserts by herself once a month, may soon be available. Nuvaring prevents conception by releasing low doses of the hormones norgestrel and ethinyl estradiol. Inserted around the cervix, the ring is worn for three weeks, and is then removed for the week of menstruation. Many women report that they can't even feel the ring when it's in place. Pending approval by the U.S. Food and Drug Administration (FDA), Nuvaring could be launched in the United States by the end of 2001.

Kinder, Gentler Implant

Implanon is a new, single-rod version of the contraceptive implant that uses a gentler form of the hormone progesterone than that found in Norplant. Like its six-rod predecessor, it is inserted under the skin of the upper arm. After a local anesthetic is administered, the slender device is placed just below the surface of the skin. No incision is necessary. When it is time for Implanon to be removed, a small cut in the skin is made at one end of the rod, which can then be extracted. Implanon is designed to last for three years.

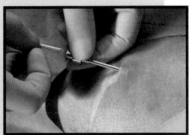

About the size of a matchstick, Implanon is inserted under the skin in about a minute.

The rod can be removed at any time at the woman's request. Fertility returns rapidly. Implanon is already available in several countries, including Great Britain and Australia, but has not yet been submitted to the FDA for U.S. approval. Side effects may include irregular bleeding and breast tenderness.

Permanent Contraception without Surgery

Women who want permanent birth control but who don't want to go under the knife may soon have another option. In the selective tubal occlusion procedure, the Essure device, a soft, flexible coil about 4 inches (10 cm) long, is used to plug the fallopian tubes so that eggs can't make it through to the uterus. A physician places the coils using a visually guided system called a hysteroscope, which is passed through the cervix and uterus to the opening of each fallopian tube; after about three months, the tubes are effectively blocked. Because general anesthesia isn't necessary and no incisions are made, the procedure can be done in a doctor's office in less than 30 minutes. Recovery is expected to be faster than with tubal ligation.

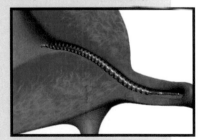

The Essure device uses small coils that are inserted into the fallopian tubes as a form of permanent contraception.

Essure is currently being tested in clinical trials and could potentially be approved in the United States in 2003. It received approval for marketing in parts of Europe in early 2001.

Drug Development
Diabetes Drug May Prevent Miscarriage in Women With Polycystic Ovary Syndrome

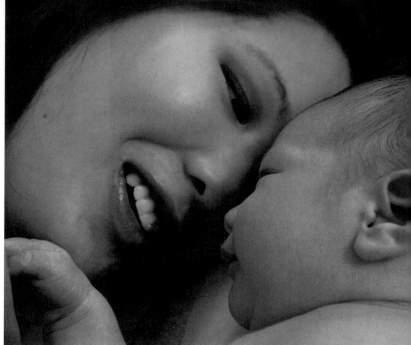

Women with a condition called polycystic ovary syndrome (PCOS) are often infertile, and when they do conceive, they have a higher rate of miscarriage than other women. In recent years, women with PCOS have been given an existing diabetes drug to treat their symptoms and help them conceive. Now, researchers at Jewish Hospital, in Cincinnati, Ohio, report that those who continue taking the medication through their pregnancy have a lower first-trimester miscarriage rate.

PCOS affects about 6 to 10 percent of women in their reproductive years. In this condition, the ovaries develop multiple, fluid-filled cysts, and ovulation may not occur. What's the connection with diabetes? Many women with PCOS are less sensitive to the hormone insulin, which puts them at higher risk for the disease. Scientists now believe that this insulin resistance may be what causes infertility indirectly, by making the body produce too much of certain male sex hormones, such as testosterone, and too little estrogen. This hormonal imbalance causes side effects ranging from acne and increased body hair to menstrual irregularity and infertility.

For women with PCOS, taking the diabetes drug metformin (brand name Glucophage) corrects the hormonal imbalance, allowing them to experience normal menstruation, conception, and pregnancy.

How it works. Metformin helps decrease insulin resistance, which in turn stops the overproduction of male hormones, allowing normal menstruation and ovulation. It also significantly reduces the incidence of first-trimester miscarriage, possibly by providing better blood flow to the placenta through its actions on various hormones and on a protein responsible for blood clotting. The drug does not appear to have any adverse effects on the development of the fetus or on the health of the mother.

▲ The diabetes drug Glucophage may help women with polycystic ovary syndrome carry a pregnancy to term.

Availability. Metformin is approved by the U.S. Food and Drug Administration only for people with type 2 diabetes. It can, however, be prescribed by doctors for a woman with PCOS as an off-label (not FDA-approved) use. Studies on metformin to curb PCOS-related miscarriage are still preliminary and more research is needed before the use of this drug during pregnancy becomes a standard practice for women with PCOS.

STAY TUNED FOR...

Male Infertility Test

A new male infertility test described in the January 2001 issue of the journal *Human Reproduction* may help identify the presence of defective sperm and spare women unnecessary tests and infertility treatment. While infertility was long considered a woman's problem, today we know that it can be traced to the man one-third of the time, to the woman one-third of the time, and to mixed reasons for the remaining one-third.

Unlike traditional semen analysis, the test looks for a protein called ubiquitin, which can indicate defects in sperm cells. Testing for high levels of ubiquitin can determine why a couple is infertile when other diagnostic tests have failed. Ubiquitin tagging might even one day be used to "tag" the defective sperm from semen samples so that only healthy sperm are used in artificial fertilization.

Key Finding

HRT May Not Protect Against Heart Disease in Postmenopausal Women

Although studies continue to pour in on the pros and cons of hormone replacement therapy (HRT) at menopause, the jury is still out. HRT, which is a combination of the hormones estrogen and progestin, has been shown to alleviate menopause symptoms such as hot flashes. For years, researchers have been trying to determine whether HRT also protects women against heart disease. Now a new study from Germany published in February 2001 suggests that HRT does not slow the progression of atherosclerosis—a buildup of fatty plaque in the arteries— in postmenopausal women who are at increased risk of heart disease.

▶ **For preventing stroke and heart attack in women, the American Heart Association now recommends lifestyle changes—not HRT.**

In fact, the evidence from recent studies that HRT may not protect women against heart disease is so compelling that in July 2001, the American Heart Association issued new guidelines cautioning doctors that heart reasons alone are not enough to warrant prescribing HRT.

According to the guidelines, doctors can consider heart protection when prescribing HRT for healthy postmenopausal women, but it should not drive the decision. And because studies have shown that HRT does not offer cardiac protection to women with established heart disease, these women should not be started on the therapy. Women with heart disease who are already receiving and doing well on HRT may choose to continue or stop treatment, based on non-coronary factors including patient preference.

More definitive answers will be provided by two large ongoing studies of healthy women randomly assigned to receive HRT. Results are expected in five to eight years.

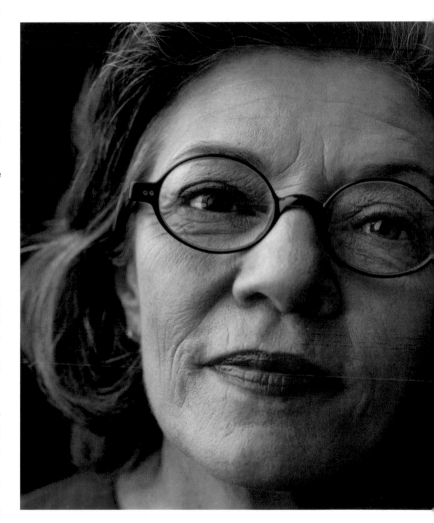

> **FAST FACTS**
> **1940** Approximate year when estrogen replacement therapy was first prescribed **51** Average age of a woman at menopause **60** Percentage of women who experience hot flashes at menopause

Alternative Answers
St. John's Wort May Ease PMS

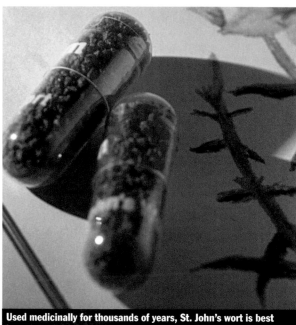

Used medicinally for thousands of years, St. John's wort is best known as an herbal antidepressant. It also alleviates anxiety.

In a study published in the July 2000 issue of the *British Journal of Obstetrics and Gynaecology*, researchers found that St. John's wort, the herbal remedy used to lift symptoms of mild to moderate depression, may give relief to women with premenstrual syndrome (PMS). St. John's wort is taken by more than 20 million Germans on a daily basis and has become quite popular worldwide. For women with PMS, researchers reported that the herb may help by easing nervous tension, anxiety, and insomnia.

In the four-month study, 19 women with PMS kept track of their daily symptoms. During months three and four, the women took 300 mg of hypericin, the active ingredient in St. John's

> ## St. John's wort is taken by more than 20 million Germans.

wort, daily. Treatment for two menstrual cycles led to significant improvements in PMS symptoms, greatly reducing nervous tension, insomnia, crying, and depression. A word of caution, though: Researchers consider the study preliminary, and not proof that St. John's wort is an effective treatment. The study does indicate that further research is warranted.

How it works. Hypericin is the principal component in St. John's wort and contains the chemicals that allevi-

ate depression. St. John's wort is thought to work very much like the antidepressant Prozac, increasing the availability of the neurotransmitter serotonin, a chemical produced by the brain that exerts a calming effect.

Availability. St. John's wort is available without a prescription. Because the herb can interact with prescription medications—especially antidepressants—talk to your doctor before taking it. And if you do start using it, speak to your doctor if you change your mind, as it may be necessary to taper off its use and not stop suddenly.

STAY TUNED FOR...

An End to Periods
A new birth control pill, Seasonale, may eliminate monthly periods altogether. Normally, women who take birth control pills take them for 21 days and have a period once a month. Seasonale, now in clinical trials, is taken for 84 consecutive days, followed by 7 days off. (Currently, some physicians may prescribe such a schedule for birth controls pills already in use, when a woman must avoid menstruating because of medical problems.) If approved by the U.S. Food and Drug Administration (FDA), it could be on the market by 2004.

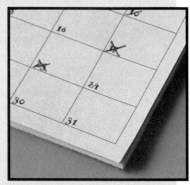

A Birth Control Pill that Relieves PMS
For women who experience water retention, moodiness, and increased appetite before or during their periods, a new birth control pill, known as Yasmin, could provide relief according to a study presented at a meeting of the American College of Obstetricians and Gynecologists in April 2001. Yasmin is a combination of two hormones—estrogen and drosperinone, a type of progestin—and acts as a diuretic, preventing water retention. It also reduces moodiness and irritability. After six months of treatment, study participants rated their premenstrual and menstrual symptoms as significantly improved. (A decrease in PMS symptoms can also occur in some women on currently available low dose birth control pills.) Future studies will evaluate the effectiveness of Yasmin in women who have more severe menstrual symptoms. Yasmin received FDA approval in May 2001.

Alternative Answers
New Heat Patch Eases Menstrual Cramps

Sometimes old folk remedies really do work. According to a new study at Health Quest Therapy and Research Institute in Austin, Texas, published in the March 2001 issue of the *Journal of Obstetrics and Gynecology*, using a heating pad may help ease menstrual cramps as effectively as taking ibuprofen.

The heat used by the women in the study was generated from a self-adhesive patch known as Thermacare. The patch has an adhesive strip that sticks to the inside of underclothing (not to the skin), where it delivers heat for eight hours.

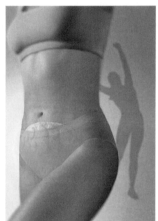

▲ The Thermacare patch delivers soothing heat that lasts for hours.

Women in the study who used both the heat patch and ibuprofen reported relief after 90 minutes; women who used ibuprofen without heat had to wait nearly three hours before they got relief. Both groups (as well as a group that used the heat patch and a placebo, or dummy pill) experienced the same amount of pain relief.

How it works. While researchers still have much to learn about the pain-reducing mechanism of heat, they do know that heat widens the blood vessels and increases blood flow. Applying heat to the abdomen may relax the uterus, and it may even counteract the activity of hormones that cause the uterus to contract.

Mark Akin, M.D., who headed the Austin research team and is currently involved in a similar study comparing the heat patch with acetaminophen, commented: "Grandma perfected this a long time ago. With modern medical research, we've finally confirmed it." Because the patch is worn under clothing, it eliminates the need to be "chained" to a hot water bottle or electric heating pad. Akin also pointed out that the pain-relieving effects of the heat patch are delivered without any of the side effects that may accompany drugs used to treat pain.

Availability. Thermacare will be on drugstore shelves in January 2002. In the meantime, it can be purchased through Procter & Gamble by calling 1-800-488-7288 or logging on to their website at www.Thermacare.com.

PATIENT PROFILE

Period Pain Begone

The first time Mary Patane, a physical therapist in her late thirties, tried the Thermacare heat patch for her menstrual cramps, she was at a medical conference two hours from home. Normally she would have used a heating pad, but that wasn't practical at the conference. As coincidence would have it, Procter & Gamble representatives were there handing out samples of Thermacare.

"It was great, because it happened to be a really heavy day for me, and I had leg pains and abdominal cramping," Patane remembers. When she put on the patch, "it started melting away the pain and was wonderful." She was impressed with "the simplicity of it and the convenience," along with the thinness of the patch, which never got uncomfortably warm. Patane reports that since she first tried the patch about a year ago, she has relied less on over-the-counter medication.

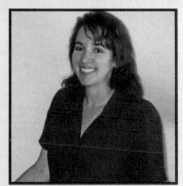

Mary Patane

[
FAST FACTS
106 Average number of periods prehistoric women had in a lifetime due to frequent pregnancy and nursing
318 Average number of periods women experience today **75** Percentage of women who have some symptoms of PMS **30–40** Percentage of women who have PMS symptoms severe enough to interfere with everyday living
]

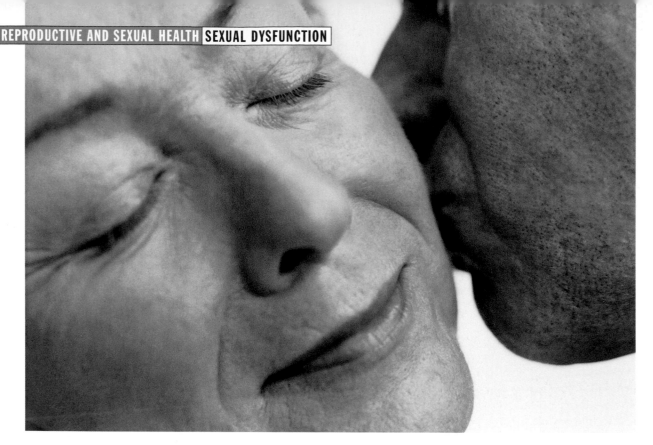

Drug Development

New Viagra-Type Drug Is for Women, Too

▲ A new drug treats both erectile dysfunction in men and sexual dysfunction in women.

Research shows that sexual dysfunction is more common in women than in men. (In women, the term sexual dysfunction covers a variety of complaints, including diminished vaginal lubrication, pain during intercourse, decreased arousal, and difficulty achieving orgasm.) But so far, there's no Viagra for women, even though the basic mechanism of sexual arousal—increased blood flow to the reproductive organs—is the same for both sexes.

Enhanced blood flow is the main effect of a new sexual dysfunction drug, phentolamine mesylate, which is being tested in both men (as Vasomax, an oral drug) and women (as Vasofem, a vaginal suppository).

How it works. Vasomax and Vasofem belong to a class of drugs known as alpha-receptor antagonists, which block the action of hormones that constrict blood vessels. Other alpha-receptor antagonists are used to treat high blood pressure (hypertension) and prostate enlargement. Whether in oral or suppository form, the drug is used before sexual activity, and it works faster than Viagra and similar drugs, taking effect within 30 to 40 minutes instead of an hour.

Availability. Vasomax is available by prescription in Mexico and Brazil (as Z-Max) and clinical studies are under way in Great Britain. But the drug's makers, at the behest of the U.S. Food and Drug Administration (FDA), are conducting further studies in animals to prove its safety before clinical studies can continue in the United States. The manufacturer has been able to continue offshore clinical trials for Vasofem while waiting for the FDA's go-ahead.

> **FAST FACTS**
> **52** Percentage of men who will be affected by impotence during their lifetime
> **64** Percentage of women who have difficulty achieving arousal or orgasm at some point in their lives

Topical Cream for Men

A new topical erectile dysfunction drug, applied directly to the penis, is showing success in clinical trials, and without the side effects of pills or injectable drugs. Topiglan is a new formulation of alprostadil, which in its old form can be administered only by injection into the penis or by insertion with a syringe-like device. The new cream is far easier and much more comfortable to use. It is heading toward the last round of clinical trials before it can be approved for marketing in the United States.

Arousal Via Nasal Spray

A new nasal spray containing the drug apomorphine is a promising treatment for women with female sexual dysfunction and men with erectile dysfunction. Apomorphine works by stimulating parts of the brain that are normally stimulated by dopamine, a messenger chemical thought to be important to erections but which may be deficient in some people. Apomorphine is also used to treat Parkinson's disease. In fact, the observation that it triggered erections in men with Parkinson's led to its study for sexual dysfunction. The nasal spray appears to produce arousal within a few minutes of its administration and is currently being tested in clinical trials by the manufacturer, the Nastech Pharmaceutical Company.

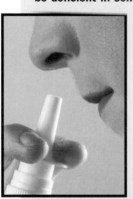

More Competition for Viagra

Two new drugs—vardenafil and Cialis—under investigation for erectile dysfunction are showing positive results and are working their way toward U.S. Food and Drug Administration approval. And with Vasomax currently in a holding pattern in the United States, these two drugs may be the next contenders to show up in pharmacies—possibly as early as 2002.

Drug Development
Promising Treatment for Erectile Dysfunction

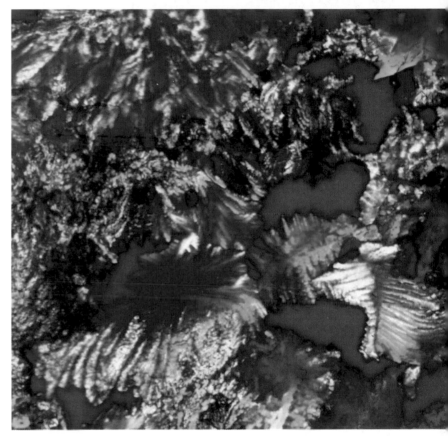

A drug being studied as a self-tanning agent was found to produce an interesting side effect: erections. Now a preliminary study published in the October 2000 issue of the journal *Urology* shows that Melanotan II, a synthetic form of the hormone DHEA, may indeed have a future as a treatment for erectile dysfunction.

▲ DHEA, a hormone produced in the adrenal glands, is converted by the body to testosterone, shown here in a polarized light micrograph.

In the study, which involved men whose erectile dysfunction was caused by conditions such as heart disease, diabetes, high blood pressure, or injury, about 60 percent of Melanotan II injections resulted in erections. The drug takes about 1½ hours to take effect, and the men experienced about 2.5 erections over the course of six hours after the injection. Researchers believe the compound acts directly on the hormone-regulating part of the brain because, after a man has received an injection, he is able to have erections without sexual stimulation.

The researchers are continuing their study of Melanotan II, which is still years away from commercial development.

RESPIRATORY SYSTEM

We've all suffered through miserable colds and other respiratory ills. But new breakthroughs may allow us to breathe a little easier in the future. Soon kids (and adults, too) may be able to receive the flu vaccine from a nasal spray instead of a shot. And while there's still no cure for the common cold, a drug is on its way that could shorten its duration and ease symptoms. For some of the most vulnerable members of our population—those in nursing homes and hospitals—pneumonia and other respiratory infections are increasingly widespread. To help control these serious problems, the first of a brand-new class of antibiotics is close to approval—a much-needed addition to the arsenal required to attack deadly drug-resistant bacteria.

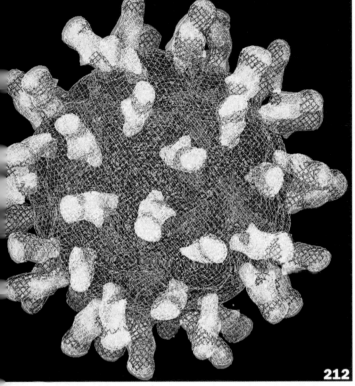

212

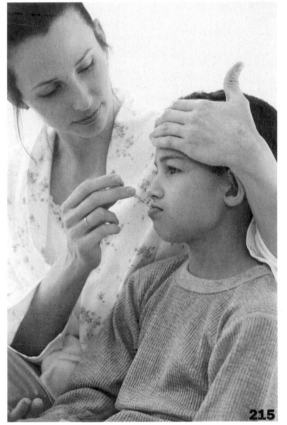

215

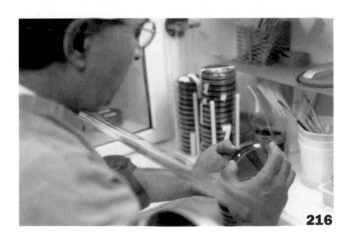

216

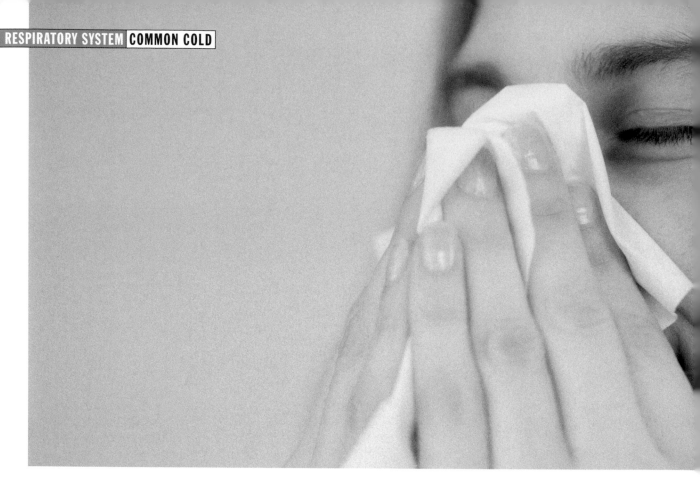

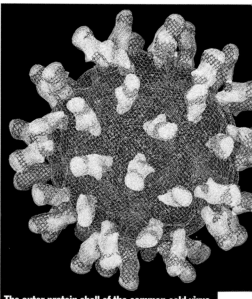

▲ COLD COMFORT Zicam, a zinc nasal spray, delivers zinc right to where most colds start: the nose.

Alternative Answers

Spray Away the Common Cold

There may be good reason for the popularity of the over-the-counter cold treatment called Zicam. This zinc nasal spray showed very promising results in a study of 213 patients, published in the *Ear, Nose, and Throat Journal* in October 2000. Symptoms were reduced by as much as 75 percent, the average time for recovery was reduced to 2 days instead of the 9 days it took for those not given the remedy, and in some cases symptoms were alleviated overnight.

The logic behind Zicam is this: Cold viruses usually enter the body through the nasal cavity, so by delivering its active ingredient, zinc gluconate, to the nose, the nasal-pump product gets at the source of the infection. Researchers believe that charged zinc atoms bind to the cold virus and prevent it from attaching to the nasal lining and multiplying, allowing the body's immune system to get rid of the virus more rapidly. In order to be effective, Zicam should be taken at the first hint of a cold. The product can be purchased over the counter across the United States. Pregnant women should consult a doctor before taking it.

The outer protein shell of the common cold virus, shown here in yellow, locks onto human cells.

Drug Development
Shortening the Life of a Cold

There's no cure yet for the common cold, but a drug is in the works that, in theory, shortens the cold's duration. In March 2001, researchers at the University of Virginia School of Medicine announced the results of two studies of an experimental drug, pleconaril (brand name Picovir), manufactured by ViroPharma. In one study, patients who took pleconaril reported that they had no cold symptoms after 6.2 days, compared with 7.1 days for patients given placebo (dummy) pills. A difference of one day isn't much, but the drug also reduced the severity of symptoms, such as fatigue, nasal congestion, runny nose, cough, and sore throat. However, the second study showed no real difference between taking pleconaril and taking a placebo. One problem with both studies is that patients were allowed to also take acetaminophen, cough syrup, or both, which may have affected the results.

Pleconaril is the first drug of its kind to be shown to decrease the duration of a cold by targeting the virus itself; in contrast, cold drugs currently on the market treat only the cold symptoms. Experts say that people who are the most endangered by colds, such as those with asthma and the elderly, will probably benefit the most from antiviral drugs like pleconaril, which could help prevent colds from leading to more serious conditions, such as sinusitis and middle ear infections.

How it works. Two pleconaril tablets are taken three times a day for five days at the first sign of a cold. Pleconaril appears to work against two common types of cold virus—rhinovirus and enterovirus, which account for about half of all colds. It disrupts the infection cycle at several stages, essentially stopping the virus from copying itself and spreading to other cells.

Availability. ViroPharma plans to submit pleconaril for marketing approval from the U.S. Food and Drug Administration by the end of 2001. If approved, the drug probably will not be covered by most health insurance plans, at least initially. And it won't come cheap: The company estimates that the drug will cost between $40 and $65 for one treatment.

A cure for the common cold?

Scientists have designed a drug that can stop picornaviruses, a large family of viruses that cause colds, meningitis, and polio.

Pleconaril

Picornavirus

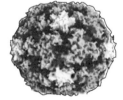

Virus shell

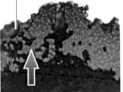

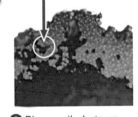

❶ Scientists determined that the viruses are 20-sided geometric forms with many crater-like areas.

❷ The viruses have pores in these craters from which they release their genes into healthy cells.

❸ Pleconaril plugs up these sites much like a broken key in a lock, preventing the virus from damaging healthy cells.

FAST FACTS
7.8 DAYS Average duration of common cold
1 BILLION Number of colds Americans suffer each year **200** Number of different viruses that can cause a cold **15** Number of seconds that a person's hands should be lathered to get rid of cold germs

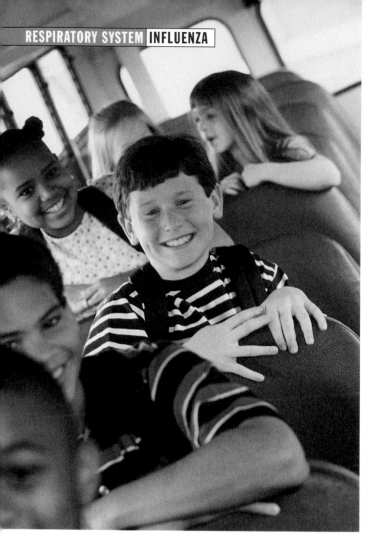

▲ STOPPING THE SPREAD BY TARGETING CHILDREN
Many scientists believe that preschoolers and schoolchildren are the main carriers of flu both in the community and at home. Stop kids from getting the flu, the thinking goes, and the rest of us will benefit. Recent studies seem to indicate that this popular theory holds true: Vaccinating children against the flu appeared to reduce the spread of the disease among other family members—and possibly protected the community at large as well. Flu vaccines are available for children and even infants. Speak to your doctor about whether getting the vaccine is a good idea for your child.

Kids getting the flu

Researchers say influenza is surprisingly common in kids. Here is a look at the number of children, by age, who go to the doctor each year due to the flu.

Doctor visits per 100 children

Less than 6 months
10

6 months to less than 1 year
14.8

1 year to less than 3 years
10.7

3 years to less than 6 years
8

6 years to less than 16 years
6.4

Drug Development
Flu Drugs Help Protect the Healthy, Too

Trying not to get sick when you live with someone who has the flu can be a losing battle, but help may be on the way. Two new prescription drugs, oseltamivir (brand name Tamiflu) and zanamivir (brand name Relenza), may help cut the risk that the flu will spread within a family.

Oseltamivir, the first flu drug in pill form, was initially approved for people who have been sick with the flu for no more than two days. But as shown in a study published in the February 14, 2001, issue of the *Journal of the American Medical Association*, healthy people may benefit too. Within 48 hours of the start of flu symptoms in a household member, study participants took either oseltamivir or a placebo (dummy) pill once a day for seven days. (The household members who actually had the flu received no treatment.) The result? Those who took oseltamivir were 89 percent less likely to develop flu symptoms than those who took the placebo, showing that the drug can, in fact, prevent outbreaks of the flu within households. The study was conducted at 76 centers in North America and Europe during the winter of 1998–1999.

In a study of zanamivir, an inhaled drug, published in the *New England Journal of Medicine* on November 2, 2000, families with two to five members (including at least one adult and at least one child who was five years of age or older) were enrolled before the 1998–1999 flu season. If a flu-like illness developed in one family member, the family was randomly assigned to receive either inhaled zanamivir or a placebo: sick members twice a day for 5 days and

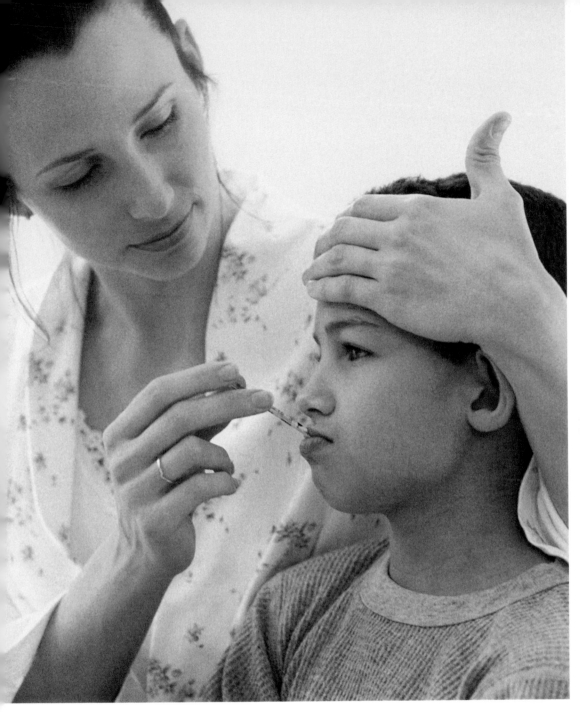

► **ALL IN THE FAMILY** Once someone in the household gets the flu, there's a good chance others will too. But researchers have discovered that two flu drugs can keep the rest of the family from getting sick.

healthy members once a day for 10 days. The rate of protection against the flu was found to be 79 percent in the entire group of healthy family members and 72 percent in the families whose lab tests proved that the illness was actually the flu.

How it works. Oseltamivir and zanamivir are in a class of drugs called neuraminidase inhibitors. Both drugs stop the flu virus from multiplying and spreading by targeting neuraminidase, a protein on the virus's surface that lets the virus break through the walls of cells. When this protein is inhibited, the multiplying virus is unable to escape the cell it has

Those who took oseltamivir were 89 percent less likely to develop flu symptoms.

infected. The drugs are not intended, however, to be substitutes for an annual flu shot.

Availability. Oseltamivir was approved by the U.S. Food and Drug Administration (FDA) in October 1999 for the treatment of flu in adults. In November 2000, it was okayed for use in adolescents aged 13 years and older, and the following month it was approved for use in children aged 1 year and older. Oseltamivir is available in both pill and liquid form. The drug also has been approved in Switzerland, Canada, Japan, and many Latin American countries. It was submitted for approval in Europe in February 2001.

Approved by the FDA in September 1999, zanamivir was the first of this type of drug to reach the market in the United States. People with asthma or a lung condition called chronic obstructive pulmonary disease should be aware that this drug may exacerbate their condition.

FAST FACTS

80 MILLION Number of flu-vaccine doses U.S. manufacturers will produce for next year's flu season **30–35 MILLION** Number of Americans who get sick with the flu yearly **20,000** Number of deaths the flu causes in the United States per year

STAY TUNED FOR...

First Nasal Spray Flu Vaccine

People who are afraid of needles may soon breathe easier with news of an experimental flu vaccine in the form of a nasal spray. At a U.S. Food and Drug Administration (FDA) expert panel meeting in July 2001, the panel agreed that the vaccine, called FluMist, works. However, safety concerns prevented the group from recommending its release. Questions about the drug's safety revolved mostly around its use by children 18 years and under. The drug's manufacturer, Aviron, is working to provide the safety data the FDA has requested and hopes for FluMist to be available for the 2002–2003 flu season. If approved, it would be the first flu vaccine delivered as a nasal mist to be commercially available in the United States.

Researchers say the nasal vaccine may provide stronger protection against the flu than the standard flu vaccine because it kills the

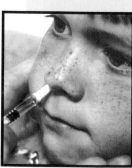

virus in the nasal passages, without ever entering the bloodstream. A drawback of the drug is that it's difficult to transport because it has to remain frozen until used. Aviron is currently working on a liquid version that could be easily shipped all over the world.

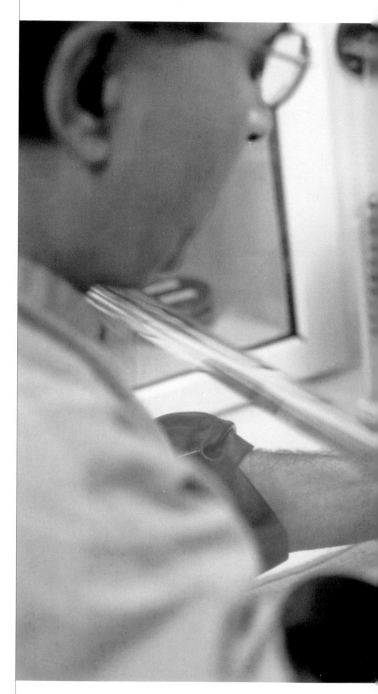

▼ By changing the structure of older antibiotics, scientists have created a new type that is effective against drug-resistant respiratory infections such as pneumonia and bronchitis.

Drug Development

New Weapon Against Drug-Resistant Bacteria

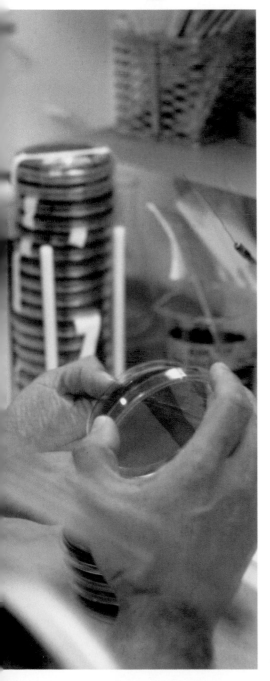

Once upon a time, penicillin was a big gun that worked every time against potentially serious infections such as pneumonia and bronchitis. Not anymore. Now, more and more strains of bacteria that cause respiratory tract infections are developing an alarming resistance to antibiotics—meaning the drugs can no longer clear the infection. In fact, according to a study presented on April 5, 2001, at the 11th European Congress of Clinical Microbiology and Infectious Diseases in Frankfurt, Germany, 39.9 percent of all pneumococci (pneumonia-causing) bacteria are resistant to penicillin. In some countries, such as South Korea and France, the levels of resistance are far higher. Resistance to another common antibiotic, called erythromycin, is also on the rise.

Now there's a family of antibiotic drugs that adds to the arsenal of weapons doctors can use against infectious diseases, including pneumonia, bronchitis, sinusitis, and other respiratory infections. The family is called ketolides, and the "first-born" drug is telithromycin (brand name Ketek). Ketolides are derived from macrolides—the current standard treatment for many bacterial infections—but they've been chemically engineered to kill bacteria that are resistant to these other drugs. There's another advantage: Telithromycin is taken just once a day instead of the three times a day that's standard for many antibiotics, and for many diseases it requires a shorter treatment period than other antibiotics.

How it works. Telithromycin interferes with the production of proteins that enable the bacteria to grow. It does this by binding to the bacteria's ribosome (a cell "organ" located inside the cell membrane that is a site of protein synthesis). Telithromycin binds to ribosomes 10 times more tightly than erythromycin.

Availability. Telithromycin was recommended for approval by the Anti-infective Drug Advisory Committee of the U.S. Food and Drug Administration (FDA) on April 26, 2001 for the treatment of community-acquired pneumonia (pneumonia acquired outside of a hospital setting) in patients aged 18 years and older. Although the FDA is not required to make its decision on the basis of the advisory committee's recommendations, it usually follows them. On July 30, 2001, the drug received approval to be sold in parts of Europe for the same type of pneumonia and for some types of bronchitis, sinusitis, tonsillitis, and pharyngitis.

FAST FACTS
90,147 Number of pneumonia-related deaths recorded in the United States in 1998 **1.4 MILLION** Number of hospitalizations caused by pneumonia in the United States in 1999 **4.8 MILLION** Number of cases of pneumonia in the United States in 1996

f looking good and feeling good go hand in hand, then millions
of people will soon be feeling a whole lot better thanks to
several recent breakthroughs. For the terrible redness, flaking,
and itching of psoriasis, two high-tech drugs have cleared the last
hurdle before they can be considered for approval. These drugs may
do more than just eliminate symptoms—they may actually cause
lasting remission of the disease. And eczema sufferers could benefit
from the first new type of eczema drug in decades, one that provides
effective relief without the dangerous side effects of steroids.

Those seeking eternal youth—or at least a way to get rid of
wrinkles—have new options as well, including a gentler type of laser
treatment that works without damaging the surface of the skin.
And women troubled by unwanted facial hair can now slow hair growth
with a pill originally developed to fight African sleeping sickness.
There's also a new way to combat gum disease so your smile will
stay as good-looking as your skin.

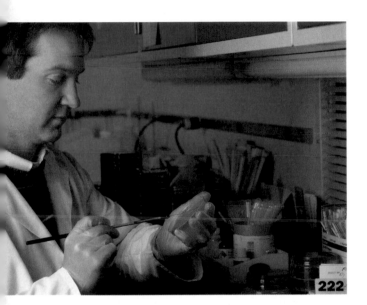

222

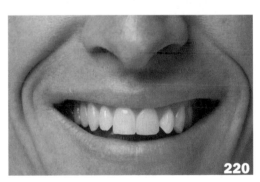

220

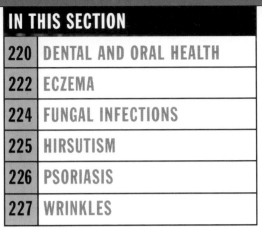

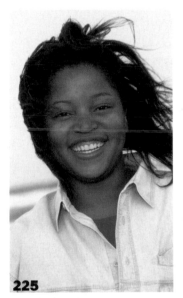

225

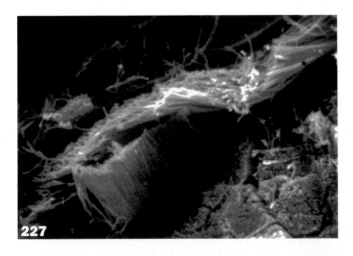

227

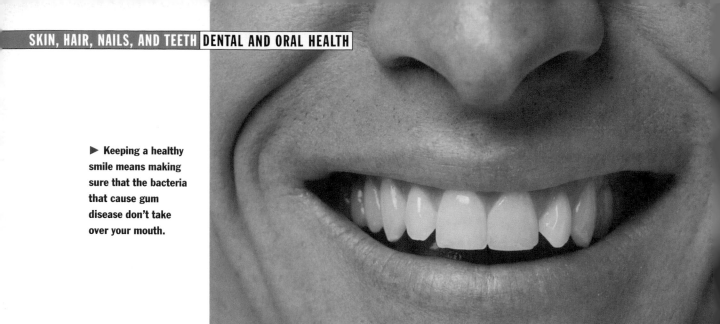

► Keeping a healthy smile means making sure that the bacteria that cause gum disease don't take over your mouth.

Drug Development
Tiny Warriors in the Fight Against Gum Disease

The mouth is home to a nasty bunch of bacteria just waiting to invade every nook and cranny. They can even create gaps between your teeth and gums. The gaps, called pockets, are quickly colonized by more bacteria and by plaque. When this happens, you have an early form of gum disease (and three out of four adults over age 35 do). Left untreated, gum disease can extend below the gums and can eat away at your jaw-bone, causing teeth to fall out. Studies even suggest a link between gum disease and other health problems, ranging from heart disease to stroke to diabetes.

Now there is a new way to counteract gum disease, with tiny self-adhesive pellets of antibiotic placed directly in the gum pocket. Called Arestin, they fight re-infection after scaling and planing, a standard deep-cleaning procedure that removes damaged and diseased tissue and bone.

Three out of four adults over 35 have some degree of gum disease.

How it works. The pellets, or microspheres, are self-sticking, so there is no need for bulky dressing to keep them in place. They release an antibiotic over time, protecting the area from re-infection long enough for the body to begin the healing process. Patients can resume normal brushing and flossing within 12 hours, and there is nothing to remove after the treatment is completed because the microspheres dissolve on their own.

Availability. Arestin was approved by the U.S. Food and Drug Administration in February 2001. A Marketing Authorization Application—the first step in the European approval process—was filed with the Swedish Medical Products Agency in December 2000. It shouldn't be long before Arestin becomes a widely used method to treat gum disease.

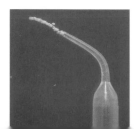

◄ A new treatment for gum disease uses a syringe to place tiny pellets of antibiotic between the tooth and the gum.

Key Finding
Cigarettes: Smoking Guns

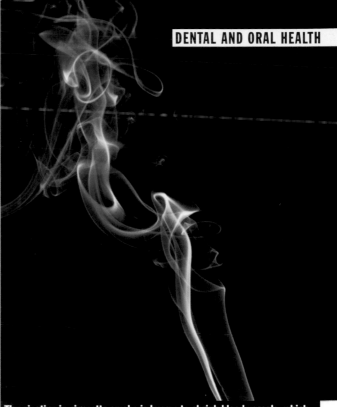

The nicotine in cigarette smoke is known to shrink blood vessels, which may be an underlying reason why smokers—and people exposed to cigarette smoke—are at increased risk for gum disease.

Not only can smoking kill you, it can also cause you to lose your teeth. That's the conclusion drawn by several recent studies that examined the connection between gum disease and smoking. Numerous reports had already shown that smoking was linked to gum disease, including one particularly authoritative study based on a nationwide health survey conducted between 1988 and 1994 in the United States. The study, published in May 2000, indicated that more than half of all cases of periodontitis (inflammation of the gum surrounding a tooth) were attributable to cigarette smoking; in smokers with periodontitis, nearly three-quarters of cases could be connected to smoking. The authors concluded that many cases of periodontitis could be prevented by quitting smoking. Now the following two studies have added to the case against smoking cigarettes:

- A study published in the February 2001 *American Journal of Public Health* found that people who lived around those who smoked—that means at home or in the workplace for as little as one hour a day—were at a 50 to 60 percent greater risk of developing gum disease than were nonsmokers who were not subjected to significant amounts of passive smoke.
- Researchers reported in the April 2001 issue of *Community Dentistry and Oral Epidemiology* that teens who smoke have three times the chance of developing gum

disease by age 26 as those of the same age who don't light up. The study looked at smoking habits at age 15, 18, 21, and 26 for 900 men and women. The results stand even after factoring in dental hygiene habits such as the frequency of flossing and brushing.

The culprit may be nicotine, the active ingredient in tobacco smoke. Nicotine is known to shrink blood vessels and impair the immune system. As a result, sensitive gums and underlying bones have a reduced blood supply and lowered immunity to the bacteria that cause gum disease.

RESEARCH ROUNDUP

■ **HONEY FOR YOUR TEETH.** A recent study out of New Zealand—a place famous for its honey—has found that the sticky stuff actually combats dental plaque and cavities. The effect is the result of an enzyme in honey that produces hydrogen peroxide, which stops cavity-causing bacteria from multiplying in the mouth.

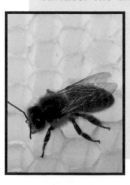

Bees may hold a key to healthier teeth; a new study shows that honey protects against plaque and cavities.

It also prevents the bacteria from producing dextran, the glue-like substance that helps them stick to teeth.

■ **BAD NEWS ABOUT BRACES.** It is becoming increasingly evident that changes to the dental arch (the curve formed by the rows of teeth in the mouth) and lower jaw continue well into adulthood. That explains why orthodontics to straighten teeth are not as lasting as we hoped. The results of a study based in Sweden raise further questions about whether a stable arrangement of teeth can be maintained after adolescence once braces have been removed.

FAST FACTS
50 MILLION Number of Americans with gum disease **20** Percentage of Americans with gum disease who receive treatment for the disease **41.3** Percentage of daily smokers over age 65 who are toothless

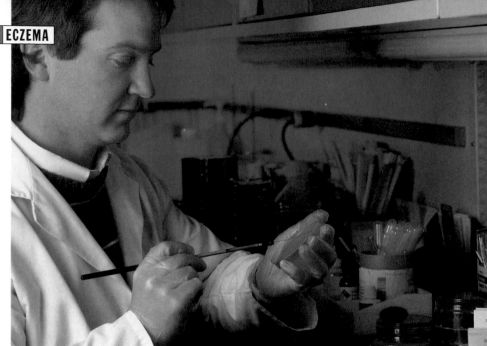

▶ **ITCH BE GONE**
Researchers have discovered a drug that targets immune cells in the skin, stopping the itch of eczema.

Drug Development
First New Eczema Drug in 40 Years

The first new type of drug for eczema in more than 40 years may finally bring relief to people who aren't helped by steroids. Called topical immunomodulators, or TIMs, they don't weaken the skin as steroids do, and studies indicate that they are highly effective for this itchy skin condition.

The first drug in this class to be approved, tacrolimus (brand name Protopic), was originally used to calm the immune system of transplant patients so that they wouldn't reject their new organs. Now it may also help interrupt the "itch-scratch cycle" of eczema.

How it works. The immune system seems to behave abnormally in people with eczema. When those who have eczema scratch, chemical messengers called cytokines are released, tricking the body into thinking it's been invaded by foreign substances. Stopping that immune reaction may be the key to preventing eczema symptoms. TIMs do this by blocking the synthesis and release of cytokines. Because they specifically target immune cells in the skin, there is less chance of the side effects seen with long-term use of steroids (such as thin skin, weak bones, and high blood sugar). However, TIMs may increase the sensitivity of skin to ultraviolet light, so people using them should limit their exposure to the sun or protect themselves by wearing sunscreen.

Availability. In December 2000, the U.S. Food and Drug Administration (FDA) approved tacrolimus ointment for people with moderate to severe eczema who cannot use other treatments because of potential risks or who have not been helped by other treatments. A new drug application for another TIM, called pimecrolimus, was submitted to the FDA in December 2000; pimecrolimus has shown promise in children as young as three months, but it has not yet been approved.

STAY TUNED FOR...

Relief from Severe Eczema
A drug that has been shown to reduce the frequency of asthma attacks is now being tested on people with eczema. These people have abnormally high levels of an antibody (specialized immune-system warriors) called immunoglobulin E (IgE), which tells the body to start an allergic reaction. The drug, a laboratory-synthesized antibody called olizumab, works by binding to IgE so that the release of inflammatory substances that can cause eczema is blocked. Olizumab is currently being studied for the treatment of moderate to severe eczema in patients aged 6 to 16.

Alternative Answers
Oolong Tea for Eczema

Many people find drinking a nice cup of hot tea to be a soothing experience. As it turns out, tea may soothe more than just your nerves; it may also help ease symptoms of stubborn eczema. In a study at Shiga University of Medical Science in Japan, patients were asked to drink about four cups of oolong tea (a type of black tea) each day while continuing their regular eczema therapy. After one month, 63 percent of the patients had either marked or moderate improvement; after six months, 54 percent were still experiencing relief.

Oolong tea is a source of antioxidant compounds called polyphenols. They have been shown to inhibit allergic reactions by neutralizing the unstable oxygen molecules known as free radicals, which can damage cells and lead to disease. Polyphenols may also help by preventing the destruction of essential fatty acids; a deficiency of these nutrients has been linked to eczema. Oolong tea contains more polyphenols than black tea does because the leaves undergo less fermentation, which destroys these antioxidants.

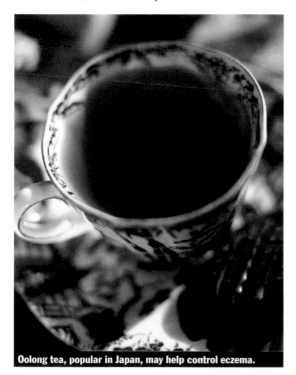

Oolong tea, popular in Japan, may help control eczema.

RESEARCH ROUNDUP

■ **SEALED FOR YOUR PROTECTION.** Mattress covers can do more than help control allergies; they may help control eczema, too. According to researchers at the Karolinska Institutet in Stockholm, Sweden, patients who covered their bedding with polyurethane-coated cotton covers found that the severity of their eczema was reduced by 45 percent. Improvement was also seen with plain cotton covers. The coverings may have reduced the amount of airborne allergens such as dust mites, pollen, mold, and pet dander present in the beds.

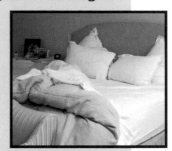

A new study shows that using a mattress cover may reduce eczema symptoms.

■ **STRESS SENSITIVE.** Stress is one of the many triggers that can cause an eczema flare-up. Now a German study has shown that stress affects people with eczema differently than it does other people. A team at Hannover Medical School induced stress in study subjects by having them give a speech or solve math problems in front of an audience. Blood samples were taken before, immediately after, and one hour and one day after the stressful event. After 10 minutes of mental stress, certain T lymphocytes—cells involved in the immune response—reacted significantly more in subjects with eczema than in the healthy subjects. These results indicate that stress has a greater effect on the immune system of people with eczema than on those without eczema. The aim of further studies will be to define the exact role this difference plays in the skin condition.

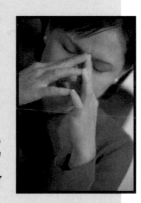

It's not news that stress can cause eczema flare-ups, but now research is showing that, in people with eczema, stress may have a greater effect on the immune system.

FAST FACTS

65 Percentage of eczema patients who develop symptoms in the first year of life **90** Percentage of patients who develop symptoms before age 5 **60** Percentage of infants and young children with eczema who continue to have symptoms into adulthood **SLEEP DISRUPTION** Side effect experienced by 80 percent of people with eczema

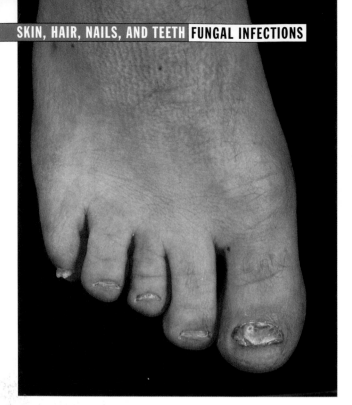

Drug Development
Nail Lacquer Proven to Kick Nail Fungus

◄ **FUNGUS AMONG US**
Nail fungus is notoriously stubborn, but a prescription nail lacquer can help.

When the first topical prescription medication for nail fungus became available more than a year ago, its success rates did not look as high as the oral treatments on the market. However, research carried out during its first year of widespread use has shown ciclopirox nail lacquer (sold under the brand name Penlac) to be effective against both toenail and fingernail fungus. The results of 15 studies conducted around the world showed cure rates of 29 percent to 69 percent for toenail fungus, with minimal side effects. The lacquer should be applied daily for up to 48 weeks. Future studies will determine whether ciclopirox is effective when used in combination with other treatments.

This is bad news for the fast-spreading onychomycosis, a contagious fungal infection of the nail bed. According to a recent large-scale study, the infection has become more common than ever in North America over the last two decades. Of more than 1,800 people tested across the continent, 13.8 percent showed signs of infection, compared with only 2 percent of people in a national survey carried out more than 20 years ago.

Some of the blame for the spread can be laid on overuse of antibiotics, which can lead to increased resistance to treatment. In addition, the aging of the population has played a part, with people becoming more vulnerable to infection as a result of changes in their immune system and circulatory system.

RESEARCH ROUNDUP

■ **RINGWORM AMONG WRESTLERS.** High school wrestlers and runners may both be in great shape, but wrestlers are less healthy in one regard: They have a much higher incidence of ringworm, a fungal infection that produces round, scaly patches on the skin that can cause itchiness. According to a study conducted at the University of Cincinnati in Ohio, 7 of 29 wrestlers tested on one high school team—nearly one in four—showed signs of the fungal infection, compared with none of the 30 tested members of the track team. The condition is particularly contagious in wrestlers— passing from one to

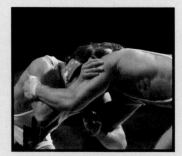

another through direct skin contact—and is so well known in these athletes that it is sometimes called tinea corporis gladiatorum, or gladiator's ringworm.

■ **GARLIC GOOD FOR ATHLETE'S FOOT.** An extract from garlic called ajoene could fight athlete's foot as effectively as a standard treatment, terbinafine cream, according to a Venezuelan study. A total of 70 soldiers with athlete's foot were treated for one week with either ajoene gel or terbinafine. When they were tested 60 days after the end of treatment, all of the subjects treated with one percent ajoene were cured, compared with 94 percent of those treated with 1 percent terbinafine. (Only 47 soldiers were available for the final evaluation, however, so other studies will be needed to confirm these findings.) Because ajoene is relatively inexpensive and easy to prepare, it could become a valuable alternative therapy in developing countries.

High-Tech Help
Better Hair-Removal Treatment for Dark Skin

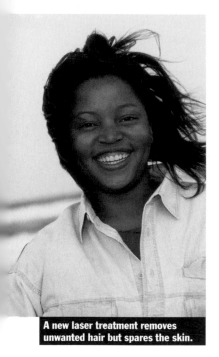

A new laser treatment removes unwanted hair but spares the skin.

Lasers have become powerful tools for hair removal, but many patients—particularly those with dark skin—have experienced considerable pain and even skin discoloration as a result of treatments. Now the Athos laser system, which was approved by the U.S. Food and Drug Administration in October 2000, uses pulses of longer-wavelength light that allow it to target the hair more precisely without harming the skin.

How it works. When a hair-removal laser is applied to skin, the beam passes through the skin and is absorbed by the pigment melanin in the hair. The wavelengths of light used by some laser systems—generally between about 700 and 800 nanometers—are easily absorbed by melanin in the skin as well as that in the hair, sometimes injuring dark skin, which contains more melanin. The Athos system uses a longer wavelength (just over 1,000 nanometers), so less light is absorbed by most types of skin.

Availability. As of July 2001, more than a dozen Athos systems had been sold to U.S. dermatologists, plastic surgeons, and other physicians who perform cosmetic surgery.

Drug Development
The Lifesaver That Became a Face-saver

When they developed a drug for African sleeping sickness, the scientists at Bristol-Myers Squibb probably never envisioned that anyone in the West would want it. The drug, eflornithine hydrochloride, was originally used to cure a deadly insect-borne disease that infects several hundred thousand people in sub-Saharan Africa each year. It is exceptionally effective against the disease, but it happens to have a side effect that makes it desirable in more developed countries as well: It significantly slows the growth of unwanted hair. In July 2000, the U.S. Food and Drug Administration approved an eflornithine facial cream (brand name Vaniqa) as the first topical prescription product to treat excess facial hair.

> **The drug was originally used to cure a deadly insect-borne disease.**

How it works. Eflornithine is thought to block an enzyme in hair follicles necessary to hair growth. The cream slows hair growth but it does not remove hair; most women will need to use a hair-removal method along with the medication.

Availability. Eflornithine is available only by prescription and should be used only on the face and under the chin. It is not meant for use by anyone under the age of 12. Women who are pregnant or breastfeeding should speak to a doctor about whether they can use the cream.

Facial hair no more

Removal of unwanted facial hair could be getting easier. Eflornithine (brand name Vaniqa), a topical cream, blocks an enzyme in the hair follicle that makes the hair grow.

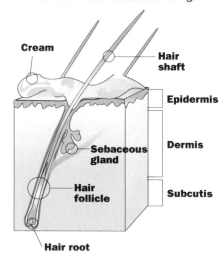

Cream · Hair shaft · Epidermis · Sebaceous gland · Dermis · Hair follicle · Subcutis · Hair root

Drug Development
Breakthrough Drugs for Psoriasis May Offer Best Treatment Yet

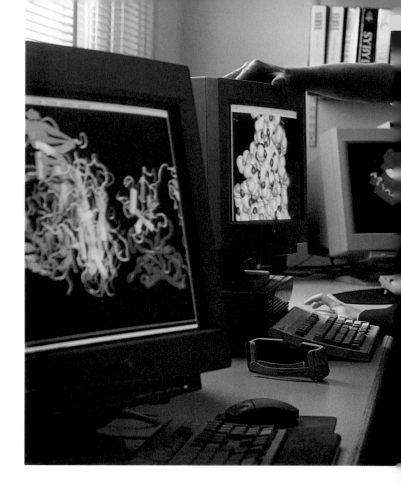

The hope attached to both drugs is for a treatment that will not just eliminate symptoms but also provide lasting remission of the disease.

Rough, dry, dead skin cells—this was once called "the heartbreak of psoriasis." The condition still troubles millions of people worldwide, causing inflammation, unsightly patches of thickened skin, discomfort, and sometimes pain. Ranging from annoying to disabling, psoriasis is a condition that has been treated with everything from creams and ointments to pills and phototherapy—with mixed success. Now, two biotech companies—Biogen and Genentech—have completed phase III clinical trials of drugs that work "smarter" than the drugs currently available and may offer more, longer-lasting relief.

How it works. Genentech's drug, Xanelim, developed in partnership with Xoma Ltd, is a monoclonal antibody—a specially engineered version of the body's own antibodies (proteins that recognize and bind to dangerous invaders). To date, monoclonal antibodies have been successful at targeting cancer cells and destroying them without the toxic effects of chemotherapy and radiation. Now Xanelim takes aim at moderate to severe psoriasis by preventing the activation of immune cells called T cells and their migration to sites of inflammation on the skin. Biogen's drug, Amevive, is a protein that targets

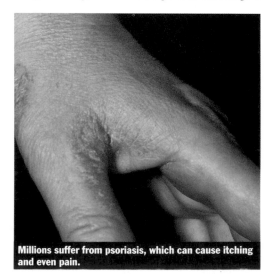

Millions suffer from psoriasis, which can cause itching and even pain.

▲ Scientists at Biogen research a new kind of drug to treat psoriasis that targets the underlying cause of the condition.

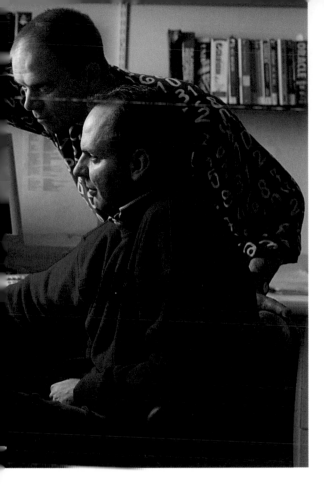

High-Tech Help

Laser Zaps Wrinkles without "Burn Victim" Results

Many people who consider having laser resurfacing to rejuvenate their skin are put off when they learn about the bruising, swelling, and crusty, oozing skin that follow the procedure, as well as the weeks of at-home recovery required. But a new, gentler type of laser, the NLite Laser Collagen Replenishment system, targets the skin layers below the surface, allowing patients to return to their normal activities immediately after treatment.

As a bonus, the skin improvements that follow a laser resurfacing session appear gradually, over the course of 30 to 90 days, so you don't suddenly show up at work looking years younger.

How it works. The NLite laser focuses its energy on layers of colla-

▼ A new laser treatment for wrinkles targets the collagen layer under the skin's surface.

only the specific T cells linked to psoriasis, leaving the rest of the immune system alone.

The hope attached to both drugs is for a treatment that will not just eliminate symptoms but also provide lasting remission of the disease. The drugs also could potentially be successful in treating a wide range of autoimmune disorders, such as rheumatoid arthritis, ulcerative colitis, Crohn's disease, and multiple sclerosis, that affect at least 10 million people in the United States, Europe, and Japan. Genentech began testing Xanelim in kidney transplant patients in early 2000 to evaluate its ability to prevent organ rejection.

Availability. Final-stage clinical trials for both Xanelim and Amevive have shown promising results against psoriasis symptoms. Biogen applied for U.S. Food and Drug Administration approval in August 2001, and Genentech will do so by early 2002.

FAST FACTS
7 MILLION Estimated number of Americans affected by psoriasis **BETWEEN 15 AND 35** Ages when psoriasis most typically first develops

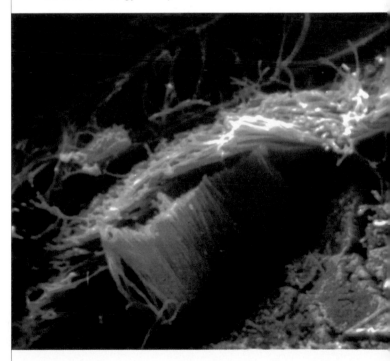

gen (a protein that gives the skin its structural support) below the surface of the skin. Unlike earlier lasers, it uses a frequency of yellow light that passes right through the outermost skin layer without harming it. The treatment takes about 30 to 60 minutes, depending on the size and number of wrinkles being treated. No anesthesia is required. The procedure stimulates the growth of new collagen to replace that damaged by the laser, leaving the wrinkles in the treated areas shallower and less noticeable.

Availability. In September 2000, the NLite became the first laser cleared by the U.S. Food and Drug Administration for nonablative treatment (one that does not destroy outer skin tissue) of wrinkles around the eyes. The treatment is available in the offices of qualified physicians.

RESEARCH ROUNDUP

■ **SMOKING WEAKENS THE SKIN.** A study may finally have explained why smokers tend to look older than nonsmokers. Skin is supported by a scaffolding of collagen, a protein in the skin's middle layer. The skin continually renews itself by breaking down and rebuilding collagen. Now, researchers at St. John's Institute of Dermatology in London have found that a gene that triggers the release of a collagen-destroying enzyme is very active in smokers. Because this enzyme is known to be involved in wrinkles induced by sunbathing, these results indicate that cigarettes damage the skin through the same pathways as sunlight.

■ **VITAMIN C MAKES OLD SKIN LOOK NEWER.** Vitamin C cream can rearrange the structure of collagen in the skin, making it look more like that of younger skin, according to a new study. Using a mold to make incredibly detailed relief images of the skin, French researchers compared the number and arrangement of skin wrinkles in 20 women before and after six months of treatment with 5 percent vitamin C cream. At the end of the treatment period, the skin of subjects treated with the cream showed wrinkles arranged in random directions rather than in similar directions, as is characteristic of older skin. In addition, the cream stimulated the production of new collagen. Vitamin C is a well-known antioxidant, but this study is the first time that scientists have shown how it works in human skin to lessen the signs of aging.

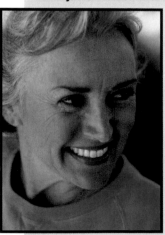

Vitamin C cream has been shown to improve the appearance of older skin.

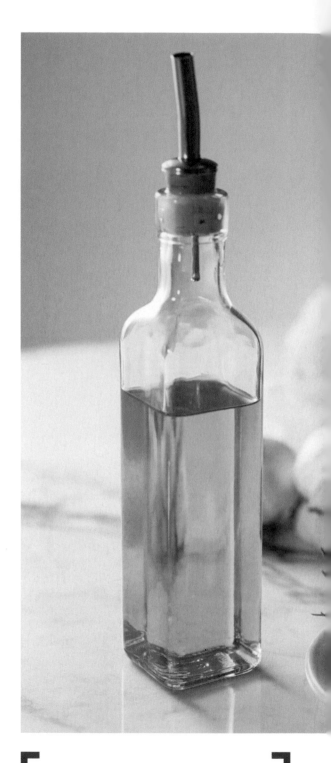

FAST FACTS
1,897,508 Number of chemical peels performed in the United States in 2000 **244,370** Number of facelifts performed in the United States in 2000 **UP TO 90** Percentage of skin damage thought to be caused by prolonged sun exposure **$800 TO $1,800** Approximate cost of the NLite laser treatment

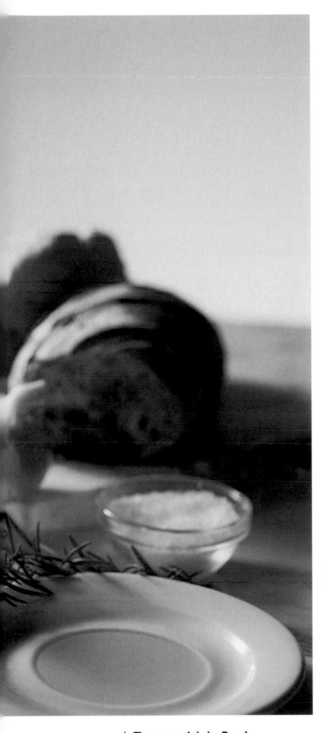

▲ The research is in: People who eat a healthy diet rich in olive oil and lean on meat have fewer wrinkles.

Nutrition Tip
Wholesome Foods Ward Off Wrinkles

A healthier diet could help prevent wrinkles, according to an international study of eating habits and skin aging published in the *Journal of the American College of Nutrition* in April 2001.

Researchers at Monash University in Melbourne, Australia studied more than 400 elderly subjects living in Australia, Greece, and Sweden, including both light-skinned Anglo-Celts and darker-skinned people born in Greece. The subjects' diets were evaluated for nutrient content, and their skin was assessed for wrinkling. Analysis showed that people who ate substantial amounts of green leafy vegetables, beans, and olive oil had significantly less skin wrinkling—regardless of age, smoking, and sun exposure—and that those who consumed a lot of meat and dairy products, including butter, had more wrinkling.

According to the study's authors, the high levels of antioxidant vitamins (such as vitamins A, C, and E) in certain foods may strengthen the skin's defenses against sun damage. Future studies will be needed to confirm the wrinkle-resistant qualities of these good-for-you foods.

STAY TUNED FOR...

Green Tea Sunblock

Drinking green tea is known to be good for you, and now we've learned that putting it on your skin may actually protect against sun damage. In a study published in the March 2001 issue of the *Journal of the American Academy of Dermatology*, extracts of powerful antioxidants called polyphenols, found in green tea, were applied to the skin of healthy subjects. After 30 minutes the skin was exposed to ultraviolet light. The treated areas developed less redness, fewer sunburn cells, and less DNA damage than normal. That means green tea products could add a natural alternative to the array of sunblocks currently on the market.

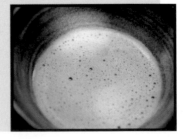

THE URINARY TRACT

I f you're over 50, there's a good chance that you'll develop some kind of urinary problem within the next 15 years. The conditions that strike most often—prostate enlargement and urinary incontinence—aren't fatal, but they can rob you of your independence. Using breakthrough techniques introduced in the past year, doctors will soon be shrinking enlarged prostates with injections of alcohol or the application of microwave energy. A new treatment for incontinence uses special tape inserted through needles only 5 mm in diameter to effectively tighten the muscles that control the bladder.

There's new hope for serious kidney conditions as well. A promising drug relieves a debilitating side effect of dialysis, the blood-filtering procedure that cleanses the blood when the kidneys shut down. And a vaccine to prevent bladder infections is on its way to approval. This key advance will prevent untreated bladder infections from advancing to kidney failure.

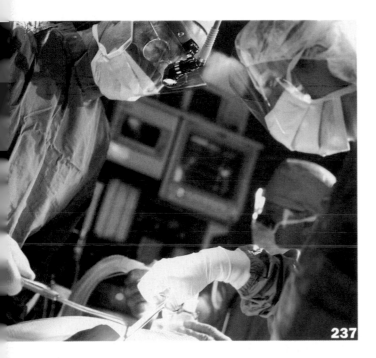

237

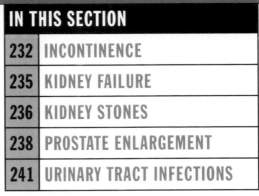

234

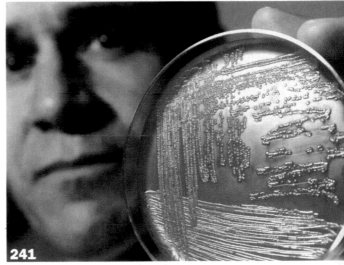

241

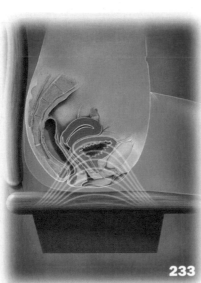

233

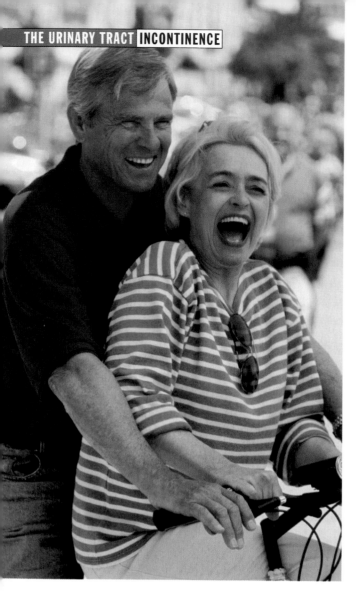

▲ A sneeze, a cough, or even a laugh can cause urine leakage in people with stress incontinence, common in older women. A new procedure makes surgery to correct the condition easier.

STAY TUNED FOR...

Stem Cells to Strengthen Weak Bladders

Someday, doctors may be able to permanently cure incontinence by using stem cells to rebuild damaged bladder muscle. Working in rats, researchers from the University of Pittsburgh in Pennsylvania took stem cells—cells that have the potential to develop into different types of tissue—from normal muscle and injected them into urethral sphincters (circular muscles that close around the bladder opening, preventing urine from leaking out) that had been deprived of their nerve supply. After two weeks, in response to electrical stimulation, the treated muscle strips had recovered most of their function. In addition, new muscle fiber was found at the site of the injection. These findings open the way to future studies in humans.

Surgical Solution

Solving a Personal Problem— Permanently

Every year, the number of operations for stress incontinence—the most common type of urinary incontinence—increases by 30 percent. Why the growing number of these operations? The aging of the population is partly responsible. As women reach middle age, they are more likely to develop stress incontinence, marked by urine leakage any time the urethra is subjected to pressure (exerted by sneezing, coughing, laughing, heavy lifting, and similar activities). More women are also opting for incontinence surgery because improved techniques have made it less invasive and less painful. A new technique uses a recently developed type of tape placed through a small incision in the vagina in order to shore up the structures that support the urethra, tightening the urinary opening so that urine cannot leak out.

How it works. In this operation, the surgeon makes two tiny incisions above the pubic bone and a third tiny incision within the vagina, just below the urethra. Two curved needles are then passed through the tissue between the urethra and vagina, creating a tunnel to the vaginal incision. The tape is placed through the tunnel and adjusted to provide optimal support of the urethra. The operation is done under a local anesthetic and usually takes about 30 minutes.

One advantage over similar operations (known as sling procedures) is that the tape, unlike other materials, does not have to be stitched or stapled into place—its size and positioning prevent it from moving. In addition, the surgical approach used in this procedure (passing the needles from above rather than below) has less risk of causing damage to the bowel or blood vessels near the bladder.

Availability. The SPARC Sling System from American Medical Systems became available in parts of Europe in the spring of 2001 and was approved by the U.S. Food and Drug Administration (FDA) for marketing in the United States in August 2001. Other sling systems are also available in the United States, including the BioSling from Prosurg, which was granted FDA approval in late May 2001.

High-Tech Help
Urinary Incontinence? Pull Up a (Magnetic) Chair

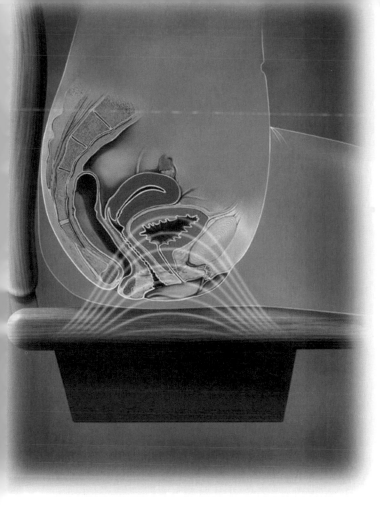

W omen whose pelvic floor muscles—the muscles that support the bladder and urethra—have been weakened by childbearing are especially susceptible to urinary incontinence as they age. Most doctors recommend simple exercises called Kegels to help strengthen these muscles, but many women have trouble getting the knack, since they find it hard to isolate the muscles involved.

◄ **The NeoControl chair uses a magnetic field to tone muscles of the so-called pelvic floor.**

Now a noninvasive device called the NeoControl Pelvic Floor Therapy System is available to make the pelvic floor muscles contract involuntarily; the muscles become conditioned in the process. The device also helps women recognize the sensation of contracting these muscles so they can eventually do Kegels on their own.

How it works. A patient sits fully clothed in a chair that has a programmable magnetic field generator positioned near the center of the seat. By inserting a customized electronic card into the control panel that is located next to the chair, the patient activates the generator to emit a highly focused magnetic field targeting the nerves that control pelvic floor contraction. The magnetic field activates nerves along the tailbone. Impulses from these activated nerves trigger involuntary contractions of the patient's pelvic floor muscles.

These treatments, which last about 20 minutes each, typically take place in a doctor's office twice a week until the patient is able to contract the muscles on her own, which is usually after eight weeks.

Availability. The NeoControl Pelvic Floor Therapy System is found in university hospitals, major medical centers, and private urologists' offices.

RESEARCH ROUNDUP

■ **BLADDER CONTROL.** Researchers from Roche Bioscience recently made a major advance in understanding how the body stores and releases urine. They isolated a receptor (a molecule that picks up hormonal signals) on the surface of bladder cells that activates nerve endings that provoke the release of urine. The discovery could pave the way for new drugs designed to block or remove the P2X3 receptor, potentially restoring urinary control. Current drug treatments for overactive bladder block acetylcholine receptors, involved in nerve-to-muscle communications throughout the body. Because these receptors are so widespread in the body, the drugs that block them in the bladder also block them elsewhere, causing a range of side effects. P2X3 receptors are found only in the bladder, so blocking them should not affect the rest of the body.

Older drugs to treat stress incontinence provide relief but come with unwanted side effects. Now a new generation of drugs that don't dry out skin is on the horizon.

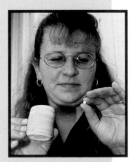

[
FAST FACTS
13 MILLION People with incontinence in the United States **85** Percentage of those with incontinence who are women **50** Percentage of nursing home residents who are incontinent
]

233

Drug Development
Blood Pressure Drug Cuts Side Effects of Dialysis

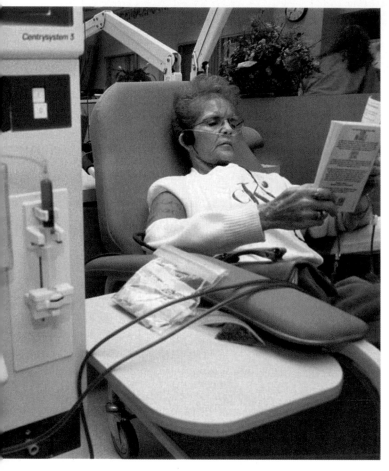

▲ During dialysis, blood pressure can drop precipitously, causing dizziness and nausea. Now researchers are discovering that a drug used to treat high blood pressure can help.

People with end-stage renal disease (defined as 85 to 90 percent loss of kidney function) must regularly undergo the blood-cleansing procedure known as dialysis in order to stay alive. One unpleasant and potentially dangerous side effect, experienced by as many as half of dialysis patients during and after each treatment, is a nose dive in blood pressure caused by the rapid loss of fluid that has accumulated in the body between dialysis sessions. This condition, known as intradialytic hypotension (IDH), can trigger life-threatening heart rhythm abnormalities as well as nausea, vomiting, and dizziness. IDH is so uncomfortable and frightening that it keeps many patients from continuing with their dialysis treatments.

Mark Perazella, M.D., associate professor of medicine and director of Acute Dialysis Services at Yale School of Medicine in New Haven, Connecticut, has found that a drug called midodrine (brand name ProAmatine) relieves IDH in people who were resistant to other therapies. And the effect of midodrine was found to be long lasting. Doctors ordinarily prescribe midodrine to treat the low blood pressure that occurs when people with weak hearts and poor circulation stand up too quickly. Perazella also noted that patients on midodrine experience few side effects.

How it works. Midodrine makes dilated arteries and veins constrict by activating a certain receptor (a molecule that picks up hormonal signals) on vessel walls. This receptor binds to hormones that tell the body to send more blood to the brain and heart. In response, the blood vessels tighten, and blood pressure rises.

Availability. Midodrine has not been approved specifically for dialysis patients in the United States, but because it has approval for treating low blood pressure, doctors are free to prescribe it for this purpose.

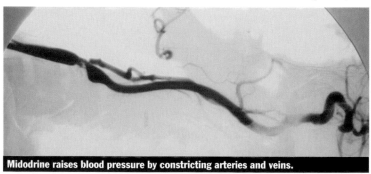

Midodrine raises blood pressure by constricting arteries and veins.

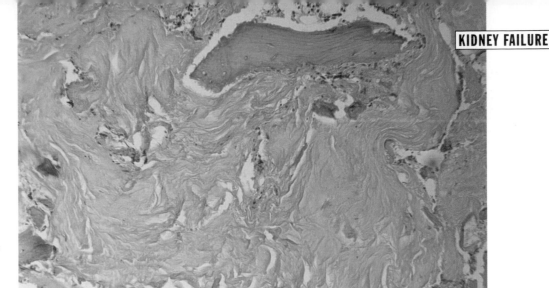

►Bone marrow cells (shown in a microscopic view) may help people with kidney transplants avoid organ rejection, without the use of drugs to suppress their immune system.

Progress in Prevention
Anti-Rejection Insurance for Transplant Patients

If you've had a kidney transplant—or any other major organ transplant—you probably expect to take immune system-suppressing medication for the rest of your life. But soon that may no longer be necessary. As Benedict Cosimi, M.D., of Massachusetts General Hospital in Boston reported at the Experimental Biology 2001 meeting, a technique called mixed chimerism could permanently trick the immune system into accepting someone else's kidney.

How it works. In this technique, the patient receives not only the kidney from the donor, but some of their bone marrow cells, too. Bone marrow produces the immune system cells that distinguish "self" from foreign tissues and mobilize an attack against anything that appears foreign. The hope is that the donor's bone marrow will reduce the risk of organ rejection without suppressing the immune system.

Availability. So far only two patients have been treated with mixed chimerism. Both of them were able to stop taking immune-suppressing drugs about three months after their transplants. Larger trials of mixed chimerism were planned for later in 2001.

About three months after their transplants, those treated with mixed chimerism no longer needed immune-suppressing drugs.

> **FAST FACTS**
> **250,000** Number of people in the United States who undergo dialysis
> **50,000** Number of people who die from kidney failure each year in the United States **30–40** Percentage of people with type 1 diabetes who develop kidney disease **10–15** Percentage of people with type 2 diabetes who develop kidney disease **35** Percentage of donor kidneys rejected by their recipients' immune system within one year of transplantation

Progress in Prevention
The New Stone-Stopping Diet

Most people who have endured a kidney stone would do just about anything never to have another one. Even a stone scarcely bigger than a grain of sand can cause excruciating pain. Doctors often give dietary advice to help people avoid stones, but new findings have changed those recommendations dramatically.

Got milk? Most kidney stones form when urinary calcium binds with substances called oxalates that crystallize in the kidney. Apart from genetic predisposition (having family members with kidney stones triples your risk), it's unclear why calcium and oxalate forge their unholy alliance in some people and spare others. Until recently, doctors advised a low-calcium diet for people susceptible to kidney stones. Studies in the past several years, however, have shown that limiting your calcium intake actually promotes the formation of stones.

Eat your vegetables. Another recommendation, to eat less protein, stemmed from the fact that the more protein you eat, the more calcium your kidneys excrete. The source of your protein seemed important as well: Studies found that meat-eaters had more new stones than did vegetarians who consumed the same amount of protein from beans, nuts, and grains. Experts concluded that animal protein promoted stone formation more than plant protein. But in the March 2001 *Journal of the American Dietetic Association,* researchers reported an experiment that challenged this conclusion. When 23 volunteers with a history of kidney stones spent two days on a diet with beef as the protein source and two more days on the same diet with beans, nuts, seeds, and grains for protein, the risk of kidney stones (based on the composition of the urine) didn't change.

The path of a kidney stone

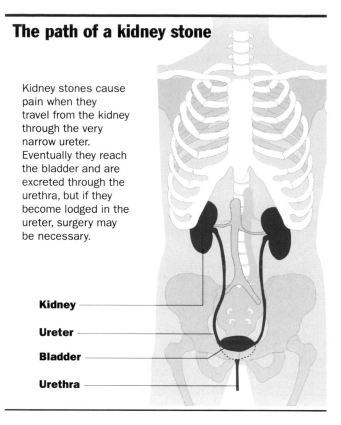

Kidney stones cause pain when they travel from the kidney through the very narrow ureter. Eventually they reach the bladder and are excreted through the urethra, but if they become lodged in the ureter, surgery may be necessary.

Kidney

Ureter

Bladder

Urethra

Studies in the past several years have shown that limiting your calcium intake actually promotes the formation of kidney stones.

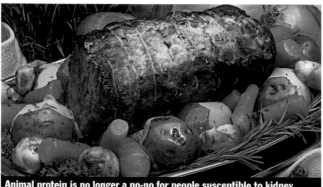

Animal protein is no longer a no-no for people susceptible to kidney stones. Just make sure you keep within recommended limits.

What does this mean? First, consuming too much protein from any source is still a bad idea both for people predisposed to kidney stones and for the population as a whole. Second, as long as you limit your intake to 43 to 50 grams per day (the lower number for women), the source of the protein doesn't matter.

And last but not least, the best thing you can do is to cut back on processed and salty foods and (surprise!) add more fruits and vegetables to your diet. The study showed that people on "real-life" diets full of convenience foods had more stone-promoting substances in their urine than people on either experimental diet.

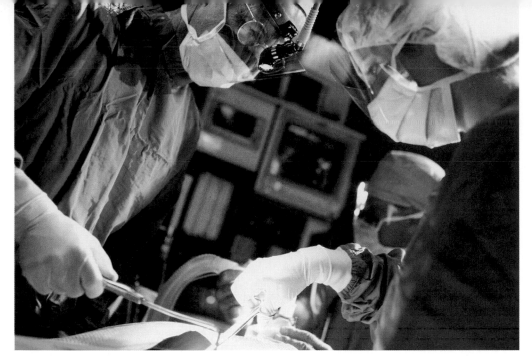

◄ In the future, surgeons may switch to a newer way to cut out kidney stones.

High-Tech Help
A Kinder Cut for Kidney Stone Surgery

Large stones lodged deep in the kidney's urine collection system may not hurt as much as small stones passing into the bladder, but they can do serious damage. Some of these stones can be removed through a noninvasive procedure that uses high-frequency sound waves to pulverize them into tiny bits that are then carried out in the urine. But some stones still require surgical removal. Unfortunately, operating on the kidney is tricky business because the organ's blood supply is so plentiful and its filtering units are packed so tightly together. Now a tissue- and blood-sparing technique called water jet resection, which was pioneered for liver surgery, is being studied for possible use in removing kidney stones and tumors as well.

How it works. Water jet resection uses an ultra-fine, pressurized jet of saline (salt water) to cut through the delicate structures of the kidney without severing blood vessels that are more than 0.3 mm in diameter. In the July 2000 issue of *European Urology*, German urologist R.F. Basting, M.D., reported successful stone and tumor removal, with minimal blood loss and short operating time (14 to 30 minutes), using the water jet system.

Availability. Water jet resection is in its earliest testing stages for kidney surgery. The technique will not be widely available for several years to come.

FAST FACTS
85 Percentage of kidney stones that are passed spontaneously
1 MILLION Number of U.S. residents who periodically have kidney stones
2.5 LITERS Amount of water kidney stone patients should drink each day to prevent recurrence

RESEARCH ROUNDUP

■ **SHIFT YOUR SLEEP POSITION AND SAY GOODBYE TO KIDNEY STONES.** A recent finding from the University of California–San Francisco suggests that you can cut the risk of kidney stone recurrence simply by shifting your sleep position every few hours during the night. Building on the observation that many people who have repeated kidney stone attacks always get them on the same side of the body, the researchers spent two years following 110 kidney stone patients who had had multiple stones on the same side. Most of the patients (84 percent) slept on the same side every night and, of that group, 75 percent consistently slept on the stone-producing side. The possible explanation: Blood circulation, already reduced during sleep, is particularly sluggish on the weight-bearing side of the body, perhaps keeping the kidney on that side from clearing itself of stone-promoting substances.

High-Tech Help
Shrinking the Prostate Without Drugs or Surgery

More than half of all men over age 60 have prostate enlargement, or benign prostatic hyperplasia (BPH), an overgrowth of tissue in the reproductive gland at the base of the bladder. This condition causes increased frequency of urination and makes it difficult to empty the bladder completely. Surgery can solve the problem by destroying excess prostate tissue, but two potential complications—urinary incontinence and impotence—make this option less than ideal. Now, two U.S. companies have found better ways to reduce the size of enlarged prostates.

One method, a procedure called microwave thermoplasty, involves heating the prostate to destroy excess tissue with microwaves delivered through a urinary catheter. It has been performed for several years, but the latest technique has a new twist: a balloon-tipped catheter. The balloon is inflated in the part of the urethra compressed by the prostate, making it possible to reduce obstruction with less heat—and less discomfort. The other procedure, ProstaJect, which is already used in other organs, involves injecting ethanol (alcohol) to destroy cells in the enlarged gland.

How it works. In the microwave thermoplasty technique, a catheter is inserted through the urethra, placed next to the prostate, and set to emit microwave energy, gradually heating the gland to a temperature of about

Surgery can solve the problem by destroying excess prostate tissue, but two potential complications— urinary incontinence and impotence— make this option less than ideal.

115°F (46°C). This causes the tissue to shrink. Unlike two similar microwave devices already approved to treat enlarged prostate, this one is effective immediately (instead of several days later) because a balloon at the tip of the catheter stretches the urethra, making it easier to pass urine. Because the device heats the prostate to a lower temperature than similar devices, there is also less pain during recovery.

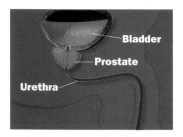

◀ When the prostate is enlarged, the urethra is constricted, making urination difficult.

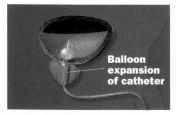

◀ A new type of catheter delivers microwave radiation to shrink the prostate and also has a balloon that, when inflated (as shown here), stretches the urethra to make urination easier.

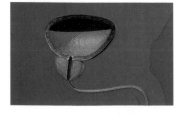

◀ After the heating procedure is complete, the catheter is withdrawn, leaving the urethra clear.

ProstaJect for prostate enlargement

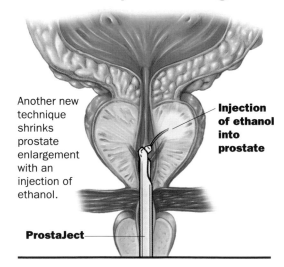

Another new technique shrinks prostate enlargement with an injection of ethanol.

Injection of ethanol into prostate

ProstaJect

The procedure is done in a doctor's office and takes about one hour.

In the second technique, Prosta-Ject delivers ethanol to the prostate through a thin tube passed through the urethra. Ethanol, a powerful solvent, draws water out of tissues. This causes cells to collapse and die. Ethanol injection has been used to destroy obstructions in the liver, esophagus, and colon, but ProstaJect is the first ethanol injection tool designed specifically for the prostate. This in-office procedure is done under a local anesthetic and mild sedation.

Availability. A study, started in New York at the end of 2000 and in nine other sites around the United States in early 2001, is comparing the microwave device (Celsion's Micro-focus BPH 800) with the drug finasteride (brand name Proscar), a first-line therapy for BPH, to determine whether one is more effective than the other. If the procedure works as well as or better than the drug, it should be available sometime in 2002.

ProstaJect went on the market in parts of Europe in April 2001. In the United States, safety trials started at 13 medical centers in January 2001. If the results are good, ProstaJect may be approved for use in the United States sometime in 2002.

STAY TUNED FOR...

A Disappearing Catheter
After minimally invasive procedures to reduce the size of the prostate, many men need a urinary catheter for several days because of swelling of the urethra. Making the catheter obsolete would meet with tremendous appreciation. American Medical Systems is on the way to creating a solution with the development of a stent (a specially designed mesh cylinder placed in a narrowed passageway, such as the urethra, to keep it open) made from materials the body will absorb within two to four weeks.

Drug Development
Next-Generation Drugs Promise Better Relief of BPH

For several years, a group of blood pressure drugs called alpha blockers has been used to treat prostate enlargement, or benign prostatic hyperplasia (BPH). Trouble is, if your problem is BPH and your blood pressure is just fine, alpha blockers will still relax your blood vessels, with the unwelcome side effects of dizziness and fatigue. A reformulation of the alpha-blocking drug doxazosin (brand name Cardura) may solve that problem. Also in the pipeline is dutasteride, a drug similar to but more potent than finasteride (brand name Proscar), a first-line drug therapy for some men with BPH.

▶ Blood pressure drugs have been used to treat prostate enlargement, but they can cause dizziness and fatigue. A new drug relieves symptoms without the side effects.

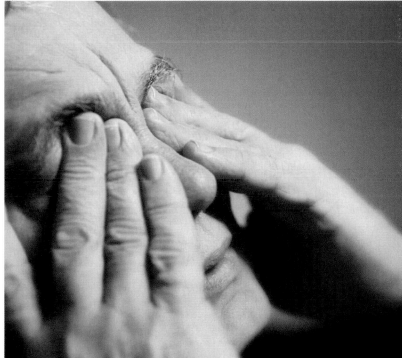

How it works. Alpha blockers relax the body's smooth muscles—including muscle fibers in the prostate gland and bladder neck. The muscles become more pliant, relieving urinary blockage. Traditional alpha blockers also relax the blood

FAST FACTS
1 BILLION Dollars spent on drug therapy for BPH **90** Percentage of men in the United States aged 70 and older with BPH **13 MILLION** Number of men in the United States with BPH

vessels. But the new formulation of Cardura, called (S)-doxazosin, has a slightly different molecular structure. It affects urinary smooth muscle without dramatically altering the tone of blood vessels, making the occurrence of side effects less common.

Finasteride and the experimental drug dutasteride both work by suppressing the hormone DHT (dihydrotestosterone), which stimulates the growth of prostate tissue. But dutasteride blocks two of the enzymes the body uses to manufacture DHT, while finasteride blocks only one. This second action may make dutasteride more effective than finasteride. In a 24-week comparison of the two drugs, DHT levels in the dutasteride group were 18 percent lower than in the finasteride group. Researchers are currently looking at whether this translates to greater reduction of BPH symptoms.

Availability. In March 2001, the makers of (S)-doxazosin started phase I clinical testing to determine its safety. The drug could be available in two to three years. Dutasteride's manufacturer is in the last phase of testing to prove the drug's efficacy before applying for regulatory approval in the United States and Europe. It could hit the market as soon as 2002.

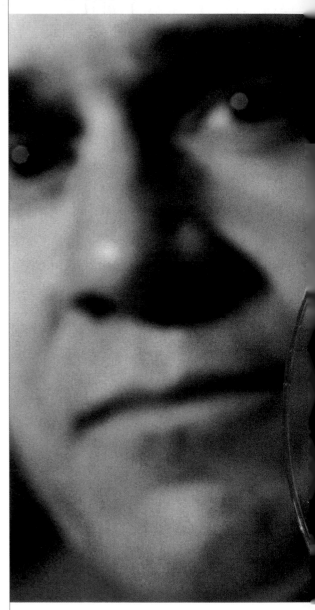

▼ TAKE AIM The bacterium *E. coli* causes the majority of urinary tract infections. A new vaccine can stop it in its tracks.

RESEARCH ROUNDUP

■ **WHO NEEDS PROSTATE SURGERY?** Some expert panels recommend surgery to reduce the size of the prostate after a single episode of acute urinary retention—in other words, being unable to urinate and requiring a catheter to drain the bladder and relieve pain. But if the prostate is not severely enlarged, it's possible to avoid surgery without suffering urinary retention again, according to a recent British study. Researchers from Leighton Hospital in Crewe, England, followed 40 men for 8 to 24 months after an episode of acute urinary retention, managed with two days of catheterization. More than half of the men did not experience a recurrence of retention. The best predictor was prostate size at the time of the initial retention episode. The men who stayed unblocked had a mean prostate weight of 15.9 grams, while the men who wound up needing surgery had a mean prostate weight of 27.5 grams.

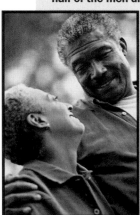

A new study shows that not all men who have suffered an episode of urinary retention will need prostate surgery.

Progress in Prevention
Vaccine Protects against Urinary Tract Infections

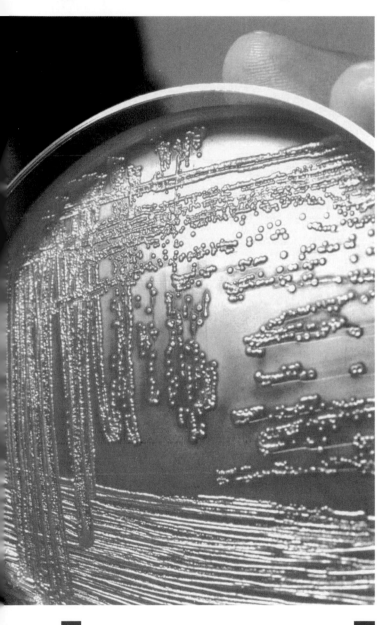

Women get urinary tract infections (UTIs) far more often than men. By age 30, about 50 percent of women have had at least one infection, and as many as 10 percent suffer recurrent infections. The culprit in more than 80 percent of cases is *Escherichia coli*, a bacterium that normally grows in the lower intestine. A vaccine now being tested in 390 women with recurrent UTIs seems to stop *E. coli* from anchoring itself to bladder cells, preventing the most common type of UTI.

How it works. The vaccine is made from a protein component of *E. coli* that promotes the organism's growth in the bladder. Once inoculated with this protein, a woman's immune system is primed to produce antibodies (specific germ-recognition proteins) against it. Thereafter, the immune system will recognize and attack that component of *E. coli*, preventing the bacterium from multiplying and colonizing the bladder.

The first and second doses of the vaccine are spaced four weeks apart, and the third dose is given five to six months after the second.

Availability. Preliminary results from trials being conducted should be available by the end of 2001. Before the U.S. Food and Drug Administration can approve the vaccine, larger trials involving a few thousand women will be necessary to strengthen the proof of its effectiveness.

The company that developed the vaccine, MedImmune, in Gaithersburg, Maryland, plans to market it in the United States and Europe pending the results of the trials.

> ## The culprit in more than 80 percent of urinary tract infections is E. coli, a bacterium that normally grows in the lower intestine.

FAST FACTS
40 Percentage of women who have had at least one UTI
20 Percentage of women who have recurrent UTIs
600,000 Number of catheter-related infections in United States hospitals per year

Resource Directory

For a wealth of information on a particular ailment or other medical topic, turn to the organizations listed here. Call, write, or log on to their websites to find out what type of news, information, and services they provide. Many offer patient guides, events listings, study enrollment, advocacy programs, support groups, newsletters, free publications, and physician referrals.

GENERAL RESOURCES

AARP
601 E Street, NW
Washington, DC 20049
(800) 424-3410
www.aarp.org

American Academy of Pediatrics
141 Northwest Point Boulevard
Elk Grove Village, IL 60007
(847) 434-4000
www.aap.org

American Medical Association
515 N. State Street
Chicago, IL 60610
(312) 464-5000
www.ama-assn.org

American Medical Women's Association
801 N. Fairfax Street
Suite 400
Alexandria, VA 22314
(703) 838-0500
www.amwa-doc.org

Center for Science in the Public Interest
1875 Connecticut Avenue, NW
Suite 300
Washington, DC 20009
(202) 332-9110
www.cspinet.org

Centers for Disease Control and Prevention
1600 Clifton Road
Atlanta, GA 30333
(800) 311-3435
(404) 639-3311
www.cdc.gov

Clinicaltrials.gov
www.clinicaltrials.gov

MEDLINEplus
U.S. National Library of Medicine
8600 Rockville Pike
Bethesda, MD 20894
www.medlineplus.gov

National Institute on Aging
Building 31, Room 5C27
31 Center Drive, MSC 2292
Bethesda, MD 20892
(301) 496-1752
www.nih.gov/nia

National Institutes of Health
Bethesda, MD 20892
www.nih.gov

National Women's Health Information Center
8550 Arlington Boulevard
Suite 300
Fairfax, VA 22031
(800) 994-9662
www.4woman.gov

U.S. Food and Drug Administration
5600 Fishers Lane
Rockville, MD 20857
(888) 463-6332
www.fda.gov

World Health Organization
Avenue Appia 20
1211 Geneva 27
Switzerland
011-41-22-791-2111
www.who.int

BRAIN AND NERVOUS SYSTEM

Alzheimer's Association
919 N. Michigan Avenue
Suite 1100
Chicago, IL 60611
(800) 272-3900
(312) 335-8700
www.alz.org

Alzheimer's Disease Education and Referral Center
P.O. Box 8250
Silver Spring, MD 20907
(800) 438-4380
www.alzheimers.org

Children and Adults with Attention Deficit Hyperactivity Disorder
8181 Professional Place
Suite 201
Landover, MD 20785
(800) 233-4050
(301) 306-7070
www.chadd.org

Epilepsy Foundation
4351 Garden City Drive
Landover, MD 20785
(800) 332-1000
(301) 459-3700
www.efa.org

National Center on Sleep Disorders Research
2 Rockledge Centre
Suite 10038
6701 Rockledge Drive
MSC 7920
Bethesda, MD 20892
(301) 435-0199
www.nhlbi.nih.gov/about/ncsdr/index.htm

CANCER

DIGESTION AND METABOLISM

EYES AND EARS

**National Institute of
Neurological Disorders
and Stroke**
P.O. Box 5801
Bethesda, MD 20892
(800) 352-9424
www.ninds.nih.gov

**National Multiple
Sclerosis Society**
733 Third Avenue
New York, NY 10017
(800) 344-4867
(212) 986-3240
www.nationalmssociety.org

**National Sleep
Foundation**
1522 K Street, NW
Suite 500
Washington, DC 20005
(202) 347-3471
www.sleepfoundation.org

**National Spinal Cord
Injury Association**
6701 Democracy Boulevard
Suite 300-9
Bethesda, MD 20817
(800) 962-9629
(301) 588-6959
www.spinalcord.org

**Parkinson's Disease
Foundation**
710 West 168th Street
New York, NY 10032
(800) 457-6676
(212) 923-4700
www.pdf.org

American Cancer Society
1599 Clifton Road NE
Atlanta, GA 30329
(800) 227-2345
(404) 320-3333
www.cancer.org

**American Society
of Clinical Oncology**
1900 Duke Street
Suite 200
Alexandria, VA 22314
(703) 299-0150
www.asco.org

National Cancer Institute
Building 31, Room 10A03
31 Center Drive, MSC 2580
Bethesda, MD 20892
(301) 435-3848
www.nci.nih.gov

**Y-ME National Breast
Cancer Organization**
212 West Van Buren
Suite 500
Chicago, IL 60607
(800) 221-2141
(312) 986-8338
www.y-me.org

**American Diabetes
Association**
1701 N. Beauregard Street
Alexandria, VA 22311
(800) 232-3472
(703) 549-1500
www.diabetes.org

**Hepatitis Foundation
International**
30 Sunrise Terrace
Cedar Grove, NJ 07009
(800) 891-0707
(973) 239-1035
www.hepfi.org

**International Foundation
for Functional
Gastrointestinal
Disorders**
P.O. Box 170864
Milwaukee, WI 53217
(888) 964-2001
(414) 964-1799
www.iffgd.org

**National Institute of
Diabetes & Digestive
& Kidney Diseases**
31 Centre Drive, MSC 2560
Bethesda, MD 20892
www.niddk.nih.gov

**Weight Control
Information Network**
1 WIN Way
Bethesda, MD 20892
(877) 946-4627
(202) 828-1028
www.niddk.nih.gov/health/
nutrit/win.htm

Better Hearing Institute
515 King Street
Suite 420
Alexandria, VA 22314
(800) 327-9355
(703) 684-3391
www.betterhearing.org

Glaucoma Foundation
116 John Street
Suite 1605
New York, NY 10038
(800) 452-8266
(212) 285-0800
www.glaucomafoundation.
org

National Eye Institute
2020 Vision Place
Bethesda, MD 20892
(301) 496-5248
www.nei.nih.gov

**National Institute
on Deafness and
Other Communications
Disorders**
31 Center Drive, MSC 2320
Bethesda, MD 20892
(301) 496-7243
www.nidcd.nih.gov

**Prevent Blindness
America**
500 E. Remington Road
Schaumburg, IL 60173
(800) 331-2020
(847) 943-2020
www.preventblindness.org

HEART AND CIRCULATION

American Heart Association
7272 Greenville Avenue
Dallas, TX 75231
(800) 242-8721
www.americanheart.org

Mended Hearts Inc.
7272 Greenville Avenue
Dallas, TX 75231
(800) AHAUSA 1
www.mendedhearts.org

National Heart, Lung, and Blood Institute
P.O. Box 20824
Bethesda, MD 20892
(301) 251-1222
www.nhlbi.nih.gov

National Stroke Association
9707 East Easter Lane
Englewood, CO 80112
(800) 787-6537
(303) 649-9299
www.stroke.org

MENTAL HEALTH

Alcoholics Anonymous
Grand Central Station
P.O. Box 459
New York, NY 10163
(212) 870-3400
www.alcoholicsanonymous.org

American Lung Association
(For smoking cessation information)
1740 Broadway
New York, NY 10019
(212) 315-8700
www.lungusa.org

American Psychiatric Association
1400 K Street NW
Washington, DC 20005
(888) 357-7924
www.psych.org

American Psychological Association
750 First Street NE
Washington, DC 20002
(800) 374-3120
www.apa.org

National Institute of Mental Health
56001 Executive Boulevard
Room 8184
MSC 8030
Bethesda, MD 20892
(301) 443-4513
www.nimh.nih.gov

National Institute on Alcohol Abuse and Alcoholism
6000 Executive Boulevard
Willco Building
Bethesda, MD 20892
(301) 496-4000
www.niaaa.nih.gov

MUSCLES, BONES, AND JOINTS

American Podiatric Medical Association
9312 Old Georgetown Road
Bethesda, MD 20814
(800) 366-8273
www.apma.org

Arthritis Foundation
P.O. Box 7669
Atlanta, GA 30357
(800) 283-7800
www.arthritis.org

Lupus Foundation of America
1300 Piccard Drive
Suite 200
Rockville, MD 20850
(800) 558-0121
(301) 670-9292
www.lupus.org

Lyme Disease Network
43 Winton Road
East Brunswick, NJ 08816
www.lymenet.org

National Chronic Fatigue Syndrome and Fibromyalgia Association
P.O. Box 18426
Kansas City, MO 64133
(816) 313-2000

National Institute of Arthritis and Musculoskeletal and Skin Diseases
1 AMS Circle
Bethesda, MD 20892
(301) 495-4484
www.niams.nih.gov

National Osteoporosis Foundation
1232 22nd Street NW
Washington, DC 20037
(800) 624-2663
(202) 223-2226
www.nof.org

REPRODUCTIVE AND SEXUAL HEALTH

AIDS.org
7985 Santa Monica Boulevard, #99
West Hollywood, CA 90046
(323) 656-0699
www.aids.org

American College of Obstetricians and Gynecologists
409 12th Street, SW
P.O. Box 96920
Washington, DC 20090
www.acog.org

National Institute of Allergy and Infectious Diseases
Building 31, Room 7A-50
31 Center Drive, MSC 2520
Bethesda, MD 20892
(301) 496-5717
www.niaid.nih.gov

Planned Parenthood Federation of America
810 Seventh Avenue
New York, NY 10019
(800) 230-7526
www.plannedparenthood.org

RESOLVE
(For infertility information)
1310 Broadway
Somerville, MA 02144
(617) 623-0744
www.resolve.org

RESPIRATORY SYSTEM

**American Lung
Association**
1740 Broadway
New York, NY 10019
(212) 315-8700
www.lungusa.org

**Asthma and Allergy
Foundation of America**
1233 20th Street, NW
Suite 402
Washington, DC 20036
(800) 727-8462
(202) 466-7643
www.aafa.org

**National Heart, Lung,
and Blood Institute**
P.O. Box 20824
Bethesda, MD 20892
(301) 251-1222
www.nhlbi.nih.gov

**National Institute of
Allergy and Infectious
Diseases**
Building 31, Room 7A-50
31 Center Drive, MSC 2520
Bethesda, MD 20892
(301) 496-5717
www.niaid.nih.gov

SKIN, HAIR, NAILS, AND TEETH

**American Academy
of Dermatology**
930 North Meacheam Road
Schaumburg, IL 60168
(847) 330-0230
www.aad.org

**American Dental
Association**
211 East Chicago Avenue
Chicago, IL 60611
(312) 440-2500
www.ada.org

**National Institute
of Arthritis and
Musculoskeletal
and Skin Diseases
Information**
1 AMS Circle
Bethesda, MD 20892
(301) 495-4484
www.niams.nih.gov

**National Institute of
Dental & Craniofacial
Research**
Bethesda, MD 20892
(301) 496-4261
www.nidr.nih.gov

**National Psoriasis
Foundation**
6600 SW 92nd Avenue
Suite 300
Portland, OR 97223
(800) 723-9166
(503) 244-7404
www.psoriasis.org

URINARY TRACT

**American Foundation
for Urologic Disease**
1120 North Charles Street
Baltimore, MD 21201
(410) 468-1800
www.afud.org

**National Institute of
Diabetes & Digestive
& Kidney Diseases**
31 Centre Drive, MSC 2560
Bethesda, MD 20892
www.niddk.nih.gov

**National Kidney
Foundation**
30 East 33 Street
Suite 1100
New York, NY 10016
(800) 622-9010
(212) 889-2210
www.kidney.org

Credits

COVER *Front, top* Comstock; *middle* ©PhotoDisc; *bottom* Comstock; *Back* Abiomed. **2** *top* ©AP/Wide World Photos; *bottom left* ©A. Liepins/Photo Researchers, Inc.; *bottom right* AP/Wide World Photos. **6** AP/Wide World Photos. **7** *left* ©PhotoDisc; *middle* ©Corbis Images/PictureQuest; *right* Curon Medical, Inc. **8** *left* ©PhotoDisc; *middle left* Abiomed; *middle right* SPL/Custom Medical Stock Photography; *right* HealthTronics, Inc. **9** *left* Ortho-McNeil; *middle left* AP/Wide World Photos; *middle right* ©EyeWire; *right* courtesy of NeoTonus, Inc. **10** ©PhotoDisc. **11** Pharmaceutical Research and Manufacturers Association/NIH. **12** *top left* AP/Wide World Photos; *top right* ©Dr. Y. Nikas, SPL/Photo Researchers, Inc.; *bottom left* ©2001 R. Friedman; *bottom right* ©PhotoDisc. **12-13** *top* P. Damiani/Advanced Cell Technology; *bottom* AP/Wide World Photos. **13** *top left* SPL/Custom Medical Stock Photography; *top right* Plant Research International; *bottom left* ©GJLP, CNRI/Photo Researchers, Inc.; *bottom right* ©A. Liepins/ Photo Researchers, Inc. **14-15** AP/Wide World Photos. **15** AP/Wide World Photos. **16** *top* ©Biophoto Associates/ Photo Researchers, Inc.; *bottom* AP/Wide World Photos. **16-17** AP/Wide World Photos. **18** AP/Wide World Photos. **19** Custom Medical Stock Photography. **20** AP/Wide World Photos. **21** AP/Wide World Photos. **22-23** AP/Wide World Photos. **24** *both* AP/Wide World Photos. **25** *top* Johns Hopkins University; *bottom* ©Dr. Y. Nikas, SPL/Photo Researchers, Inc. **26** AP/Wide World Photos. **26-27** AP/Wide World Photos. **27** J. Carson/Custom Medical Stock Photography. **28-29** AP/Wide World Photos. **30** P. Damiani/Advanced Cell Technology. **31** AP/Wide World Photos. **32** *bottom* ©D. Phillips/Photo Researchers, Inc. **32-33** *top* ©Roslin Institute. **33** AP/Wide World Photos. **34-35** SPL/Custom Medical Stock Photography. **35** SIU BioMed/Custom Medical Stock Photography. **36** *top* ©Quest/Photo Researchers, Inc.; *bottom* AP/Wide World Photos. **37** SPL/Custom Medical Stock Photography. **38-39** Plant Research International. **40** *top* SIU BioMed/ Custom Medical Stock Photography; *bottom* Carlos Bustamente Laboratory. **41** Mark B. Roth/Joseph G. Gall, Carnegie Institution. **42-43** ©2001 R. Friedman. **44** *top* SIU BioMed/Custom Medical Stock Photography; *bottom* SPL/Custom Medical Stock Photography. **45** *top* Altea Development Corporation; *bottom* Inhale Therapeutic Systems, Inc. **46** ©W. and D. McIntyre/Photo Researchers, Inc. **47** *top* MIT/D. Coveney. **48-49** ©PhotoDisc. **50** *top* ©J. King-Holmes/Photo Researchers, Inc.; *bottom* Custom Medical Stock Photography. **51** ©L. Mulvehill/Photo Researchers, Inc. **52-53** AP/Wide World Photos. **53** AP/Wide World Photos. **54-55** adapted from Newsweek– K. Hand ©2001 Newsweek, Inc. All rights reserved. Reprinted by permission. **56** AP/Wide World Photos. **57** AP/Wide World Photos. **58-59** ©GJLP, CNRI/Photo Researchers, Inc. **60** *top* P. Barber/Custom Medical Stock Photography; *bottom* J. Meyer/Custom Medical Stock Photography. **61** *top* Millennium Imaging; *bottom* ©GJLP, CNRI/Photo Researchers, Inc. **62** *both* Virtual Physical™. **63** *both* OmniCorder Technologies. **64** *top* Cadx; *both bottom* Lehigh Magnetic Imaging Center. **65** R2 Technology. **66-67** Art & Science/Custom Medical Stock Photography. **67** ©M. Chris and P. Clark/Photo Researchers, Inc. **68** ©A. Liepins/Photo Researchers, Inc. **69** *left* Therion Biologics; *right* ©C. Fox/Photo Researchers, Inc. **70** *top* ©PhotoDisc; *middle left* Optobionics Corporation; *middle right* Abiomed; *bottom left* Ortho-McNeil; *bottom right* AP/Wide World Photos. **71** *top left* N. Rowan/Custom Medical Stock Photography; *top right* Given Imaging, Ltd.; *middle left* SPL/Custom Medical Stock Photography; *middle right* AP/Wide World Photos; *bottom left* ©PhotoDisc; *bottom right* AP/Wide World Photos. **73** *top left* ©PhotoDisc; *middle left* ©EyeWire; *bottom left* PhotoTake; *right* AP/Wide World Photos. **74** *top* ©PhotoDisc; *bottom* AP/Wide World Photos. **75** PhotoTake. **76-77** ©EyeWire. **77** AP/Wide World Photos. **78** ©PhotoDisc. **79** *both* ©PhotoDisc. **80** ©EyeWire. **81** AP/Wide World Photos. **82-83** ©PhotoDisc. **83** *both* ©PhotoDisc. **84** ©PhotoDisc. **85** adapted from Alexion Pharmaceuticals/J. Springhorn. **86** ©PhotoDisc. **87** AP/Wide World Photos. **88-89** ©PhotoDisc. **88** ©PhotoDisc. **89** Influ-ENT. **90** AP/Wide World Photos. **90-91** AP/Wide World Photos. **91** ©PhotoDisc. **93** *top left* ©PhotoDisc; *bottom left* AP/World Wide Photos; *right* Myriad Genetics, Inc. **94** *both* ©PhotoDisc. **95** N. Rowan/Custom Medical Stock Photography. **96** *both* ©PhotoDisc. **97** *left* Pro-Duct Health, Inc.; *right* AP/Wide World Photos. **98-99** ©PhotoDisc. **99** *left* ©The StayWell Company; *right* SPL/Custom Medical Stock Photography. **100** *top* ©Eye of Science/ Photo Researchers, Inc.; *bottom* SIU BioMed/Custom Medical Stock Photography. **101** *top* ©Eye of Science/ Photo Researchers, Inc.; *bottom* AP/Wide World Photos. **102-103** AP/Wide World Photos. **103** AP/Wide World Photos. **104** Courtesy of P. Russell. **105** ©PhotoDisc. **106-107** ©Corbis Images/PictureQuest.

107 *both* ©PhotoDisc. **108** ©EyeWire. **109** R. Becker/ Custom Medical Stock Photography. **110-111** AP/Wide World Photos. **111** ©PhotoDisc. **112** Myriad Genetics, Inc. **113** *left* ©PhotoDisc; *right* SIU BioMed/Custom Medical Stock Photography. **114** AP/Wide World Photos. **115** *top* AP/Wide World Photos; *bottom* ©PhotoDisc. **116** ©PhotoDisc. **117** *top* ©PhotoDisc; *bottom* ©D. Phillips/ Photo Researchers, Inc. **119** *top left* Given Imaging, Ltd.; *bottom left* ©PhotoDisc; *top right* SIU BioMed/Custom Medical Stock Photography; *bottom right* BioEnterics. **120** *both* AP/Wide World Photos. **121** ©PhotoDisc. **122** *left* ©EyeWire; *right* ©The StayWell Company. **123** Curon Medical, Inc. **124** ©Corbis Images/Picture-Quest. **125** SIU BioMed/Custom Medical Stock Photography. **126** *left* AP/Wide World Photos; *right* Given Imaging, Ltd. **127** Given Imaging, Ltd. **128** ©PhotoDisc. **129** *left* ©PhotoDisc; *right* Agricultural Research Service/USDA/M. Thompson. **130** BioEnterics. **131** *top* Desert Tropicals; *bottom* Courtesy of B. Barber. **133** *top left* ©PhotoDisc; *bottom left* National Eye Institute, NIH; *top right* Cochlear Corporation; *bottom right* University of Arizona Health Sciences Center. **134** *top* ©PhotoDisc; *bottom* Courtesy of J. Doddick, M.D. **135** *both* ©PhotoDisc. **136** *top* ©PhotoDisc; *bottom* National Eye Institute, NIH. **137** *both* Symphonix Devices, Inc. **138** *left* ©EyeWire. **138-139** Cochlear Corporation. **140** *both* Optobionics Corporation. **141** Optobionics Corporation. **142** National Eye Institute, NIH. **143** *top* Adaptive Eyecare, Ltd.; *bottom* University of Arizona Health Sciences Center. **145** *top left* ©S. Camazine/S. Trainor/Photo Researchers, Inc.; *bottom left* Abiomed; *top right* ©EyeWire; *bottom right* Cordis Corporation. **146** AP/Wide World Photos. **147** AP/Wide World Photos. **148** *top* Cardio-Genesis Corporation; *bottom* Courtesy of R. Reed. **149** *top* ©C. Howe 2000; *bottom* Courtesy of L.VAD Technology. **150** *left* AP/Wide World Photos; *right* Acorn Cardiovascular, Inc. **151** ©PhotoDisc. **152** *top* AP/Wide World Photos; *bottom* ©PhotoDisc. **153** Abiomed. **154-155** *both* Cordis Corporation. **156** ©EyeWire. **157** AP/Wide World Photos. **158** ©EyeWire. **159** Embolic Protection, Inc. **160** Embolic Protection, Inc. **161** InterCure, developers of RespeRate. **163** ©S. Camazine/S. Trainor/Photo Researchers, Inc. **164** Courtesy of E. Taub, Ph.D. **165** ©EyeWire. **166** *top* University of Florida photo by Ray Carson; *bottom* ©A. Leonard/Photo Researchers, Inc. **167** *both* Diomed, Ltd. **169** *top left* ©W. and D. McIntyre/Photo Researchers, Inc.; *bottom left* ©PhotoDisc; *top right* SPL/Custom Medical Stock Photography; *bottom right* ©PhotoDisc. **170** ©PhotoDisc. **171** *left* SPL/Custom Medical Stock Photography; *right* ©PhotoDisc. **172** AP/Wide World Photos. **173** *both* AP/Wide World Photos. **174** ©EyeWire. **175** *left* ©PhotoDisc; *right* SPL/Custom Medical Stock Photography. **176-177** ©PhotoDisc. **177** SPL/Custom Medical Stock Photography. **178** *both* ©PhotoDisc. **178-179** ©W. and D. McIntyre/Photo Researchers, Inc. **179** © PhotoDisc. **180-181** ©PhotoDisc. **181** *both* ©PhotoDisc. **183** *top left* Kyphon, Inc.; *bottom left* AP/Wide World Photos; *top right* HealthTronics, Inc.; *bottom right* ©PhotoDisc. **184** AP/Wide World Photos. **185** AP/Wide World Photos. **186** *both* ©PhotoDisc. **187** AP/Wide World Photos. **188** *both* ©PhotoDisc. **189** HealthTronics, Inc. **190** *top* ©PhotoDisc; *bottom* Roseman/Custom Medical Stock Photography. **190-191** ©PhotoDisc. **191** AP/Wide World Photos. **192** *top* J. Carson/ Custom Medical Stock Photography; *bottom* ©PhotoDisc. **193** *top* ©PhotoDisc; *bottom* Agricultural Research Service/USDA/S. Bauer. **194** Kyphon, Inc. **195** ©PhotoDisc. **197** *top left* ©PhotoDisc; *bottom right* ©PhotoDisc; *top right* ©EyeWire; *bottom right* Ortho-McNeil. **198** ©PhotoDisc. **199** AP/Wide World Photos. **200** *top* AP/Wide World Photos; *bottom* Reprinted with permission from Science Magazine. © 2001 American Association for the Advancement of Science. **201** ©2001 Berlex Laboratories. **202** ©EyeWire. **203** *left* Ortho-McNeil; *top* BioMed/ Custom Medical Stock Photography; *bottom* Conceptus. **204** ©EyeWire. **205** ©PhotoDisc. **206** *both* ©PhotoDisc. **207** *top* Procter & Gamble; *bottom* Courtesy of M. Patane. **208** ©PhotoDisc. **209** *left* ©PhotoDisc; *right* Custom Medical Stock Photography. **211** *top left* AP/Wide World Photos; *bottom left* ©PhotoDisc; *right* ©EyeWire. **212** *top* ©PhotoDisc; *bottom* AP/Wide World Photos. **213** AP/Wide World Photos. **214** *top* ©EyeWire; *bottom* AP/Wide World Photos. **215** ©EyeWire. **216** AP/Wide World Photos. **216-217** ©PhotoDisc. **219** *top left* ©Royalty Free/Corbis; *bottom left* ©PhotoDisc; *top right* ©EyeWire; *bottom right* Hossler Ph.D./Custom Medical Stock Photography. **220** *top* ©PhotoDisc; *bottom* OraPharma, Inc., makers of Arestin. **221** *both* ©PhotoDisc. **222** ©Royalty Free/Corbis. **223** *left* ©EyeWire; *top* ©PhotoDisc; *bottom* ©EyeWire. **224** *top* Custom Medical Stock Photography; *bottom* ©PhotoDisc. **225** *top* ©EyeWire; *bottom* AP/Wide World Photos. **226** *bottom* Custom Medical Stock Photography. **226-227** Biogen, Inc. **227** Hossler Ph.D./Custom Medical Stock Photography. **228** ©PhotoDisc. **228-229** ©PhotoDisc. **229** ©PhotoDisc. **231** *top left* ©EyeWire; *bottom left* Courtesy of NeoTonus, Inc.; *top right* ©PhotoDisc; *bottom right* AP/Wide World Photos. **232** ©PhotoDisc. **233** *top* Courtesy of NeoTonus, Inc.; *bottom* AP/Wide World Photos. **234** *top* AP/Wide World Photos; *bottom* ©PhotoDisc. **235** ©PhotoDisc. **236** *top* AP/Wide World Photos; *bottom* ©EyeWire. **237** ©EyeWire. **238** *left* ©2001 LifeHouse Productions, LLC/Celsion; *right* ProstaJect™ Ethanol Injection System, For International Use Only, courtesy of American Medical Systems, Inc., Minnetonka, Minnesota. **239** ©PhotoDisc. **240** ©EyeWire. **240-241** AP/Wide World Photos.

Index

Bladder, incontinence of, 232–33

Bladder infections, vaccine for, 240–41

Blindness
artificial retina for, 140–41
verteporfin for prevention of, 142

Blood clot prevention and treatment
contraceptive pill and factor V Leiden, 20–21, 51
in heart attack, tenecteplase for, 158
low-dose warfarin for, 157
robotic surgery for, 57

Blood pressure control, 161–62
deep breathing for, 161–62
during dialysis, 234
stress management in, 181

B lymphocyte stimulator inhibitors, for lupus, 190–91

BLyS protein inhibitors, for lupus, 190–91

Bone loss (osteoporosis), 194–95

Bone marrow transplants
adult stem cells and, 24, 27
chemotherapy and, 109, 117

Borreliosis (Lyme disease), 192–93

Braces, dental, 221

Brachytherapy, for prostate cancer, 113

Brain cancer, 94–96
dendritic cell vaccine for, 94–95
environmental causes of, 96
genetics and, 95–96

Brain damage, after stroke, 162–66

Brain waves, in ADHD, 78

Breast cancer, 96–97
biochip for detection of, 41

ductal lavage test for, 96–97
mammography for, 64–65, 97
monoclonal antibodies for, 37
mutated BRCA genes and, 18
vaccines for, 69

Bupropion, for smoking cessation, 179

Burns, stem cell therapy for, 25

C

CAD. See Coronary artery disease

Calcium, kidney stone formation and, 236

Camera-in-a-pill, 126–27

Campral (acamprosate), alcoholic relapse and, 171

Cancer, 92–117. See also specific types
BioScanIR imaging system and, 63–64
chemotherapy (See Chemotherapy)
monoclonal antibodies and, 35
PET scans and, 106
stem cell therapy for, 25, 117
vaccines for (See Vaccines)

Capecitabine (Xeloda), for colon cancer, 101

Carbohydrates, for breakfast, 83

Cardiac jacket, for heart failure, 150

CardioVad system, for congestive heart failure, 149

Cardura (doxazosin), for benign prostatic hyperplasia, 239–40

Cataracts, 134–35

CAT scans. See CT scans

Cavities, dental, 221

Celecoxib (Celebrex)
for Alzheimer's disease, 75
for prostate cancer, 114

Cell behavior, stem cell research and, 25

Cerebrovascular accident. See Stroke

Cervical cancer, 98–99

Cetuximab (IMC-C225), for colon cancer, 101

Chemicals
brain cancer and, 96
Parkinson's disease and, 88–89

Chemotherapy
for brain cancer, 95–96
for colon cancer, 101
effects of, 36
individualized by molecular markers, 100
for leukemia, 102–4
response to, 95–96
and stem cell treatments, 109, 117

Chest pain
clopidegrel for, 148
laser surgery for, 147–48

Children
ADHD in, 76–78
bipolar disorder treatment for, 175
braces, for teeth in, 221
epilepsy, behavioral problems and, 79
IBS in, 129
influenza vaccines for, 214
Lyme disease vaccine for, 193
obsessive-compulsive disorder in, 175

Chimerism, mixed, for organ rejection prevention, 235

Chinese medicine, 105

Cholesterol
coronary artery disease prevention guidelines, 151–52
personalized medicine for, 50–51

Chondroitin, for arthritis, 185

Choroidal neovascularization, verteporfin for, 142

Chromosomes, 16, 30

Chronic fatigue syndrome, 187

Chronic myelogenous leukemia, 21, 102–4

Chronotherapeutics, 46–47

Cialis, for erectile dysfunction, 209

Ciclopirox (Penlac), for nail fungus, 224

Cigarette smoking. See Smoking

Clinical trials, phases of, 200

Clonidine, for smoking cessation, 179

Cloning, 28–33
Dolly (sheep), 28
ethics of, 28, 30
mouse studies, 32–33
process, 30–31
reasons for, 31–32
sexual reproduction vs., 30
therapeutic, 32, 33

Clopidegrel (Plavix), for angina, 148

Clot prevention and treatment
in heart attack, 158
low-dose warfarin for, 157

Clozapine (Clozaril), for schizophrenia, 176

Codeine, individual response to, 50

Cognitive-behavioral therapy
for obsessive-compulsive disorder, 175
for panic disorder, 172

Colds, 212–13

Colitis, 127

Collagen, in skin
smoking effects on, 228
vitamin C effects on, 228
wrinkle removal procedure and, 227–28

Colon cancer, 100–101
aspirin and, 111
breast cancer drug for, 101
IMC-C225 (cetuximab) for, 101

Colon imaging
camera-in-a-pill, 126–27
conventional colonoscopy, 61–62